Pulmonary Rehabilitation: Role and Advances

Editors

LINDA NICI
RICHARD L. ZUWALLACK

CLINICS IN
CHEST MEDICINE

www.chestmed.theclinics.com

June 2014 • Volume 35 • Number 2

ELSEVIER

1600 John F. Kennedy Boulevard • Suite 1800 • Philadelphia, Pennsylvania, 19103-2899

http://www.theclinics.com

CLINICS IN CHEST MEDICINE Volume 35, Number 2
June 2014 ISSN 0272-5231, ISBN-13: 978-0-323-29917-6

Editor: Patrick Manley
Developmental Editor: Casey Jackson

Clinics in Chest Medicine (ISSN 0272-5231) is published quarterly by Elsevier Inc., 360 Park Avenue South, New York, NY 10010-1710. Months of issue are March, June, September, and December. Periodicals postage paid at New York, NY and additional mailing offices. Subscription prices are $345.00 per year (domestic individuals), $556.00 per year (domestic institutions), $165.00 per year (domestic students/residents), $380.00 per year (Canadian individuals), $690.00 per year (Canadian institutions), $470.00 per year (international individuals), $690.00 per year (international institutions), and $230.00 per year (international and Canadian students/residents). International air speed delivery is included in all Clinics subscription prices. All prices are subject to change without notice. **POSTMASTER:** Send address changes to Clinics in Chest Medicine, Elsevier Health Sciences Division, Subscription Customer Service, 3251 Riverport Lane, Maryland Heights, MO 63043. **Customer Service: Telephone: 1-800-654-2452** (U.S. and Canada); **1-314-447-8871** (outside U.S. and Canada). **Fax: 1-314-447-8029. E-mail: journalscustomerservice-usa@elsevier.com** (for print support); **journalsonlinesupport-usa@elsevier.com** (for online support).

Reprints. For copies of 100 or more of articles in this publication, please contact the Commercial Reprints Department, Elsevier Inc., 360 Park Avenue South, New York, NY 10010-1710. Tel.: 212-633-3874; Fax: 212-633-3820; E-mail: reprints@elsevier.com.

Clinics in Chest Medicine is covered in *MEDLINE/PubMed (Index Medicus), Current Contents/Clinical Medicine, EMBASE/ Excerpta Medica, Science Citation Index,* and *ISI/BIOMED.*

Contributors

EDITORS

LINDA NICI, MD
Pulmonary Medicine/Critical Care Section, Providence VA Medical Center; Professor of Medicine, Brown University, Providence, Rhode Island

RICHARD L. ZUWALLACK, MD
Associate Chief, Pulmonary and Critical Care, St. Francis Hospital and Medical Center; Professor of Clinical Medicine; University of Connecticut School of Medicine, Hartford, Connecticut

AUTHORS

VASILEIOS ANDRIANOPOULOS, MSc
Department of Research & Education, CIRO+, Centre of Expertise for Chronic Organ Failure, Horn, The Netherlands

JEAN BOURBEAU
Montreal Chest Institute, McGill University Health Centre, Montréal, Québec, Canada

DINA BROOKS, PhD, PT
Senior Scientist; Department of Respiratory Medicine, West Park Healthcare Centre; Professor of Physical Therapy; University of Toronto; CIHR Chair in COPD Research; Graduate Department of Rehabilitation Science, Faculty of Medicine, Toronto, Ontario, Canada

CARLOS A. CAMILLO, MSc, PT
KU Leuven, Department of Rehabilitation Sciences, Faculty of Kinesiology and Rehabilitation Sciences, Leuven, Belgium

BRIAN CARLIN, MD
Assistant Professor of Medicine; Drexel University School of Medicine, Philadelphia, Pennsylvania; Medical Director, Lifeline Pulmonary Rehabilitation and Therapy, Pittsburgh, Pennsylvania

REBECCA H. CROUCH, PT, DPT, MS, CCS, FAACVPR
Clinical Director of Pulmonary Rehabilitation; Duke University Medical Center, Durham, North Carolina

HELEEN DEMEYER, MSc, PT
KU Leuven, Department of Rehabilitation Sciences, Faculty of Kinesiology and Rehabilitation Sciences; Respiratory Rehabilitation and Respiratory Division, University Hospital Leuven, Leuven, Belgium

RACHAEL A. EVANS, MBChB, MRCP (UK), PhD
Department of Respiratory Medicine, Glenfield Hospital, Leicester, United Kingdom

BONNIE F. FAHY, RN, MN, CNS
Clinical Documentation Specialist, Mayo Clinic Hospital, Phoenix, Arizona

CARL FAIRBURN, PT, DPT
Cardiovascular and Pulmonary Physical Therapy Resident, Duke University Medical Center, Durham, North Carolina

VINCENT S. FAN, MD, MPH
Staff Physician, Veterans Affairs Puget Sound Health Care System and Associate Professor of Medicine, Department of Medicine, University of Washington, Seattle, Washington

FRITS M.E. FRANSSEN, PhD, MD
Department of Research & Education, CIRO+, Centre of Expertise for Chronic Organ Failure, Horn, The Netherlands

JUDITH GARCIA-AYMERICH, MD, PhD
Associate Research Professor, Centre for
Research in Environmental Epidemiology
(CREAL), Barcelona, Spain

CHRIS GARVEY, FNP, MSN, MPA
Cardiopulmonary Rehabilitation, Seton
Medical Center, Daly City, UCSF Sleep
Disorders, San Francisco, California

ROGER GOLDSTEIN, MB ChB, FRCP
Senior Scientist, Department of Respiratory
Medicine, West Park Healthcare Centre;
Professor of Medicine and Physical Therapy;
University of Toronto; NSA-University of
Toronto Chair in Respiratory Rehabilitation
Research; Graduate Department of
Rehabilitation Science, Faculty of Medicine,
Toronto, Ontario, Canada

KYLIE HILL, PhD
Associate Professor, School of Physiotherapy
and Exercise Science, Faculty of Health
Science, Curtin University; Lung Institute of
Western Australia, Centre for Asthma, Allergy
and Respiratory Research, University of
Western Australia; Physiotherapy Department,
Royal Perth Hospital, Perth, Western Australia,
Australia

ANNE E. HOLLAND, PhD
Associate Professor, Department of
Physiotherapy, La Trobe University;
Department of Physiotherapy, Alfred Health;
Institute for Breathing and Sleep, Melbourne,
Victoria, Australia

MIEK HORNIKX, MSc, PT
KU Leuven, Department of Rehabilitation
Sciences, Faculty of Kinesiology and
Rehabilitation Sciences; Respiratory
Rehabilitation and Respiratory Division,
University Hospital Leuven, Leuven,
Belgium

DAISY J.A. JANSSEN, MD, PhD
Program Development Centre, CIRO+,
Centre of Expertise for Chronic Organ
Failure, Horn; Centre of Expertise for
Palliative Care, Maastricht University
Medical Centre+ (MUMC+), Maastricht,
The Netherlands

WIM JANSSENS, MD, PhD
KU Leuven, Pneumology, Faculty of Medicine
and Respiratory Rehabilitation and Respiratory
Division, University Hospital Leuven, Leuven,
Belgium

PETER KLIJN, PhD
Department of Pulmonology, Merem Asthma
Center Heideheuvel, Hilversum, The
Netherlands

SUZANNE C. LAREAU, RN, MS
Senior Instructor, College of Nursing,
University of Colorado, Aurora, Colorado

RODERICK MACDONALD, MS
Minneapolis VA Health Care System,
Minneapolis, Minnesota

JAMES R. McCORMICK, MD, FCCP
Division of Pulmonary, Critical care, and
Sleep Medicine, University of Kentucky
Medical School, Lexington, Kentucky

PAULA M. MEEK, RN, PhD
Professor, College of Nursing, University
of Colorado, Colorado

**MICHAEL D.L. MORGAN, MB BChir, MA,
MD, FRCP**
Professor, Department of Respiratory
Medicine, Glenfield Hospital, Leicester,
United Kingdom

LINDA NICI, MD
Pulmonary Medicine/Critical Care Section,
Providence VA Medical Center; Professor
of Medicine, Brown University, Providence,
Rhode Island

FABIO PITTA, PT, PhD
Adjunct Professor, Laboratory of Research in
Respiratory Physiotherapy (LFIP),
Departamento de Fisioterapia, Londrina, Brazil

MILO A. PUHAN, MD, PhD
Professor of Epidemiology and Public Health;
Institute of Social and Preventive Medicine,
University of Zurich, Zurich, Switzerland

JONATHAN RASKIN, MD
Pulmonary Rehabilitation, Beth Israel Medical
Center, New York, New York

KATHRYN RICE, MD
Minneapolis VA Health Care System,
Minneapolis, Minnesota

CAROLYN L. ROCHESTER, MD, FCCP
Medical Director, Clinical COPD Program;
Associate Professor of Medicine; Section
of Pulmonary, Critical Care and Sleep, Yale
University School of Medicine, New Haven,
Connecticut; Medical Director, Pulmonary
Rehabilitation Program, VA Connecticut
Healthcare System, West Haven, Connecticut

SALLY SINGH, FCSP, PhD
Centre for Exercise and Rehabilitation Science,
University Hospitals of Leicester NHS Trust,
Leicester, United Kingdom

MARTIJN A. SPRUIT, PhD
Department of Research & Education, CIRO+,
Centre of Expertise for Chronic Organ Failure,
Horn, The Netherlands; Faculty of Medicine

and Life Sciences, REVAL-Rehabilitation
Research Center, BIOMED-Biomedical
Research Institute, Hasselt University,
Diepenbeek, Belgium

THIERRY TROOSTERS, PT, PhD
KU Leuven, Department of Rehabilitation
Sciences, Faculty of Kinesiology and
Rehabilitation Sciences; Respiratory
Rehabilitation and Respiratory Division,
University Hospital Leuven, Leuven, Belgium

TIMOTHY J. WILT, MD, MPH
Minneapolis VA Health Care System,
Minneapolis, Minnesota

RICHARD L. ZUWALLACK, MD
Associate Chief, Pulmonary and Critical Care,
St. Francis Hospital and Medical Center;
Professor of Clinical Medicine; University
of Connecticut School of Medicine, Hartford,
Connecticut

Contents

Pulmonary rehabilitation is a complex intervention for which it is difficult to craft a succinct yet inclusive definition. Pulmonary rehabilitation should be considered for all patients with chronic obstructive pulmonary disease (COPD) who remain symptomatic or have decreased functional status despite otherwise optimal medical management. The essential components of pulmonary rehabilitation are exercise training and self-management education, tailored to the needs of the individual patient and integrated into the course of the disease trajectory. Emerging data support a role for pulmonary rehabilitation in nontraditional contexts, such as during exacerbation in the non-COPD patient and in the home setting.

The systemic effects and comorbidities of chronic respiratory disease such as COPD contribute substantially to its burden. Symptoms in COPD do not solely arise from the degree of airflow obstruction as exercise limitation is compounded by the specific secondary manifestations of the disease including skeletal muscle impairment, osteoporosis, mood disturbance, anemia, and hormonal imbalance. Pulmonary rehabilitation targets the systemic manifestations of COPD, the causes of which include inactivity, systemic inflammation, hypoxia and corticosteroid treatment. Comorbidities are common, including cardiac disease, obesity, and metabolic syndrome and should not preclude pulmonary rehabilitation as they may also benefit from similar approaches.

The aim of this article is to appraise the quality of evidence reported for important outcomes in pulmonary rehabilitation using the approach of the Grading of Recommendations Assessment, Development and Evaluation Working Group. This appraisal was carried out by identifying Cochrane systematic reviews and systematic reviews that have been subsequently reported since the last Cochrane report. The focus of this appraisal was to determine the effectiveness of pulmonary rehabilitation programs versus control therapy in chronic obstructive pulmonary disease patients. This analysis did not evaluate other aspects of the pulmonary rehabilitation intervention.

Pulmonary rehabilitation programs vary in terms of duration and location. Differences also exists in the patients who are judged eligible for rehabilitation. This article reviews the options clinicians have to organize programs in terms of who should be referred, when, where, and for how long. There are several risk factors for lack of uptake and non-adherence to programs. Logistical aspects are also an important barrier. In terms of election, patients with muscle dysfunction are likely the best candidates for exercise training. Patients with exercise-induced symptoms and those after exacerbations should also be referred.

Exercise training remains a cornerstone of pulmonary rehabilitation (PR) in patients with chronic respiratory disease. The choice of type of exercise training depends on the physiologic requirements and goals of the individual patient as well as the available equipment at the PR center. Current evidence suggests that, at ground walking exercise training, Nordic walking exercise training, resistance training, water-based exercise training, tai chi, and nonlinear periodized exercise are all feasible and effective in (subgroups) of patients with chronic obstructive pulmonary disease. In turn, these exercise training modalities can be considered as part of a comprehensive, interdisciplinary PR program.

Despite the well-established benefits of exercise training in people with chronic respiratory disease, there are a group of people in whom it confers minimal gains. Furthermore, there is increasing recognition of the prevalence of comorbid conditions among people with chronic obstructive pulmonary disease and other respiratory diseases, such as musculoskeletal disorders, which make participation in traditional exercise training programs challenging. This article focuses on several adjuncts or strategies that may be implemented by clinicians during exercise training, with the goal of optimizing the proportion of pulmonary rehabilitation participants who achieve significant and meaningful gains on program completion.

Behavioral change is critical for improving health outcomes in patients with chronic obstructive pulmonary disease. An educational approach alone is insufficient; changes in behavior, especially the acquisition of self-care skills, are also required. There is mounting evidence that embedding collaborative self-management (CSM) within existing health care systems provides an effective model to meet these needs. CSM should be integrated with pulmonary rehabilitation programs, one of the main goals of which is to induce long-term changes in behavior. More research is needed to evaluate the effectiveness of assimilating CSM into primary care, patient-centered medical homes, and palliative care teams.

A comprehensive assessment is the foundation of a successful pulmonary rehabilitation programme. There is a broad selection of outcome measures that tend to be categorized into measures of exercise performance (including measures of strength) quality of life (health status), psychological well-being, nutritional status and more recently knowledge and self-efficacy. There is a growing interest in the measurement of physical activity too, although this is a current line of research activity. A sophisticated suite of outcomes allows the rehabilitation program to be personalised to the individual and deliver effective rehabilitation.

Patients with chronic respiratory diseases are usually physically inactive, which is an important negative prognostic factor. Therefore, promoting regular physical activity is of key importance in reducing morbidity and mortality and improving the quality of life in this population. A current challenge to pulmonary rehabilitation is the need to develop strategies that induce or facilitate the enhancement of daily levels of physical activity. Because exercise training alone, despite improving exercise capacity, does not consistently generate similar improvements in physical activity in daily life, there is also a need to develop behavioral interventions that help to promote activity.

Pulmonary rehabilitation (PR) is an important therapeutic intervention that should no longer be considered suitable only for patients with chronic obstructive pulmonary disease (COPD). A strong rationale exists for providing PR to persons with a broad range of respiratory disorders other than COPD. Evidence shows that PR for these patients is feasible, safe and effective. A disease-relevant approach should be undertaken, based on individual patients' needs. Further research is needed to better understand the optimal program content, duration and outcomes measures, to enable diverse patients to achieve maximal benefits of PR.

Pulmonary rehabilitation (PR) is associated with improvements in exercise capacity, health related quality of life, psychological symptoms and response to utilization. Acute exacerbations threaten these improvements. An awareness of the clinical sequelae of acute exacerbation of chronic obstructive pulmonary disease enables approaches, such as early post exacerbation rehabilitation to mitigate its negative effects.

In this article, the prevalence of depression, anxiety, and cognitive impairment in persons with chronic obstructive pulmonary disease, and the impact of these psychological and cognitive factors on clinical outcomes in COPD is reviewed. Methods for screening and identification of these conditions in COPD are described. The extent to which depression, anxiety or cognitive impairment limit or modify the effectiveness of pulmonary rehabilitation, and whether pulmonary rehabilitation may ameliorate these psychological and cognitive impairments are discussed.

Numerous barriers exist to the timely introduction of palliative care in patients with advanced chronic obstructive pulmonary disease (COPD). The complex needs of patients with advanced COPD require the integration of curative-restorative care and palliative care. Palliative care and pulmonary rehabilitation are both important components of integrated care for patients with chronic respiratory diseases. Pulmonary rehabilitation provides the opportunity to introduce palliative care by implementing education about advance care planning. Education about advance care planning addresses the information needs of patients and can be an effective strategy to promote patient-physician discussion about these issues.

Variable aspects of pulmonary rehabilitation (PR) programs include staff composition, setting, structure, and duration. Longer PR programs generally translate into greater improvements in outcomes and (perhaps) prolonged maintenance of benefits. Barriers to PR include transportation issues, inconvenience for the patient, cost and insurance coverage problems, lack of perceived benefit, concurrent illness, and influence of the provider. PR settings include inpatient and outpatient environments. PR has been shown to improve health care utilization during or immediately following chronic obstructive pulmonary disease exacerbations. Challenges to providing PR may be partially addressed by technological developments.

The importance of exercise for pulmonary patients is unquestioned. Decreased functional status has been attributed to increased hospitalizations, leading to further decreases in functionality, decreased quality of life and increased mortality. Despite known benefits of pulmonary rehabilitation, recruitment and retention of program participants can be a challenge. Alternatives to traditional pulmonary rehabilitation are reviewed with an emphasis on physical activity, exacerbation awareness and a reduction in hospital admissions.

Pulmonary rehabilitation is now an established standard of care for patients with chronic obstructive pulmonary disease (COPD). Although pulmonary rehabilitation has no appreciable direct effect on static measurements of lung function, it arguably provides the greatest benefit of any available therapy across multiple outcome areas important to the patient with respiratory disease, including dyspnea, exercise performance, and health-related quality of life. It also appears to be a potent intervention that reduces COPD hospitalizations, especially when given in the periexacerbation period. The role of pulmonary rehabilitation within the larger schema of integrated care represents a fruitful area for further research.

CLINICS IN CHEST MEDICINE

RELATED INTEREST

Clinics in Laboratory Medicine, Vol. 34, No. 2 (June 2014)
Respiratory Infections
Michael Loeffelholz, *Editor*

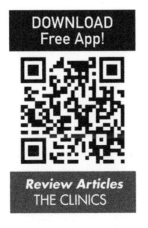

NOW AVAILABLE FOR YOUR iPhone and iPad

Preface

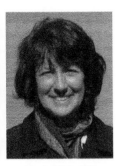
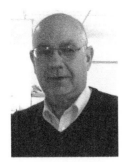

Linda Nici, MD   Richard L. ZuWallack, MD
Editors

Pulmonary rehabilitation, with major components of exercise therapy and behavioral intervention, has really come of age over the past four decades! We have witnessed its impressive rise in status from that of an intervention that had only common sense (but no real science) behind it to its current status and widespread recognition as a gold standard of care for chronic obstructive pulmonary disease (COPD). Pulmonary rehabilitation complements other forms of therapy, including pharmacologic therapy, for patients with chronic airways disease: further improvement in dyspnea, exercise performance, and quality of life can be reasonably expected when pulmonary rehabilitation is given to a patient who remains symptomatic despite what would be considered standard medical care. Furthermore, optimization of treatment with bronchodilators can be expected to allow a patient to achieve more benefit from the exercise training component of pulmonary rehabilitation. It is indeed a good marriage of two forms of therapy. New and exciting developments in pulmonary rehabilitation include emerging evidence that it may play an important role in reducing health care utilization in COPD, especially when given near the time of an exacerbation. Emerging evidence is also beginning to point to a role for the potential usefulness of pulmonary rehabilitation in other forms of chronic respiratory disease. We are proud to present, in this issue of *Clinics in Chest Medicine*, the collective wisdom and professional experience of 36 experts in the fields of pulmonary rehabilitation and the clinical management of chronic lung disease. Like pulmonary rehabilitation itself, this has truly been a multidisciplinary effort to provide the latest science and concepts behind this complex intervention.

Linda Nici, MD
Pulmonary Medicine/Critical Care Section
Providence VA Medical Center
830 Chalkstone Avenue
Providence, RI 02908, USA

Richard L. ZuWallack, MD
Pulmonary Medicine, Critical Care–Medical
Saint Francis Medical Group, Inc
Department of Pulmonary Medicine
114 Woodland Street
Hartford, CT 06105, USA

E-mail addresses:
linda_nici@brown.edu (L. Nici)
rzuwalla@stfranciscare.org (R.L. ZuWallack)

http://dx.doi.org/10.1016/j.ccm.2014.03.001
0272-5231/14/$ – see front matter © 2014 Published by Elsevier Inc.

chestmed.theclinics.com

Pulmonary Rehabilitation
Definition, Concept, and History

Linda Nici, MD[a],*, Richard L. ZuWallack, MD[b]

KEYWORDS

- Pulmonary rehabilitation • Chronic obstructive pulmonary disease • Exercise training
- Behavioral change

KEY POINTS

- Pulmonary rehabilitation is a comprehensive intervention including exercise training, education, and behavior change, which improves the physical and emotional condition of people with chronic respiratory disease.
- Pulmonary rehabilitation can and should be delivered at multiple times in the disease trajectory of chronic respiratory disease.
- Pulmonary rehabilitation, by its essential nature, is designed to provide the right therapy for the right patient at the right time and therefore, fits perfectly into the concept of integrated care.

DEFINITION AND CONCEPT

Pulmonary rehabilitation is a complex intervention whose implementation varies widely among pulmonary rehabilitation centers worldwide, and indeed often varies considerably within a center, depending on the needs and goals of a particular respiratory patient. Furthermore, individual elements of the comprehensive pulmonary rehabilitation intervention, such as the promotion of exercise and self-management, are often applied in isolation as part of good medical care. Consequently, it is difficult to craft a succinct yet inclusive definition of pulmonary rehabilitation.

The 2013 American Thoracic Society/European Respiratory Society Statement on Pulmonary Rehabilitation perhaps comes closest to a workable definition of pulmonary rehabilitation: pulmonary rehabilitation is a comprehensive intervention based on a thorough patient assessment followed by patient-tailored therapies which include, but are not limited to, exercise training, education, and behavior change, designed to improve the physical and emotional condition of people with chronic respiratory disease and to promote the long-term adherence to health-enhancing behaviors.[1]

To better understand what pulmonary rehabilitation is, some amplification of this definition is necessary.

1. *Pulmonary rehabilitation.* Although combining different therapies, pulmonary rehabilitation is an entity on its own. Although each of its components could, and often should, be given as part of good medical care, these components are conveniently bundled into a package and delivered by professionals with expertise and experience in this area. Pulmonary rehabilitation is much more than the sum of its parts.[2]
2. *Comprehensive intervention.* Pulmonary rehabilitation can be delivered at multiple times in the disease trajectory of any individual patient with chronic respiratory disease. Its focus and components vary depending on the patient's goals, functional impairments, and disabilities. This approach requires a dedicated interdisciplinary team, which may include physicians, nurses, nurse practitioners, respiratory therapists, physiotherapists, occupational therapists, psychologists, behaviorists, exercise physiologists, nutritionists, and social workers. The composition of any particular pulmonary

[a] Pulmonary Medicine/Critical Care Section, Providence VA Medical Center, 830 Chalkstone Avenue, Providence, RI 02908, USA; [b] Pulmonary Medicine, Critical Care - Medical, Department of Pulmonary Medicine, Saint Francis Medical Group, Inc, 114 Woodland Street, Hartford, CT 06105, USA
* Corresponding author.
E-mail address: linda_nici@brown.edu

Clin Chest Med 35 (2014) 279–282
http://dx.doi.org/10.1016/j.ccm.2014.02.008
0272-5231/14/$ – see front matter Published by Elsevier Inc.

rehabilitation program will depend on available resources.

3. *Thorough patient assessment.* To effectively treat the often complex and unique morbidities of the individual patient with chronic respiratory disease, these must be first identified. For instance, exercise limitation in a patient with chronic obstructive pulmonary disease (COPD) often reflects multiple factors, such as ventilatory constraints, ambulatory muscle dysfunction, cardiovascular limitation, joint disease, and psychological and cognitive problems. Their identification will allow for a targeted and thereby more effective and efficient intervention.

4. *Patient-tailored therapies.* The intervention must be individualized to the unique therapeutic requirements of the patient, which result from the respiratory disease itself, comorbidities, treatments, and their psychological and social consequences. These therapies should be integrated to provide a seamless intervention throughout the course of a patient's disease.

5. *Exercise training, education, and behavior change.* The comprehensive pulmonary rehabilitation intervention includes multiple therapies. However, exercise training and education aimed at behavior change are its essential components. Although exercise training remains the cornerstone of pulmonary rehabilitation, in itself it is not sufficient to provide optimal and long-term benefits. It must be coupled with educational efforts aimed at promoting self-management skills and positive change in health behavior.

6. *Designed to improve the physical and emotional condition of people with chronic respiratory disease.* Pulmonary rehabilitation leads to substantial benefits in dyspnea, exercise capacity, health-related quality of life, and health care utilization. These benefits, which are often of greater magnitude than those from other medical therapies such as bronchodilators, are achieved without concurrent improvements in traditional measures of physiologic impairment, such as the forced expiratory volume in 1 second. This apparent paradox is explained by the fact that rehabilitation targets the often treatable systemic manifestations of chronic respiratory disease, such as peripheral muscle dysfunction, maladaptive health behaviors, and anxiety and depression. To fully delineate the beneficial effects of pulmonary rehabilitation, a comprehensive, patient-centered outcome assessment is necessary.

7. *Promote the long-term adherence to health-enhancing behaviors.* It would be naïve to think that an isolated, 6- to 12-week intervention such as exercise training would have a substantial long-term impact on a chronic disease, a point that underscores the need to include interventions that promote true health-behavior change so as to maintain long-term benefits. This aspect has become an important focus in the implementation of pulmonary rehabilitation.

Optimal treatment of the often complex patient with chronic respiratory disease ideally requires seamless care across settings and providers, over the course of the disease: the concept of integrated care.[3] Pulmonary rehabilitation, by its essential nature, is designed to provide the right therapy for the right patient at the right time. These therapies may include providing smoking-cessation therapy when necessary, promoting regular exercise and physical activity in the home and community settings, fostering collaborative self-management strategies, optimizing pharmacotherapy and medication adherence, and, when needed, offering palliative care and hospice services. This approach requires partnering, communication, and coordination among health care providers, patients, and their families. Because pulmonary rehabilitation encompasses all of these strategies, it fits perfectly into this concept of integrated care.

HISTORY
Early Years

Components of pulmonary rehabilitation have been provided as part of good medical care for centuries. However, in the 1960s and 1970s clinicians became aware that organizing these components into a comprehensive program could lead to substantial benefits for their patients.[4] Such components included breathing techniques, walking exercise, supplemental oxygen therapy, and bronchial hygiene techniques. These bundled interventions were first trialed, after which results were presented in the form of noncontrolled before-after studies or historically controlled studies.[5–7] In 1974, pulmonary rehabilitation was first given an official definition by the American College of Chest Physicians, and in 1981 the American Thoracic Society published its first official statement on pulmonary rehabilitation.[4]

Development in 2 general outcome areas fueled the growing popularity of pulmonary rehabilitation among clinicians: the development of the timed walk test in 1976, and the creation of the Chronic Respiratory Questionnaire, a patient-centered, health-related quality of life questionnaire for COPD, in 1987.[8] Pulmonary rehabilitation led to often striking improvements in these outcome areas.

Randomized Controlled Trials Demonstrating Global Benefit from Pulmonary Rehabilitation

In 1991, Casaburi and colleagues[9] demonstrated that patients with COPD had a dose-dependent physiologic effect from exercise training. Before this, conventional thought had been that these patients were ventilatory pump limited and could not achieve physiologic benefits from exercise training. In 1994, Reardon and colleagues[10] demonstrated that exertional dyspnea improved following pulmonary rehabilitation. In that same year, Goldstein and colleagues[11] demonstrated that pulmonary rehabilitation resulted in improved health-related quality of life. In 1995 Ries and colleagues,[12] in the largest trial to date (N = 119 subjects) demonstrated that, compared with education alone, comprehensive pulmonary rehabilitation led to significant improvements in exercise tolerance, symptoms, and self-efficacy for walking. In 1996, Maltais and colleagues[13] showed that COPD was a disease of the muscles and was therefore treatable by the exercise component of pulmonary rehabilitation. In 2000, Griffiths and colleagues,[14,15] in a trial of 200 patients with COPD, showed that in comparison with usual care, pulmonary rehabilitation not only improved the traditional outcomes of exercise capacity and quality of life but also reduced subsequent health care utilization.

Acceptance as a Gold Standard of Care

In 2001 the Global Initiative for Obstructive Lung Disease (GOLD) endorsed pulmonary rehabilitation as a standard therapy for COPD, and in 2003 placed this intervention prominently in their treatment algorithm for stable COPD.[16] In addition, in 2003 the National Emphysema Treatment Trial (NETT) was published[17]; this incorporated pulmonary rehabilitation as required care for emphysema patients referred for lung-volume reduction surgery, and compared the surgical outcome against the gold standard, pulmonary rehabilitation.

The Rise of Self-Management as an Integral Component of Pulmonary Rehabilitation

The trend of transforming pulmonary rehabilitation education from didactic teaching to collaborative self-management was well under way by the early 2000s, but this was given a big boost in 2003 when Bourbeau and colleagues[18] provided strong evidence that self-management education centered around an action plan for the exacerbation led to a substantial reduction in health care utilization. This report led to the concept of the 2 pillars of pulmonary rehabilitation, exercise training and self-management education.

Funding as a Specific Entity in the United States by the Centers for Medicare and Medicaid Services

In 2010, the Centers for Medicare and Medicaid Services began funding pulmonary rehabilitation. Although many pulmonary rehabilitation providers consider this funding to be insufficient to cover costs, it reflects acceptance of pulmonary rehabilitation by this important health care system in the United States.

Broadening the Scope of Pulmonary Rehabilitation

Pulmonary rehabilitation has traditionally been provided to stable patients with moderate to severe COPD, typically in an outpatient setting. Over the past decade this somewhat narrow application has been challenged. Pulmonary rehabilitation for COPD provided in the peri-exacerbation period produces a strong signal in reduced hospital readmissions and even, perhaps, reduced mortality.[19] Moreover, COPD patients with less severe disease also stand to benefit,[20] perhaps to a similar degree as those with more advanced disease. New and growing evidence now supports the effectiveness and often equivalent benefits of pulmonary rehabilitation in the non-COPD respiratory patient.[21] Carefully structured pulmonary rehabilitation given in the home setting can result in reductions in dyspnea similar to those achieved in center-based programs.[22]

SUMMARY

Pulmonary rehabilitation should be considered for all patients with chronic respiratory disease who remain symptomatic or have decreased functional status despite otherwise optimal medical management, and thus is part of their standard management. Pulmonary rehabilitation has proven benefits in decreasing dyspnea and in improving exercise tolerance, health-related quality of life, and health care utilization. Furthermore, emerging evidence supports a beneficial effect on the number and severity of exacerbations, and on mortality. The essential components of pulmonary rehabilitation are exercise training and self-management education; however, this intervention must be tailored to the unique needs of the individual patient and integrated into the course of the disease trajectory.

Emerging data support a role for pulmonary rehabilitation in nontraditional contexts, such as during exacerbation in the non-COPD patient and in the home setting. Clinicians should look forward to applying the basic tenets of pulmonary rehabilitation to all clinical situations in which respiratory disease causes significant morbidity and mortality, and whereby the ability to improve patient-centered outcomes and optimize the outlay of precious health care dollars is anticipated.

REFERENCES

1. Spruit MA, Singh SJ, Garvey C, et al. An official American Thoracic Society/European Respiratory Society statement: key concepts and advances in pulmonary rehabilitation. Am J Respir Crit Care Med 2013;188:e13–64.
2. Nici L, Lareau S, ZuWallack R. Pulmonary rehabilitation in the treatment of chronic obstructive pulmonary disease. Am Fam Physician 2010;82:655–60.
3. Nici L, ZuWallack R. An official American Thoracic Society workshop report: the integrated care of the COPD patient. Proc Am Thorac Soc 2012;9:9–18.
4. Casaburi R. A brief history of pulmonary rehabilitation. Respir Care 2008;53:1185–9.
5. Petty TL, Nett LM, Finigan MM, et al. A comprehensive care program for chronic airway obstruction. Methods and preliminary evaluation of symptomatic and functional improvement. Ann Intern Med 1969;70:1109–20.
6. Petty TL. Ambulatory care for emphysema and chronic bronchitis. Chest 1970;58(Suppl 2):441–8.
7. Hodgkin JE, Balchum OJ, Kass I, et al. Chronic obstructive airway diseases. Current concepts in diagnosis and comprehensive care. JAMA 1975;232:1243–60.
8. Zuwallack R. A history of pulmonary rehabilitation: back to the future. Pneumonol Alergol Pol 2009;77:298–301.
9. Casaburi R, Patessio A, Ioli F, et al. Reductions in exercise lactic acidosis and ventilation as a result of exercise training in patients with obstructive lung disease. Am Rev Respir Dis 1991;143:9–18.
10. Reardon J, Awad E, Normandin E, et al. The effect of comprehensive outpatient pulmonary rehabilitation on dyspnea. Chest 1994;105:1046–52.
11. Goldstein RS, Gort EH, Stubbing D, et al. Randomised controlled trial of respiratory rehabilitation. Lancet 1994;344:1394–7.
12. Ries AL, Kaplan RM, Limberg TM, et al. Effects of pulmonary rehabilitation on physiologic and psychosocial outcomes in patients with chronic obstructive pulmonary disease. Ann Intern Med 1995;122:823–32.
13. Maltais F, LeBlanc P, Simard C, et al. Skeletal muscle adaptation to endurance training in patients with chronic obstructive pulmonary disease. Am J Respir Crit Care Med 1996;154:442–7.
14. Griffiths TL, Burr ML, Campbell IA, et al. Results at 1 year of outpatient multidisciplinary pulmonary rehabilitation: a randomised controlled trial. Lancet 2000;355:362–8.
15. Griffiths TL, Phillips CJ, Davies S, et al. Cost effectiveness of an outpatient multidisciplinary pulmonary rehabilitation programme. Thorax 2001;56:779–84.
16. Global Initiative for Chronic Obstructive Lung Disease. Global strategy for diagnosis, management, and prevention of COPD. 2008. Available at: www.goldcopd.com.
17. Fishman A, Martinez F, Naunheim K, et al. A randomized trial comparing lung-volume-reduction surgery with medical therapy for severe emphysema. N Engl J Med 2003;348:2059–73.
18. Bourbeau J, Julien M, Maltais F, et al. Reduction of hospital utilization in patients with chronic obstructive pulmonary disease: a disease-specific self-management intervention. Arch Intern Med 2003;163:585–91.
19. Puhan MA, Gimeno-Santos E, Scharplatz M, et al. Pulmonary rehabilitation following exacerbations of chronic obstructive pulmonary disease. Cochrane Database Syst Rev 2011;(10):CD005305.
20. van Wetering CR, Hoogendoorn M, Mol SJ, et al. Short- and long-term efficacy of a community-based COPD management programme in less advanced COPD: a randomised controlled trial. Thorax 2010;65:7–13.
21. Spruit MA, Singh SJ, Garvey C, et al. Key concepts and advances in pulmonary rehabilitation based on the official 2013 American Thoracic Society/European Respiratory Society statement on pulmonary rehabilitation. Amer J Respir Crit Care Med 2013;188(8):e13–64.
22. Maltais F, Bourbeau J, Shapiro S, et al. Effects of home-based pulmonary rehabilitation in patients with chronic obstructive pulmonary disease: a randomized trial. Ann Intern Med 2008;149:869–78.

The Systemic Nature of Chronic Lung Disease

Rachael A. Evans, MBChB, MRCP (UK), PhD*, Michael D.L. Morgan, MB BChir, MA, MD, FRCP

KEYWORDS

- Chronic obstructive pulmonary disease • Pulmonary rehabilitation • Systemic manifestations
- Dyspnea • Comorbidity • Exercise

KEY POINTS

- Chronic obstructive pulmonary disease (COPD) can be considered as a multisystem syndrome rather than solely a disease of the lungs.
- Systemic manifestations include skeletal muscle impairment, osteoporosis, mood disturbance, anemia, and hormonal imbalance.
- Pulmonary rehabilitation targets the secondary consequences (systemic manifestations) of COPD.
- The causes of these secondary consequences include inactivity, systemic inflammation, hypoxia, and corticosteroid treatment.
- Individuals with COPD often have a wide range of comorbidities including cardiac disease, obesity, and metabolic syndrome, but this should not prevent referral or acceptance for pulmonary rehabilitation.
- Exercise training is also usually indicated for these comorbidities, but the assessments for safety may need some attention.
- Pulmonary rehabilitation is the only therapy that targets all aspects of the COPD syndrome, and access to the key components of exercise training and education should be equitable, although how this is delivered may vary across the spectrum of disease.

INTRODUCTION

Dyspnea on exertion is the commonest symptom of chronic lung disease. Chronic obstructive pulmonary disease (COPD) is the commonest chronic lung disease, and serves as an illustrative example of how progressive airflow limitation contributes to an inability to match the ventilatory demands of exercise. This inability is due to hypoxia, gas trapping and dynamic hyperinflation,[1] and increased mechanical disadvantage of the respiratory muscles. However, in severe disease the degree of airflow obstruction correlates poorly with exercise ability.[2]

Early trials of rehabilitation were deemed to be unsatisfactory by many because they did not improve lung function.[3,4] The first appropriately designed randomized controlled trial of pulmonary rehabilitation to gain attention compared exercise performance and quality of life with normal care.[5] The degree of dyspnea was reduced and the walking distance increased in patients undergoing pulmonary rehabilitation, but there was no difference in the degree of airflow obstruction. This finding led to the recognition over the next couple of decades that COPD was not solely a disease of the lungs but also was associated with significant systemic alterations, including skeletal muscle impairment, mood disturbance, hormonal imbalance, osteoporosis, and anemia (**Box 1**).

It is now understood that the benefits of pulmonary rehabilitation come from the improvements that can be made on these secondary effects. There is ongoing debate about the exact mechanisms causing these alterations, but physical

Department of Respiratory Medicine, Glenfield Hospital, Groby Road, Leicester LE3 9QP, UK
* Corresponding author.
E-mail address: rachael.evans@uhl-tr.nhs.uk

Clin Chest Med 35 (2014) 283–293
http://dx.doi.org/10.1016/j.ccm.2014.02.009
0272-5231/14/$ – see front matter © 2014 Elsevier Inc. All rights reserved.

> **Box 1**
> **Systemic manifestations of COPD**
>
> - Skeletal muscle
> - Mood disturbance
> - Hormonal imbalance
> - Others: osteoporosis and anaemia

inactivity leading to deconditioning, systemic inflammation, hypoxia, and medication have all been implicated. COPD is a heterogeneous disease that can be thought of as a syndrome, and it is likely that causes vary between individuals in their predominance.

Pulmonary rehabilitation programs are traditionally composed of hospital-based supervised programs aimed at patients with noticeable dyspnea. However, recent evidence suggests that these secondary manifestations can occur early in the disease,[6] so perhaps physical inactivity should be targeted earlier in the disease to prevent future disablement.

Apart from the secondary manifestations of the disease, patients with COPD may also have multiple comorbidities,[7] which can cause reluctance to refer for rehabilitation. Cardiac disease (ischemic heart disease and chronic heart failure) is more prevalent in COPD than in the rest of the population even after confounding factors have been addressed. Other comorbidities such as abdominal aortic aneurysm can lead to debate over whether exercise training is safe. Obesity and metabolic syndrome are highly prevalent in COPD, perhaps even to a greater extent than in the rest of the population. There is evidence that some comorbidities may be also be part of the secondary consequences of the disease, but for the purposes of this article they are discussed separately.

SYSTEMIC MANIFESTATIONS OF COPD
Skeletal Muscle Impairment

One of the first randomized trials of pulmonary rehabilitation versus normal care noted that despite the improvement in walking distance, the degree of airflow obstruction was unchanged.[5] At a similar time leg fatigue was shown to be a very common limiting symptom to a maximal incremental cardiopulmonary exercise test on a cycle ergometer.[8] Subsequently, several studies have demonstrated that the structure of the quadriceps muscle is altered with a reduction in muscle mass and strength in COPD,[9] and is associated with a higher mortality[10,11] and morbidity, in addition to increased hospital admissions.[12] The muscle quality is also impaired; there is preferential reduction in the type I fiber cross-sectional area in the quadriceps muscle in COPD, and reduced oxidative enzyme concentration,[13-15] mitochondrial density,[16] and capillary density.[14] These adaptations reflect a loss of the aerobic profile of the muscle, which is exemplified during cycling exercise whereby individuals with moderate COPD achieve an earlier anaerobic threshold,[17] and muscle-energy requirements are unable to be met with a resultant decline in phosphocreatine and adenosine triphosphate at very low absolute power.[18] These metabolic impairments of the muscle demand an increase in ventilation on an already burdened system, causing the termination of exercise. Other supporting evidence of a peripheral muscle contribution to exercise limitation in COPD includes quadriceps contractile fatigue after whole-body exercise[19,20] and worsening exercise performance with "prefatigue" of the quadriceps muscles.[21] Lower limb aerobic and strength training are therefore essential components of a pulmonary rehabilitation program.[22,23]

Although most evidence for skeletal muscle impairment has been concentrated on the lower limbs, there is also evidence that the upper limb muscles, both proximal and distal, are weaker than healthy controls.[24]

There is debate about whether there is true weakness of the respiratory muscles in COPD. Inspiratory muscle strength measured by maximal inspiratory pressure is reduced in COPD, but the expiratory muscle strength can be preserved or reduced.[25] Isolated diaphragmatic strength has been shown to be preserved in COPD assessed by twitch transdiaphragmatic pressure when corrected for lung volume.[26] Hyperinflation leads to the muscles being put at a mechanical disadvantage. Regarding fiber type proportion, the opposite phenomenon is seen in the diaphragm muscle fibers compared with the quadriceps fibers as the type one fibers are increased compared with healthy controls.[27] In COPD, diaphragmatic strength is not fatigued by either endurance exercise to symptom limitation or hyperventilation suggesting that it is not a major limiting factor to exercise capacity.[28-30]

Mood Disturbance

Mood disturbance is very common in COPD and is a major contributing factor to morbidity.[31] Anxiety heightens the sensation of breathlessness and compounds the reduced exercise capacity. In itself this can lead to low mood and frustration. Although the symptom of dyspnea can lead directly to anxiety, there may also be a predilection for patients with COPD to suffer from anxiety, as it is more common in smokers. Pulmonary rehabilitation often improves the symptoms of anxiety when present, and patients exhibiting anxiety derive benefit from rehabilitation.[32] Depressive symptoms are also very common in COPD and should be distinguished from a clinical diagnosis of depression, which should be managed according to clinical guidelines. True depression can lead to lower motivation, loss of work and hobbies, social isolation, and impaired relationships, further worsening symptoms and health status. Similar to anxiety, symptoms of low mood are improved with pulmonary rehabilitation, are not associated with poorer completion; patients with low mood at baseline gained similar benefits in exercise performance.[32]

Hormonal Imbalance

The balance between catabolic and anabolic steroids is disrupted in COPD.[33] Testosterone levels in male patients with COPD have been shown to be consistently low in 9 trials.[34] A meta-analysis involving 5 randomized controlled trials of testosterone replacement therapy demonstrated improvement in muscle strength and peak power on an incremental exercise test, but no statistical improvement in peak oxygen uptake.[34] Supplementation with other hormones has been investigated in COPD, such as growth hormone which, although leading to weight gain, did not translate to worthwhile improvements in either muscle strength or exercise capacity.[35]

Osteoporosis

Prevalence studies have reported osteoporosis in 24% to 69% of patients with COPD, which is approximately 3 times greater than occurs in age-matched healthy controls.[36] Risk factors for osteoporosis in patients with COPD include advanced age, female sex, postmenopausal status, more severe lung-function impairment, malnutrition, low body mass index (BMI) and fat-free mass, vitamin D deficiency, smoking, excessive alcohol consumption, inactivity, and use of corticosteroids.[37] A recent study concluded that for patients with COPD, osteoporosis should be diagnosed by lumbar and hip dual x-ray absorptiometry (DEXA) scanning rather than whole-body DEXA, to achieve better detection rates.[38]

Anemia

Anemia is underrecognized but common in COPD. A prospective cohort study described 17% of patients as being anemic (hemoglobin <13.0 d/L)[39]; this was associated with a reduced median survival and an independent predictor of functional capacity (assessed by the 6-minute walk test distance). A retrospective analysis has shown anemia to be present in 33% of patients with COPD, and this was associated with increased health care utilization.[40]

MECHANISMS AND CAUSES OF THE SYSTEMIC MANIFESTATIONS OF COPD

There is ongoing debate about the major contributing factors to the systemic manifestations of COPD, but physical inactivity, systemic inflammation, hypoxia, poor nutrition, and corticosteroids are all implicated (**Box 2**). It is likely that the predominance of these factors varies between individuals and between the different systemic manifestations.

Physical Inactivity

Human skeletal muscle exhibits plasticity (ie, demonstrates hyperplasia and hypertrophy to exercise, or atrophy in the presence of disuse).[41] It is established that patients with COPD are less active than their age-matched controls across the spectrum of disease severity.[42] Although inactivity is associated with loss of quadriceps strength and endurance,[43] longitudinal studies are needed to fully understand the nature of the relationship. The differential involvement between muscle groups supports inactivity as a major cause. Even when quadriceps strength is reduced, both adductor pollicis and diaphragmatic strength may be preserved in comparison with healthy subjects.[26,44] The difference in fiber-type changes in COPD between the diaphragm and quadriceps also supports inactivity as a contributing factor.

Systemic Inflammation

COPD is associated with low-grade systemic inflammation, particularly in those with higher resting energy expenditure and lower fat-free mass.[45,46] This inflammatory process, when assessed by circulating interleukin (IL)-6, has a small

> **Box 2**
> **Causes of systemic manifestations of COPD**
>
> - Inactivity leading to deconditioning
> - Systemic inflammation
> - Nutritional abnormalities
> - Others: hypoxia and corticosteroids

influence on prognosis beyond a multicomponent disease severity index.[47] There are several theories regarding the mechanisms and implications of this systemic inflammatory process. It was previously thought that there might be spill-over from airway inflammation, but more recent evidence has shown that COPD may result from accelerated lung aging[48] secondary to oxidative stress. Telomere length is shorter in leukocytes of patients with COPD than in healthy controls, and is associated with systemic inflammation.[49]

It is not clear precisely how systemic inflammation relates to the secondary impairments. In skeletal muscle, levels of tumor necrosis factor α alpha have been contradictory.[50–53] Physical inactivity, which is a major contributing factor to skeletal muscle impairment, is associated with increased levels of systemic inflammation. Therefore, these processes are likely to be interrelated. The anemia of chronic disease is thought to be mediated through inflammatory processes. In a cohort of 101 patients with COPD, those who were anemic (13%) were associated with higher levels of C-reactive protein and IL-6 and increased levels of erythropoietin resistance, supporting an inflammatory process as the cause.[54] A recent association was described between anemia, osteoporosis, and systemic inflammation.[55] Further work is needed to investigate the mechanisms and prove causality rather than association.

Although comorbidities are discussed separately in this article, there is increasing evidence that an inflammatory process may be the common link. Data from a large multinational trial showed that heart disease, hypertension, and diabetes were associated with increased systemic inflammation.[56] An association has been reported between arterial stiffness and systemic inflammation in COPD.[57] A further report separated comorbidities into 5 groups, but each had similar levels of systemic inflammation.[58] There are now many trials indicating the relationship between systemic inflammation, systemic manifestations, some comorbidities and COPD, but as yet therapy with various anti-inflammatories has been unsuccessful.

Hypoxia

Hypoxia induced by prolonged exposure to high altitude causes skeletal muscle wasting in healthy adults and loss of muscle oxidative capacity with a reduction in mitochondria.[59] In an experiment in healthy subjects in which altitude was simulated in a hyperbaric chamber, the reduced muscle mass was associated with a significant reduction in type I fiber by 25%, and a nonsignificant reduction in type II fibers.[60] However, patients with severe COPD with and without respiratory failure have a similar reduction in type I fibers.[61] Hypoxia is unlikely to be the major contributing factor, as skeletal muscle dysfunction is demonstrated in the absence of either chronic or intermittent hypoxemia.

Corticosteroids

It is well recognized that steroids cause a proximal myopathy. Although long-term steroids are no longer recommended for most patients, people who frequently exacerbate can still be prescribed multiple courses of steroids per year. Most studies investigating skeletal muscle dysfunction excluded patients who were on long-term steroids and still found abnormalities. In a comparative trial, there was no difference in energy metabolism or oxidative and glycolytic enzyme level between patients on long-term steroids or those who were not, but there was impairment of both energy metabolism and decreased oxidative and increased glycolytic enzymes in comparison with healthy controls.[62]

ROLE OF PULMONARY REHABILITATION FOR THE SECONDARY MANIFESTATIONS

Pulmonary rehabilitation (predominantly composed of exercise training and education) targets the secondary manifestations to improve dyspnea, exercise performance, and health-related quality of life. Early studies identified that airflow obstruction was unchanged with physical training, whereas exercise tolerance was improved.[5]

The training adaptations are specific to the type of training prescribed. Aerobic high-intensity progressive exercise training improves the oxidative capacity of the muscle by increasing the cross-sectional area of type I fibers, oxidative enzymes, mitochondrial number, and capillarization, leading to improvement in exercise performance.[63] Strength training improves muscle strength, but when this is added to endurance training no further improvements in exercise tolerance or health-related quality of life are seen. Strength training is recommended in health for bone protection.[64] In a recent survey of patients with COPD undergoing pulmonary rehabilitation, the presence of osteoporosis was an independent predictor of a poorer outcome.[65]

Pulmonary rehabilitation has been shown to improve anxiety and depressive symptoms. This process is multifactorial and can be improved via physiologic and psychological pathways, and is described in more detail in an article elsewhere in this issue.

The effect of hormonal and nutritional supplementation in addition to pulmonary rehabilitation has been evaluated. Testosterone supplementation with resistance training in male patients with COPD and low levels of testosterone led to further improvements in quadriceps strength in comparison with resistance training or testosterone supplementation alone.[66] Nutritional supplementation in combination with pulmonary rehabilitation has been extensively evaluated; overall, however, neither calorie nor creatine supplementation enhance the effects of pulmonary rehabilitation in terms of exercise performance or health-related quality of life.[67,68]

COMORBIDITIES IN COPD AND PULMONARY REHABILITATION
Multiple Comorbidities

Comorbidities negatively affect exercise tolerance and health-related quality of life in patients with COPD, and can lead to hesitance to refer and accept patients for pulmonary rehabilitation. For many studies evaluating pulmonary rehabilitation, the exclusion of patients with comorbidities does not reflect the real-life situation. A prospective trial showed that nearly two-thirds of patients with COPD have at least 1 comorbid condition.[65] The commonest were systemic hypertension (35%), dyslipidemia (13%), diabetes (12%), coronary disease (11%), chronic heart failure (9%), and osteoporosis (9%) (**Box 3**). Of these, only osteoporosis was associated with a poorer outcome; however, skeletal muscle strength was not assessed so it may be that osteoporosis was merely a marker of skeletal muscle dysfunction. The number of comorbidities did not affect outcome, and there was no indication that there were more adverse events in these patients. Although patients with

---

Box 3
Most common comorbid conditions in COPD patients

Hypertension (35%)

Dyslipidemia (13%)

Diabetes (12%)

Coronary disease (11%)

Chronic heart failure (9%)

Osteoporosis (9%)

Data from Crisafulli E, Gorgone P, Vagaggini B, et al. Efficacy of standard rehabilitation in COPD outpatients with comorbidities. Eur Respir J 2010;36(5): 1042–8.

---

comorbidities may derive benefit from pulmonary rehabilitation, staffing levels may need to be increased to reflect the frailty of the population being treated.

Cardiac Disease

COPD frequently coexists with cardiovascular diseases, particularly coronary artery disease[28] and chronic heart failure.[69–72] Some overlap is to be expected, as these conditions increase in prevalence with age and have smoking as a common risk factor. The percentage of patients with both diseases ranges from 10% to 30%, and the risk ratio of developing chronic heart failure in COPD is 4.5 in comparison with age-matched controls.[73]

The presence of systemic inflammation reported in patients with coronary heart disease,[74,75] chronic heart failure,[76,77] and COPD[78,79] may be an important pathologic mechanism contributing to cardiovascular complications, a common cause of death in individuals with COPD.[80,81] Cardiovascular events increase in frequency as airflow obstruction progresses.[82,83] The coexistence of heart and lung diseases is important, as the combination is associated with a worse prognosis,[84–86] a worse outcome after hospital admissions,[87] more symptoms,[88] and lower exercise capacity.[89] In a large multicenter trial of exercise training versus usual care in patients with heart failure, the coexistence of COPD was associated with increased cardiovascular mortality and hospitalization for heart failure, but a similar response to exercise training.[90]

There is sometimes reluctance to include patients with COPD with known cardiac disease in pulmonary rehabilitation programs, but exercise has been shown to be beneficial in stable ischemic heart disease and chronic heart failure[91] and is part of the management strategy for these conditions. There are some adjustments needed to the usual rehabilitation assessment for safety as per cardiac rehabilitation guidelines, and an initial exercise test should be performed with electrocardiography and blood pressure monitoring. This approach does not necessarily entail performing a full laboratory cardiopulmonary exercise test, as field testing can be performed with telemetry for cardiac monitoring. Aspects of disease education may need individualizing to incorporate management of cardiac disease, or this may be performed outside of the rehabilitation program.

Two small studies reported a reduction in blood pressure, aortic stiffness, and cholesterol in patients with COPD after pulmonary rehabilitation,[92,93] supporting the concept that pulmonary rehabilitation provides comprehensive therapy for comorbidities.

Obesity

Obesity is a common comorbidity in COPD, more so than cachexia. In many pulmonary rehabilitation programs more than half of the population is overweight or obese,[94] and in large, randomized controlled trials the mean BMI is 27 kg/m^2.[95] Obesity is associated with worse survival in the general population,[96] but there is a paradox in COPD whereby patients who are overweight and obese appear to have a survival advantage over those who are of normal weight.[97] This finding is derived mainly from epidemiologic data, so causality has not been established. Obesity is associated with reduced exercise performance[94,98] in COPD. Of note, obesity is associated with improved incremental exercise testing with reduced dynamic hyperinflation when the weight is supported on a cycle ergometer.[99]

Many pulmonary rehabilitation programs are generally unaltered for obese individuals. In a retrospective analysis, patients with COPD gained similar benefits in terms of walking performance and health-related quality of life across the BMI spectrum.[94] However, more formal dietary advice and support may be needed, as standard pulmonary rehabilitation is not associated with weight loss. There is increasing evidence that exercise can improve insulin resistance in prediabetic obese individuals, supporting exercise rehabilitation for this group.

Metabolic Syndrome

Of several definitions of metabolic syndrome (association between obesity, hypertension, abnormal lipid profile, and/or diabetes), the most recent comes from the International Diabetes Federation, which defines the syndrome as the presence of central obesity and 2 of either raised triglycerides, reduced high-density lipoprotein cholesterol, raised blood pressure, or raised fasting glucose. A recent study from Germany reported metabolic syndrome to be present in nearly half of patients with COPD across the GOLD stages, with a slightly lower occurrence in severe disease.[100] Metabolic syndrome was associated with systemic inflammation and physical inactivity. A further population-based study showed that the risk of airflow obstruction was higher in those with metabolic syndrome,[101] supporting results from the Framingham Heart study showing that diabetes is independently associated with airflow obstruction. An inflammatory mechanism has been postulated.[102,103]

Investigation is ongoing to determine the mechanisms and relationships between COPD, adipose tissue inflammation, systemic inflammation, and metabolic syndrome. One of the most successful interventions to delay the onset of diabetes in a group at risk (prediabetes) was a lifestyle intervention aimed at weight loss and an increase in physical activity.[104] Pulmonary rehabilitation should therefore benefit features of the metabolic syndrome in COPD, but this needs formal evaluation. It has already been demonstrated that the usual benefits of pulmonary rehabilitation on exercise and quality of life can be achieved in this group.[65]

Overall, exercise and increasing daily activity are likely to benefit most comorbidities associated with COPD (**Box 4**), and should therefore remain a core part of management for this group.

VERY SEVERE DISEASE AND REHABILITATION

Patients with the most severe disability have, in many cases, much to gain from rehabilitation, although practical issues of access may often prohibit their participation. Those patients with respiratory failure represent a particular challenge. Initially it was thought that people with severe disability (Medical Research Council dyspnea rating of 5 out of 5) would not benefit from rehabilitation[105]; however, it is clear that carefully supervised programs can result in useful benefits in the same manner as those with less disability.[2] If patients require supplementary oxygen for their regular treatment, they can undertake exercise training using oxygen throughout. Ventilatory support with noninvasive ventilation may also help increase the ability to train at effective workloads. Reducing the impact of the training burden by interval training or reducing ventilatory demand by training with one leg at a time may allow more severely disabled patients to gain benefit.[106,107] One recent article suggests that training techniques borrowed from professional athletes may also be beneficial.[108] Alternatives to physical exercise training, such as transcutaneous neuromuscular stimulation, may produce positive results in patients who are too weak to train volitionally.[109] For people with severe disability who are unintentionally admitted to hospital with exacerbation,

---

Box 4
Comorbidities that might be improved with pulmonary rehabilitation

- Cardiac disease
- Obesity
- Metabolic syndrome

early rehabilitation soon after discharge may be beneficial. In general, these principles apply to all patients with chronic lung disease; however, there does seem to be an exception for those with advanced pulmonary fibrosis, in whom the extreme oxygen demands and poor prognosis may make physical training impractical.[110]

SUMMARY

The systemic effects and comorbidities of chronic respiratory disease such as COPD contribute substantially to its burden. Symptoms in COPD do not solely arise from the degree of airflow obstruction, particularly in more advanced disease, as exercise limitation is compounded by the specific secondary manifestations of the disease. Pulmonary rehabilitation is effective because it improves these secondary manifestations. Comorbid conditions may also benefit from similar approaches to rehabilitation.

REFERENCES

1. O'Donnell DE, Revill SM, Webb KA. Dynamic hyperinflation and exercise intolerance in chronic obstructive pulmonary disease. Am J Respir Crit Care Med 2001;164(5):770–7.
2. Evans RA, Singh SJ, Collier R, et al. Pulmonary rehabilitation is successful for COPD irrespective of MRC dyspnoea grade. Respir Med 2009; 103(7):1070–5.
3. Cockcroft AE, Saunders MJ, Berry G. Randomised controlled trial of rehabilitation in chronic respiratory disability. Thorax 1981;36(3):200–3.
4. McGavin CR, Gupta SP, Lloyd EL, et al. Physical rehabilitation for the chronic bronchitic: results of a controlled trial of exercises in the home. Thorax 1977;32(3):307–11.
5. Goldstein RS, Gort EH, Stubbing D, et al. Randomised controlled trial of respiratory rehabilitation. Lancet 1994;344(8934):1394–7.
6. Seymour JM, Spruit MA, Hopkinson NS, et al. The prevalence of quadriceps weakness in COPD and the relationship with disease severity. Eur Respir J 2010;36(1):81–8.
7. Crisafulli E, Costi S, Luppi F, et al. Role of comorbidities in a cohort of patients with COPD undergoing pulmonary rehabilitation. Thorax 2008;63(6): 487–92.
8. Hamilton AL, Killian KJ, Summers E, et al. Symptom intensity and subjective limitation to exercise in patients with cardiorespiratory disorders. Chest 1996; 110(5):1255–63.
9. Debigare R, Cote CH, Maltais F. Peripheral muscle wasting in chronic obstructive pulmonary disease. Clinical relevance and mechanisms. Am J Respir Crit Care Med 2001;164(9):1712–7.
10. Swallow EB, Reyes D, Hopkinson NS, et al. Quadriceps strength predicts mortality in patients with moderate to severe chronic obstructive pulmonary disease. Thorax 2007;62(2):115–20.
11. Marquis K, Debigare R, Lacasse Y, et al. Midthigh muscle cross-sectional area is a better predictor of mortality than body mass index in patients with chronic obstructive pulmonary disease. Am J Respir Crit Care Med 2002;166(6):809–13.
12. Decramer M, Gosselink R, Troosters T, et al. Muscle weakness is related to utilization of health care resources in COPD patients. Eur Respir J 1997; 10(2):417–23.
13. Maltais F, Sullivan MJ, LeBlanc P, et al. Altered expression of myosin heavy chain in the vastus lateralis muscle in patients with COPD. Eur Respir J 1999;13(4):850–4.
14. Whittom F, Jobin J, Simard PM, et al. Histochemical and morphological characteristics of the vastus lateralis muscle in patients with chronic obstructive pulmonary disease. Med Sci Sports Exerc 1998; 30(10):1467–74.
15. Maltais F, Simard AA, Simard C, et al. Oxidative capacity of the skeletal muscle and lactic acid kinetics during exercise in normal subjects and in patients with COPD. Am J Respir Crit Care Med 1996;153(1):288–93.
16. Gosker HR, Hesselink MK, Duimel H, et al. Reduced mitochondrial density in the vastus lateralis muscle of patients with COPD. Eur Respir J 2007;30(1):73–9.
17. Casaburi R, Patessio A, Ioli F, et al. Reductions in exercise lactic acidosis and ventilation as a result of exercise training in patients with obstructive lung disease. Am Rev Respir Dis 1991;143(1): 9–18.
18. Steiner MC, Evans R, Deacon SJ, et al. Adenine nucleotide loss in the skeletal muscles during exercise in chronic obstructive pulmonary disease. Thorax 2005;60(11):932–6.
19. Saey D, Debigare R, LeBlanc P, et al. Contractile leg fatigue after cycle exercise: a factor limiting exercise in patients with chronic obstructive pulmonary disease. Am J Respir Crit Care Med 2003; 168(4):425–30.
20. Man WD, Soliman MG, Gearing J, et al. Symptoms and quadriceps fatigability after walking and cycling in chronic obstructive pulmonary disease. Am J Respir Crit Care Med 2003;168(5): 562–7.
21. Gagnon P, Saey D, Vivodtzev I, et al. Impact of preinduced quadriceps fatigue on exercise response in chronic obstructive pulmonary disease and healthy subjects. J Appl Physiol (1985) 2009; 107(3):832–40.

22. Bolton CE, Bevan-Smith EF, Blakey JD, et al. British Thoracic Society guideline on pulmonary rehabilitation in adults. Thorax 2013;68(Suppl 2):ii1–30.

23. Spruit MA, Singh SJ, Garvey C, et al. An official American Thoracic Society/European Respiratory Society statement: key concepts and advances in pulmonary rehabilitation. Am J Respir Crit Care Med 2013;188(8):e13–64.

24. Pitta F, Troosters T, Spruit MA, et al. Activity monitoring for assessment of physical activities in daily life in patients with chronic obstructive pulmonary disease. Arch Phys Med Rehabil 2005;86(10):1979–85.

25. Rochester DF. The respiratory muscles in COPD. State of the art. Chest 1984;85(Suppl 6):47S–50S.

26. Man WD, Soliman MG, Nikoletou D, et al. Non-volitional assessment of skeletal muscle strength in patients with chronic obstructive pulmonary disease. Thorax 2003;58(8):665–9.

27. Levine S, Kaiser L, Leferovich J, et al. Cellular adaptations in the diaphragm in chronic obstructive pulmonary disease. N Engl J Med 1997;337(25):1799–806.

28. Polkey MI, Kyroussis D, Keilty SE, et al. Exhaustive treadmill exercise does not reduce twitch transdiaphragmatic pressure in patients with COPD. Am J Respir Crit Care Med 1995;152(3):959–64.

29. Polkey MI, Kyroussis D, Hamnegard CH, et al. Diaphragm performance during maximal voluntary ventilation in chronic obstructive pulmonary disease. Am J Respir Crit Care Med 1997;155(2):642–8.

30. Mador MJ, Kufel TJ, Pineda LA, et al. Diaphragmatic fatigue and high-intensity exercise in patients with chronic obstructive pulmonary disease. Am J Respir Crit Care Med 2000;161(1):118–23.

31. Hill K, Geist R, Goldstein RS, et al. Anxiety and depression in end-stage COPD. Eur Respir J 2008;31(3):667–77.

32. Harrison SL, Greening NJ, Williams JE, et al. Have we underestimated the efficacy of pulmonary rehabilitation in improving mood? Respir Med 2012;106(6):838–44.

33. Debigare R, Marquis K, Cote CH, et al. Catabolic/anabolic balance and muscle wasting in patients with COPD. Chest 2003;124(1):83–9.

34. Atlantis E, Fahey P, Cochrane B, et al. Endogenous testosterone level and testosterone supplementation therapy in chronic obstructive pulmonary disease (COPD): a systematic review and meta-analysis. BMJ Open 2013;3(8). pii:e003127.

35. Burdet L, de Muralt B, Schutz Y, et al. Administration of growth hormone to underweight patients with chronic obstructive pulmonary disease. A prospective, randomized, controlled study. Am J Respir Crit Care Med 1997;156(6):1800–6.

36. Graat-Verboom L, Wouters EF, Smeenk FW, et al. Current status of research on osteoporosis in COPD: a systematic review. Eur Respir J 2009;34(1):209–18.

37. Biskobing DM. COPD and osteoporosis. Chest 2002;121(2):609–20.

38. Graat-Verboom L, Spruit MA, van den Borne BE, et al. Whole-body versus local dxa-scan for the diagnosis of osteoporosis in COPD patients. J Osteoporos 2010;2010:640878.

39. Cote C, Zilberberg MD, Mody SH, et al. Haemoglobin level and its clinical impact in a cohort of patients with COPD. Eur Respir J 2007;29(5):923–9.

40. Shorr AF, Doyle J, Stern L, et al. Anemia in chronic obstructive pulmonary disease: epidemiology and economic implications. Curr Med Res Opin 2008;24(4):1123–30.

41. Booth FW, Gollnick PD. Effects of disuse on the structure and function of skeletal muscle. Med Sci Sports Exerc 1983;15(5):415–20.

42. Pitta F, Troosters T, Spruit MA, et al. Characteristics of physical activities in daily life in chronic obstructive pulmonary disease. Am J Respir Crit Care Med 2005;171(9):972–7.

43. Serres I, Gautier V, Varray A, et al. Impaired skeletal muscle endurance related to physical inactivity and altered lung function in COPD patients. Chest 1998;113(4):900–5.

44. Man WD, Hopkinson NS, Harraf F, et al. Abdominal muscle and quadriceps strength in chronic obstructive pulmonary disease. Thorax 2005;60(9):718–22.

45. Schols AM, Buurman WA, Staal van den Brekel AJ, et al. Evidence for a relation between metabolic derangements and increased levels of inflammatory mediators in a subgroup of patients with chronic obstructive pulmonary disease. Thorax 1996;51(8):819–24.

46. Broekhuizen R, Wouters EF, Creutzberg EC, et al. Raised CRP levels mark metabolic and functional impairment in advanced COPD. Thorax 2006;61(1):17–22.

47. Celli BR, Locantore N, Yates J, et al. Inflammatory biomarkers improve clinical prediction of mortality in chronic obstructive pulmonary disease. Am J Respir Crit Care Med 2012;185(10):1065–72.

48. Lee J, Sandford A, Man P, et al. Is the aging process accelerated in chronic obstructive pulmonary disease? Curr Opin Pulm Med 2011;17(2):90–7.

49. Savale L, Chaouat A, Bastuji-Garin S, et al. Shortened telomeres in circulating leukocytes of patients with chronic obstructive pulmonary disease. Am J Respir Crit Care Med 2009;179(7):566–71.

50. Montes de Oca M, Torres SH, De Sanctis J, et al. Skeletal muscle inflammation and nitric oxide in patients with COPD. Eur Respir J 2005;26(3):390–7.

51. Rabinovich RA, Figueras M, Ardite E, et al. Increased tumour necrosis factor-alpha plasma levels during moderate-intensity exercise in COPD patients. Eur Respir J 2003;21(5):789–94.

52. Petersen AM, Penkowa M, Iversen M, et al. Elevated levels of IL-18 in plasma and skeletal muscle in chronic obstructive pulmonary disease. Lung 2007;185(3):161–71.

53. Barreiro E, Schols AM, Polkey MI, et al. Cytokine profile in quadriceps muscles of patients with severe COPD. Thorax 2008;63(2):100–7.

54. John M, Lange A, Hoernig S, et al. Prevalence of anemia in chronic obstructive pulmonary disease: comparison to other chronic diseases. Int J Cardiol 2006;111(3):365–70.

55. Rutten EP, Franssen FM, Spruit MA, et al. Anemia is associated with bone mineral density in chronic obstructive pulmonary disease. COPD 2013; 10(3):286–92.

56. Miller J, Edwards LD, Agusti A, et al. Comorbidity, systemic inflammation and outcomes in the ECLIPSE cohort. Respir Med 2013;107(9): 1376–84.

57. Sabit R, Bolton CE, Edwards PH, et al. Arterial stiffness and osteoporosis in chronic obstructive pulmonary disease. Am J Respir Crit Care Med 2007;175(12):1259–65.

58. Vanfleteren LE, Spruit MA, Groenen M, et al. Clusters of comorbidities based on validated objective measurements and systemic inflammation in patients with chronic obstructive pulmonary disease. Am J Respir Crit Care Med 2013;187(7): 728–35.

59. Howald H, Hoppeler H. Performing at extreme altitude: muscle cellular and subcellular adaptations. Eur J Appl Physiol 2003;90(3–4):360–4.

60. MacDougall JD, Green HJ, Sutton JR, et al. Operation Everest II: structural adaptations in skeletal muscle in response to extreme simulated altitude. Acta Physiol Scand 1991;142(3):421–7.

61. Jakobsson P, Jorfeldt L, Brundin A. Skeletal muscle metabolites and fibre types in patients with advanced chronic obstructive pulmonary disease (COPD), with and without chronic respiratory failure. Eur Respir J 1990;3(2):192–6.

62. Pouw EM, Koerts-de Lang E, Gosker HR, et al. Muscle metabolic status in patients with severe COPD with and without long-term prednisolone. Eur Respir J 2000;16(2):247–52.

63. Man WD, Kemp P, Moxham J, et al. Exercise and muscle dysfunction in COPD: implications for pulmonary rehabilitation. Clin Sci (Lond) 2009; 117(8):281–91.

64. Kmietowicz Z. NICE publishes osteoporosis guidance after more than six years of consultation. BMJ 2008;337:a2397.

65. Crisafulli E, Gorgone P, Vagaggini B, et al. Efficacy of standard rehabilitation in COPD outpatients with comorbidities. Eur Respir J 2010;36(5):1042–8.

66. Casaburi R, Bhasin S, Cosentino L, et al. Effects of testosterone and resistance training in men with chronic obstructive pulmonary disease. Am J Respir Crit Care Med 2004;170(8):870–8.

67. Steiner MC, Barton RL, Singh SJ, et al. Nutritional enhancement of exercise performance in chronic obstructive pulmonary disease: a randomised controlled trial. Thorax 2003;58(9):745–51.

68. Deacon SJ, Vincent EE, Greenhaff PL, et al. Randomized controlled trial of dietary creatine as an adjunct therapy to physical training in chronic obstructive pulmonary disease. Am J Respir Crit Care Med 2008;178(3):233–9.

69. Hawkins NM, Jhund PS, Simpson CR, et al. Primary care burden and treatment of patients with heart failure and chronic obstructive pulmonary disease in Scotland. Eur J Heart Fail 2010;12(1):17–24.

70. Rutten FH, Moons KG, Cramer MJ, et al. Recognising heart failure in elderly patients with stable chronic obstructive pulmonary disease in primary care: cross sectional diagnostic study. BMJ 2005; 331(7529):1379.

71. Mascarenhas J, Lourenco P, Lopes R, et al. Chronic obstructive pulmonary disease in heart failure. Prevalence, therapeutic and prognostic implications. Am Heart J 2008;155(3):521–5.

72. Macchia A, Rodriguez Moncalvo JJ, Kleinert M, et al. Unrecognised ventricular dysfunction in COPD. Eur Respir J 2012;39(1):51–8.

73. Curkendall SM, DeLuise C, Jones JK, et al. Cardiovascular disease in patients with chronic obstructive pulmonary disease, Saskatchewan Canada cardiovascular disease in COPD patients. Ann Epidemiol 2006;16(1):63–70.

74. Lavie CJ, Milani RV, Verma A, et al. C-reactive protein and cardiovascular diseases–is it ready for primetime? Am J Med Sci 2009;338(6):486–92.

75. Willerson JT. Systemic and local inflammation in patients with unstable atherosclerotic plaques. Prog Cardiovasc Dis 2002;44(6):469–78.

76. Wisniacki N, Taylor W, Lye M, et al. Insulin resistance and inflammatory activation in older patients with systolic and diastolic heart failure. Heart 2005; 91(1):32–7.

77. Torre-Amione G. Immune activation in chronic heart failure. Am J Cardiol 2005;95(11A):3C–8C.

78. Garcia-Rio F, Miravitlles M, Soriano JB, et al. Systemic inflammation in chronic obstructive pulmonary disease: a population-based study. Respir Res 2010;11(1):63.

79. Higashimoto Y, Iwata T, Okada M, et al. Serum bio-markers as predictors of lung function decline in chronic obstructive pulmonary disease. Respir Med 2009;103(8):1231–8.

80. Calverley PM, Anderson JA, Celli B, et al. Salmeterol and fluticasone propionate and survival in chronic obstructive pulmonary disease. N Engl J Med 2007;356(8):775–89.

81. Sin DD, Man SF. Why are patients with chronic obstructive pulmonary disease at increased risk of cardiovascular diseases? the potential role of systemic inflammation in chronic obstructive pulmonary disease. Circulation 2003;107(11):1514–9.

82. Hole DJ, Watt GC, Davey-Smith G, et al. Impaired lung function and mortality risk in men and women: findings from the Renfrew and Paisley prospective population study. BMJ 1996; 313(7059):711–5.

83. Sin DD, Man SF. Chronic obstructive pulmonary disease as a risk factor for cardiovascular morbidity and mortality. Proc Am Thorac Soc 2005;2(1):8–11.

84. Boudestein LC, Rutten FH, Cramer MJ, et al. The impact of concurrent heart failure on prognosis in patients with chronic obstructive pulmonary disease. Eur J Heart Fail 2009;11(12):1182–8.

85. De Blois J, Simard S, Atar D, et al. COPD predicts mortality in HF: the Norwegian Heart Failure Registry. J Card Fail 2010;16(3):225–9.

86. Macchia A, Monte S, Romero M, et al. The prognostic influence of chronic obstructive pulmonary disease in patients hospitalised for chronic heart failure. Eur J Heart Fail 2007;9(9):942–8.

87. Dunlay SM, Redfield MM, Weston SA, et al. Hospitalizations after heart failure diagnosis a community perspective. J Am Coll Cardiol 2009;54(18): 1695–702.

88. Staszewsky L, Wong M, Masson S, et al. Clinical, neurohormonal, and inflammatory markers and overall prognostic role of chronic obstructive pulmonary disease in patients with heart failure: data from the Val-HeFT heart failure trial. J Card Fail 2007;13(10):797–804.

89. Sirak TE, Jelic S, Le Jemtel TH. Therapeutic update: non-selective beta- and alpha-adrenergic blockade in patients with coexistent chronic obstructive pulmonary disease and chronic heart failure. J Am Coll Cardiol 2004;44(3):497–502.

90. Mentz RJ, Schulte PJ, Fleg JL, et al. Clinical characteristics, response to exercise training, and outcomes in patients with heart failure and chronic obstructive pulmonary disease: findings from Heart Failure and A Controlled Trial Investigating Outcomes of Exercise TraiNing (HF-ACTION). Am Heart J 2013;165(2):193–9.

91. O'Connor CM, Whellan DJ, Lee KL, et al. Efficacy and safety of exercise training in patients with chronic heart failure: HF-ACTION randomized controlled trial. JAMA 2009;301(14):1439–50.

92. Gale NS, Duckers JM, Enright S, et al. Does pulmonary rehabilitation address cardiovascular risk factors in patients with COPD? BMC Pulm Med 2011; 11:20.

93. Vivodtzev I, Minet C, Wuyam B, et al. Significant improvement in arterial stiffness after endurance training in patients with COPD. Chest 2010; 137(3):585–92.

94. Greening NJ, Evans RA, Williams JE, et al. Does body mass index influence the outcomes of a Waking-based pulmonary rehabilitation programme in COPD? Chron Respir Dis 2012;9(2):99–106.

95. Celli BR, Thomas NE, Anderson JA, et al. Effect of pharmacotherapy on rate of decline of lung function in chronic obstructive pulmonary disease: results from the TORCH study. Am J Respir Crit Care Med 2008;178(4):332–8.

96. Padwal RS, Pajewski NM, Allison DB, et al. Using the Edmonton obesity staging system to predict mortality in a population-representative cohort of people with overweight and obesity. CMAJ 2011; 183(14):E1059–66.

97. Cao C, Wang R, Wang J, et al. Body mass index and mortality in chronic obstructive pulmonary disease: a meta-analysis. PLoS One 2012;7(8): e43892.

98. Sava F, Laviolette L, Bernard S, et al. The impact of obesity on walking and cycling performance and response to pulmonary rehabilitation in COPD. BMC Pulm Med 2010;10:55.

99. Ora J, Laveneziana P, Ofir D, et al. Combined effects of obesity and chronic obstructive pulmonary disease on dyspnea and exercise tolerance. Am J Respir Crit Care Med 2009; 180(10):964–71.

100. Watz H, Waschki B, Kirsten A, et al. The metabolic syndrome in patients with chronic bronchitis and COPD: frequency and associated consequences for systemic inflammation and physical inactivity. Chest 2009;136(4):1039–46.

101. Lam KB, Jordan RE, Jiang CQ, et al. Airflow obstruction and metabolic syndrome: the Guangzhou Biobank Cohort Study. Eur Respir J 2010; 35(2):317–23.

102. van den BB, Gosker HR, Zeegers MP, et al. Pulmonary function in diabetes: a meta-analysis. Chest 2010;138(2):393–406.

103. Walter RE, Beiser A, Givelber RJ, et al. Association between glycemic state and lung function: the Framingham Heart Study. Am J Respir Crit Care Med 2003;167(6):911–6.

104. Knowler WC, Barrett-Connor E, Fowler SE, et al. Reduction in the incidence of type 2 diabetes with lifestyle intervention or metformin. N Engl J Med 2002;346(6):393–403.

105. Wedzicha JA, Bestall JC, Garrod R, et al. Random-ized controlled trial of pulmonary rehabilitation in severe chronic obstructive pulmonary disease pa-tients, stratified with the MRC dyspnoea scale. Eur Respir J 1998;12(2):363–9.

106. Dolmage TE, Goldstein RS. Effects of one-legged exercise training of patients with COPD. Chest 2008;133(2):370–6.

107. Bjorgen S, Hoff J, Husby VS, et al. Aerobic high in-tensity one and two legs interval cycling in chronic obstructive pulmonary disease: the sum of the parts is greater than the whole. Eur J Appl Physiol 2009;106(4):501–7.

108. Klijn P, van Keimpema A, Legemaat M, et al. Nonlinear exercise training in advanced chronic obstructive pulmonary disease is superior to tradi-tional exercise training. A randomized trial. Am J Respir Crit Care Med 2013;188(2):193–200.

109. Maddocks M, Gao W, Higginson IJ, et al. Neuro-muscular electrical stimulation for muscle weak-ness in adults with advanced disease. Cochrane Database Syst Rev 2013;(1):CD009419.

110. Johnson-Warrington V, Williams J, Bankart J, et al. Pulmonary rehabilitation and interstitial lung dis-ease: aiding the referral decision. J Cardiopulm Rehabil Prev 2013;33(3):189–95.

Evidence-Based Outcomes from Pulmonary Rehabilitation in the Chronic Obstructive Pulmonary Disease Patient

Milo A. Puhan, MD, PhD[a], Suzanne C. Lareau, RN, MS[b],*

KEYWORDS

- Chronic obstructive pulmonary disease • Pulmonary rehabilitation • Quality of life
- Self-management • Quality of evidence

KEY POINTS

- Pulmonary rehabilitation consists of exercise, education, and support in self-management behaviors.
- The quality of evidence is high for patient-centered outcomes such as health-related quality of life and exercise capacity in stable patients.
- Pulmonary rehabilitation after an exacerbation has strong effects, and the evidence for most outcomes at this time demonstrates moderate to high quality of evidence.

INTRODUCTION

Pulmonary rehabilitation consists of exercise, education, and support in self-management behaviors. Those completing pulmonary rehabilitation have shown measureable improvement in quality of life, symptoms, exercise performance, depression and anxiety, and health care utilization. Although it is obvious why an exercise program would improve the individual's exercise capacity, the reasons why improvement occurs in other outcome areas are not as clear.[1] The purpose of this article however, is not to provide details on the reasons for these improvements, but to describe the strength of the evidence demonstrating these changes in outcomes.

Historically, attempts were made to link rehabilitation outcomes with improvements in lung function, a common goal in many trials, in particular pharmaceutical trials. However, lung function has only occasionally been found to improve following pulmonary rehabilitation, suggesting that other changes resulting from pulmonary rehabilitation may underlie these beneficial effects. Any improvements in lung function, such as prolonged time to hyperinflation with exercise, is likely due to multiple factors, including physical deconditioning and reduction in anxiety related to dyspnea. However, given the body of evidence, one is able to make some conclusions about changes in outcomes based on the quality of evidence currently available.

Outcomes that will be the focus of this article include quality of life, symptoms, exercise capacity, hospitalizations, exacerbations, and mortality. Quality-of-life outcomes that have been consistently shown to improve have usually been measured with 2 common chronic obstructive pulmonary disease (COPD) instruments, the Chronic

[a] Institute of Social and Preventive Medicine, University of Zurich, Hirschengraben 84, Zurich CH-8001, Switzerland; [b] College of Nursing, University of Colorado, Mail Stop C288, 13120 East 19th Avenue, Aurora, CO 80045, USA
* Corresponding author.
E-mail address: Suzanne.Lareau@ucdenver.edu

Clin Chest Med 35 (2014) 295–301
http://dx.doi.org/10.1016/j.ccm.2014.02.001
0272-5231/14/$ – see front matter © 2014 Elsevier Inc. All rights reserved.

Respiratory Disease Questionnaire (CRQ)[2] and the Saint George's Respiratory Questionnaire (SGRQ).[3] Several symptoms have also been shown to improve with rehabilitation, with dyspnea, fatigue, depression, and anxiety being the most common and relevant to patients, and therefore most frequently measured and reported. Dyspnea and fatigue were among the earliest symptoms measured as outcomes in the rehabilitation setting, having been demonstrated to improve using the dyspnea and fatigue subscales on the CRQ. Symptoms relating to mood have also been responsive to rehabilitation, as measured by depression and anxiety scales such as the Hospital Anxiety and Depression Score (HADS),[4] the Center for Epidemiological Studies Depressions Scale (CES-D),[5] and the Revised Symptom Checklist (SCL-90-R).[6] Improvements in exercise capacity have been measured with field tests (the 6-minute walk distance [6MWD][7] and shuttle walk test [SWT])[8] or tests of maximal exercise capacity by either treadmill or bicycle. The latter tests of exercise capacity can determine peak exercise capacity or endurance exercise capacity. Although there are other measures that have been used to evaluate quality of life and symptoms, those noted were most frequently used in meta-analysis.[9] In the last decade, the capacity to expand areas of study has occurred, and more programs are delving into assessing other outcomes of rehabilitation. Consequently, outcome researchers now also assess the effects of pulmonary rehabilitation on exacerbations,[10] hospital utilization, and mortality.

The aim of this article is to systematically appraise the quality of evidence reported for important outcomes in pulmonary rehabilitation using the approach of the Grading of Recommendations Assessment, Development and Evaluation (GRADE) Working Group. This appraisal was carried out by identifying Cochrane systematic reviews and systematic reviews that have been subsequently reported since the last Cochrane report. The focus of this appraisal was to determine the effectiveness of pulmonary rehabilitation programs versus control therapy (usually otherwise standard care) in COPD patients. This analysis did not evaluate other aspects of the pulmonary rehabilitation intervention, such as which programs provided the most benefit (eg, inpatient vs outpatient) or how long the programs should be held (program duration).

METHODS

The approach of the GRADE Working Group[11,12] is one of several approaches to evaluate the quality of evidence in a systematic way. This approach has been adopted by over 70 organizations, including the World Health Organization (WHO), the Cochrane Collaboration, the National Institute of Health and Clinical Excellence in the UK (NICE), the American College of Physicians, and UpToDate. In brief, the GRADE approach evaluates the confidence in the estimates of effects for each outcome of interest as a function of the quality of the evidence. The result is the GRADE rating from high to low that can be used to gauge how well the estimates can be trusted. A rating of high means one can be confident that: (1) the true effect (eg, odds ratio for hospitalization in treated vs untreated patients or the difference in quality of life between treatment groups) lies close to the estimates from the available evidence, and (2) that additional evidence is unlikely to change the estimate. Very low means one should have very little confidence in the effect estimate and that the true effect estimate is likely to be substantially different when more data become available. Rating of the confidence in the effect estimates (if based on randomized trials) begins at the highest level and is rated down (if there are reasons to lose confidence in the effect estimates). For example, if there are serious concerns regarding risk of bias[13] (eg, failure to conceal random allocation or blind participants to the study intervention), then the quality of evidence is rated down from high to moderate. Other criteria that may lead to a downrating are inconsistency[14] of effect estimates across studies and indirectness[15] in cases where surrogate outcomes (such as inflammatory biomarkers) are used instead of patient-important outcomes (such as exacerbations). Another example is if patients are recruited from an intensive care setting, there is a good chance that the estimates of effect are unlikely to apply to a broader COPD population. Also, imprecision[16] (a wide confidence interval) may lead to down rating in that it makes decision making challenging. Other biases that may lead to a downgrading are publication bias[17] or outcome reporting bias, if, for example, only positive results were presented when clearly there must have been negative findings.

RESULTS
Health-Related Quality of Life

Health-related quality of life as measured by the SGRQ and the CRQ in stable COPD patients following pulmonary rehabilitation is shown in **Tables 1** and **2**. These tables identify

  The subscales and total scores
  The minimal important difference (MID) (defined as "the smallest difference in score in the

Table 1
Summary of findings in stable COPD patients following pulmonary rehabilitation

Pulmonary Rehabilitation in Patients with Stable COPD

Participants: Patients with Stable COPD (No Exacerbations Within 4 wk of Enrollment)
Intervention: Pulmonary Rehabilitation with At Least 4 wk of Exercise Training
Setting: Out- or Inpatient

Outcomes	Systematic Review	Minimal Important Difference	Effect (95% Confidence Interval), P-value Between Group Difference of Change	No of Participants (RCTs)	Quality of the Evidence (GRADE)
Total HRQL (SGRQ)	Lacasse	4	−6.11 (−8.98, −3.24), P = .00003	388 (6)	High ⊕⊕⊕⊕[a]
Symptoms (SGRQ)	Lacasse	4	−4.68 (−9.61, 0.25), P = .06	388 (6)	Moderate ⊕⊕⊕O[a,b]
Dyspnea (CRQ)	Lacasse	0.5	1.06 (0.85, 1.26), P<.00001	610 (11)	High ⊕⊕⊕⊕[a]
Fatigue (CRQ)	Lacasse	0.5	0.92 (0.71, 1.13), P<.00001	618 (11)	High ⊕⊕⊕⊕[a]
Depression	Coventry	0.2	−0.47 (−0.79, −0.16), P = .003	338 (5)	Low ⊕⊕OO[c,d]
Anxiety	Coventry	0.2	−0.38 (−0.60, −0.16), P = .006	338 (5)	Low ⊕⊕OO[c,d]
Emotional function (CRQ)	Lacasse	0.5	0.76 (0.52, 1.00), P<.00001	618 (11)	High ⊕⊕⊕⊕[a]
Activity (SGRQ)	Lacasse	4	−4.78 (−7.83, −1.72), P = .002	388 (6)	High ⊕⊕⊕⊕[a]
Physical activity	Ng	NA	No pooled estimate	472 (7)	Lack of evidence[e]
Mastery (CRQ)	Lacasse	0.5	0.97 (0.74, 1.20), P<.00001	618 (11)	High ⊕⊕⊕⊕[a]
Impacts (SGRQ)	Lacasse	4	−6.27 (−10.08, −2.47), P = .001	388 (6)	High ⊕⊕⊕⊕[a]
6-minute walk distance	Lacasse	30 m	48 m (32, 65), P<.00001	669 (16)	Moderate ⊕⊕⊕O[f]
Maximum exercise capacity	Lacasse	4 W	8.4 W (3.5, 13.4), P = .0009	511 (13)	Moderate ⊕⊕⊕O[f]

GRADE Working Group grades of evidence.

High quality: Further research is very unlikely to change one's confidence in the estimate of effect.

Moderate quality: Further research is likely to have an important impact on one's confidence in the estimate of effect and may change the estimate.

Low quality: Further research is very likely to have an important impact on one's confidence in the estimate of effect and is likely to change the estimate.

Very low quality: One should be very uncertain about the estimate.

[a] Blinding of outcome assessors not a reason for downgrading because not necessary for patient reported outcomes.

[b] Downgrade −1 for imprecision.

[c] Downgrade −1 for indirectness. Patients were enrolled based on their pulmonary status and not on their psychological status. There is uncertainty about the presence and type of depression and anxiety at baseline.

[d] Downgrade −1 for risk of bias. One of the 5 studies was likely not truly randomized, and groups were different in terms of the levels of symptoms of depression and anxiety at baseline. Method of randomization and concealment of random allocation not described in some trials.

[e] Downgrade −1 for risk of bias. In most studies outcome assessors were not blinded.

[f] Different activity monitors and questionnaires used, and MID not established for most measures of physical activity.

Table 2
Summary of findings in unstable COPD patients following pulmonary rehabilitation

Pulmonary Rehabilitation in Patients with Unstable COPD

Participants: Patients After Experiencing a COPD Exacerbations
Intervention: Pulmonary Rehabilitation with At Least 4 wk of Exercise Training
Setting: Out- or Inpatient

Outcomes	Systematic Review	Minimal Important Difference	Effect (95% Confidence Interval), P-value Between Group Difference of Change	No of Participants (RCTs)	Quality of the Evidence (GRADE)
Total HRQL (SGRQ)	Puhan	4	−9.9 (−14.4, −5.4), P<.00001	128 (3)	High ⊕⊕⊕⊕
Symptoms (SGRQ)	Puhan	4	0.9 (−6.8, 8.5), P = .83	128 (3)	Moderate ⊕⊕⊕O[a]
Dyspnea (CRQ)	Puhan	0.5	0.97 (0.35, 1.58), P = .002	259 (5)	Moderate ⊕⊕⊕O[b,c,d]
Fatigue (CRQ)	Puhan	0.5	0.81 (0.16, 1.45), P = .01	259 (5)	Moderate ⊕⊕⊕O[b,c,d]
Emotional function (CRQ)	Puhan	0.5	0.94 (0.46, 1.42), P = .0001	259 (5)	Moderate ⊕⊕⊕O[b,c,d]
Activity (SGRQ)	Puhan	4	−9.9 (−16.0, −3.9), P = .001	128 (3)	High ⊕⊕⊕⊕
Mastery (CRQ)	Puhan	0.5	0.93 (−0.13, 1.99), P = .09	259 (5)	Low ⊕⊕OO[a,b,c,d]
Impacts (SGRQ)	Puhan	4	−13.9 (−20.4, −7.5), P<.00001	128 (3)	High ⊕⊕⊕⊕
6-minute walk distance	Puhan	30 m	78 m (12, 143), P = .02	299 (6)	Low ⊕⊕OO[b,c]
Incremental shuttle walk test	Puhan	48 m	64 (41, 87), P<.00001	128 (3)	High ⊕⊕⊕⊕
Hospitalization	Puhan	NA	Odds ratio: 0.22 (0.08, 0.58), P = .002 In the control group 40 people out of 100 had hospital admission over 25 wk, compared with 13 (95% confidence interval 5–28) out of 100 for the active treatment group; this represents an NNT(B) of 4 (95% confidence interval 3–8) over 25 wk	250 (5)	Moderate ⊕⊕⊕O[c]

(continued on next page)

domain of interest which patients perceive as beneficial and which would mandate, in the absence of troublesome side effects and excessive cost, a change in the patient's management"[18]) for the subscales (in order to understand if the 95% confidence interval meets the MID)

The number of participants in the studies upon which the review was based

The quality of evidence (GRADE)

Table 2
(continued)

			Pulmonary Rehabilitation in Patients with Unstable COPD		

Participants: Patients After Experiencing a COPD Exacerbations
Intervention: Pulmonary Rehabilitation with At Least 4 wk of Exercise Training
Setting: Out- or Inpatient

Outcomes	Systematic Review	Minimal Important Difference	Effect (95% Confidence Interval), P-value Between Group Difference of Change	No of Participants (RCTs)	Quality of the Evidence (GRADE)
Mortality	Puhan	NA	Odds ratio: 0.28 (0.10, 0.84), $P = .02$ In the control group 29 people out of 100 had mortality over 107 wk, compared to 10 (95% confidence interval 4–26) out of 100 for the active treatment group; this represents an NNT(B) of 6 (95% confidence interval: 5–30) over 107 wk	111 (3)	Moderate ⊕⊕⊕O[c]

GRADE Working Group grades of evidence.
   High quality: Further research is very unlikely to change one's confidence in the estimate of effect.
   Moderate quality: Further research is likely to have an important impact on one's confidence in the estimate of effect and may change the estimate.
   Low quality: Further research is very likely to have an important impact on one's confidence in the estimate of effect and is likely to change the estimate.
   Very low quality: One should be very uncertain about the estimate.
   Abbreviation: NNT(B), Number needed to treat for one patient to benefit.
   [a] Downgraded −1 for imprecision.
   [b] Downgraded −1 for risk of bias. Generation of the random sequence, concealment of random allocation, or blinding of outcome assessors in some studies not described.
   [c] Downgraded −1 for heterogeneity.
   [d] Upgraded +1 for large effect.

As seen from these tables, there is a high quality of evidence that pulmonary rehabilitation improves the quality of life of COPD patients after pulmonary rehabilitation. The symptom subscale of the SGRQ was the only subscale on these quality-of-life instruments that was not rated with high confidence. The imprecision of the effect estimates led to downgrading of the quality of evidence to moderate for the symptom subscale, because it is possible that additional evidence might change the estimate of effect. The symptoms scale on the SGRQ is a composite score, evaluating 4 symptoms (cough, sputum, dyspnea, and wheezing), all of which may not be present in a patient with COPD and therefore may not be affected by an intervention such as rehabilitation. With the exception of this subscale, the 6 other scales and a total score provide high-quality evidence for a strong effect of rehabilitation on quality of life.

Symptoms

Symptoms were measured by the CRQ, SGRQ (previously described) and in a systematic review for depression and anxiety.[19] Dyspnea and fatigue have been consistently shown to improve with pulmonary rehabilitation. The dyspnea subscale of the CRQ, however, measures only 1 aspect of dyspnea (ie, the impact of pulmonary rehabilitation on dyspnea with specific activities). There are other aspects of dyspnea besides the impact of dyspnea (eg, intensity of dyspnea with activities), such as an affective component (distress with dyspnea) and sensory–perceptual impact (what breathing feels like).[20]

Mood-specific measures of depression and anxiety, as well as the more general emotional function subscale of the CRQ, have been reported to improve following pulmonary rehabilitation. The quality of evidence varies from low (for depression and anxiety) to high (on emotional function of CRQ) at this time. Reasons for downgrading the evidence are described in **Table 1**. For example, the quality of evidence was downgraded 1 point for the results in the systematic reviewed mentioned previously[18] because of indirectness (enrollment was based on the patients' lung function status, not their psychological status) and 1 point for risk of bias (one of the studies was likely not randomized; the groups were different in terms of the level of depression at baseline, and important features of a randomized clinical trial [RCT] were not reported for some studies).

Activity and Exercise Capacity

Activity following pulmonary rehabilitation measured by activity monitors or physical activity questionnaires has not, to date, been sufficiently evaluated. A recent meta-analysis of physical activity[21] is an example of the challenge that occurs when both objective and subjective measures are included. In this meta-analysis, one could not adequately evaluate activity due to the variation in measures of activity (activity monitors, questionnaires) and lack of established MID for many of these measures. There is, however, moderate quality of evidence (downgraded because of risk of bias) that pulmonary rehabilitation has a strong effect on exercise capacity as measured by the 6-minute walk distance (6MWD) or maximum exercise capacity.

Exacerbations

Meta-analyses are not currently available on the effect of pulmonary rehabilitation for stable outpatients with COPD on hospitalizations, exacerbations, or mortality. There is however, emerging evidence that pulmonary rehabilitation can successfully be provided to COPD patients following an exacerbation.

Exacerbations are a fairly common occurrence in COPD patients. Those experiencing an exacerbation run a high risk of morbidity, mortality, and increased health care utilization. One systematic review[10] evaluated studies for quality of life, symptoms, activity, hospitalization, and mortality among individuals undergoing pulmonary rehabilitation following an exacerbation of COPD. There is moderate quality evidence that pulmonary rehabilitation after an exacerbation substantially lowers the risk of both future exacerbations and mortality. There is also high quality of evidence that pulmonary rehabilitation improves health-related quality of life following an exacerbation. Improvement in symptoms showed moderate quality of evidence for improvement. Downrating was related to risk of bias and the heterogeneity of the estimates

across studies but uprated to moderate quality of evidence due to the large effect size. Similarly, a disparity existed between field tests. The shuttle walk test (a field test) was rated as high quality of evidence, but the 6MWD was rated low for improvement following rehabilitation. This may reflect the fact that the shuttle walk test is externally-paced, while the 6MWT is self-paced.

SUMMARY

Patients with both stable and unstable COPD demonstrate many important benefits following pulmonary rehabilitation. The quality of evidence is high for patient-centered outcomes such as health-related quality of life and exercise capacity in stable patients. Pulmonary rehabilitation after an exacerbation has strong effects too, and the evidence for most outcomes at this time demonstrates, moderate to high quality of evidence.

REFERENCES

1. Lareau S, Meek P, ZuWallack R. Chapter 14; the effect of pulmonary rehabilitation on dyspnea. In: Mahler D, O'Donnell D, editors. Dyspnea: mechanisms, measurement, and management, third edition. Boca Raton, FL: CRC Press, Taylor & Francis; 2014. p. 196.
2. Guyatt GH, Berman LB, Townsend M, et al. A measure of quality of life for clinical trials in chronic lung disease. Thorax 1987;42:773–8.
3. Jones PW, Quirk FH, Baveystock CM, et al. A self-complete measure of health status for chronic airflow limitation: the St. George's Respiratory Questionnaire. Am Rev Respir Dis 1992;145:1321–7.
4. Zigmond AS, Snaith RP. The Hospital anxiety and depression scale. Acta Psychiatr Scand 1983;67: 361–70.
5. Radloff LS. The CES-D scale: a self-report depression scale for research in the general population. Appl Psychol Meas 1977;1:385–401.
6. Derogatis LR, Lipman RS, Covi L. SCL-90: an outpatient psychiatric rating scale—preliminary report. Psychopharmacol Bull 1973;9:13–28.
7. Butland RJ, Pang J, Gross ER, et al. Two-, six-, and 12-minute walking tests in respiratory disease. Br Med J (Clin Res Ed) 1982;284:1607–8.
8. Singh SJ, Morgan MD, Scott S, et al. Development of a shuttle walking test of disability in patients with chronic airways obstruction. Thorax 1992;47:1019–24.
9. Lacasse Y, Goldstein R, Lasserson TJ, et al. Pulmonary rehabilitation for chronic obstructive pulmonary disease. Cochrane Database Syst Rev 2006;(4):CD003793.
10. Puhan MA, Gimeno-Santos E, Scharplatz M, et al. Pulmonary rehabilitation following exacerbations of chronic obstructive pulmonary disease. Cochrane Database Syst Rev 2011;(10):CD005305.

11. Guyatt GH, Oxman AD, Kunz R, et al. GRADE: going from evidence to recommendations. BMJ 2008;336: 1049–51.

12. Schünemann HJ, Jaeschke R, Cook DJ, et al. An official ATS statement: grading the quality of evidence and strength of recommendations in ATS guidelines and recommendations. Am J Respir Crit Care Med 2006;174:605–14.

13. Guyatt GH, Oxman AD, Vist G, et al. GRADE guidelines: 4. Rating the quality of evidence–study limitations (risk of bias). J Clin Epidemiol 2011;64:407–15.

14. Guyatt GH, Oxman AD, Kunz R, et al. GRADE guidelines: 7. Rating the quality of evidence–inconsistency. J Clin Epidemiol 2011;64:1294–302.

15. Guyatt GH, Oxman AD, Kunz R, et al. GRADE guidelines: 8. Rating the quality of evidence–indirectness. J Clin Epidemiol 2011;64:1303–10.

16. Guyatt GH, Oxman AD, Kunz R, et al. GRADE guidelines 6. Rating the quality of evidence–imprecision. J Clin Epidemiol 2011;64:1283–93.

17. Guyatt GH, Oxman AD, Montori V, et al. GRADE guidelines: 5. Rating the quality of evidence–publication bias. J Clin Epidemiol 2011;64:1277–82.

18. Jaeschke R, Singer J, Guyatt GH. Measurement of health status. Ascertaining the minimal clinically important difference. Control Clin Trials 1989;10: 407–15.

19. Coventry PA. Does pulmonary rehabilitation reduce anxiety and depression in chronic obstructive pulmonary disease? Curr Opin Pulm Med 2009;15: 143–9.

20. Parshall MB, Schwartzstein RM, Adams L, et al. An official American Thoracic Society statement: update on the mechanisms, assessment, and management of dyspnea. Am J Respir Crit Care Med 2012; 185:435–52.

21. Ng KW, Mackney J, Jenkins S, et al. Does exercise training change physical activity in people with COPD? A systematic review and meta-analysis. Chron Respir Dis 2012;9:17–26.

Pulmonary Rehabilitation
Timing, Location, and Duration

Thierry Troosters, PT, PhD[a,b,*], Miek Hornikx, MSc, PT[a,b], Heleen Demeyer, MSc, PT[a,b], Carlos A. Camillo, MSc, PT[b], Wim Janssens, MD, PhD[a]

KEYWORDS

- Pulmonary rehabilitation • Timing • Duration • Location • Muscle dysfunction • Exacerbation

KEY POINTS

- From a group perspective, pulmonary rehabilitation has produced positive and clinically meaningful effects across multiple outcome areas in patients with chronic respiratory diseases.
- Although enthusiasm has been increased among clinicians and third party payers, and pulmonary rehabilitation is advised as a therapy for COPD in international guidelines, reimbursement remains a challenge in many regions leading to large variability in program design, duration and patient selection.
- There are several risk factors for lack of uptake and nonadherence to rehabilitation programs and logistical aspects (transportation) seem to be an important barrier.

INTRODUCTION

This issue of *Clinics in Chest Medicine* elaborates on the benefits of pulmonary rehabilitation. The effects of following a rehabilitation program cannot be stressed enough. Patients typically experience benefits in exercise capacity, functional performance, symptoms, disease mastery, and health-related quality of life. Promising, although less consistent, results are observed in increased physical activity levels of patients with chronic obstructive pulmonary disease (COPD).[1,2] The mechanisms underlying these improvements across multiple outcome areas are various[3] and are complementary to the mechanisms through which pharmacotherapy enhances lung function and patient-centered outcomes. As a consequence, pharmacotherapy and pulmonary rehabilitation exert additive or even synergistic effects.

The improvements in outcomes realized by rehabilitation can be categorized by the World Health Organization (WHO) model into areas of bodily function, activity, and participation. Not only do the interventions and beneficial effects differ considerably among various pulmonary rehabilitation programs but the importance that individual patients attribute to a particular improvement also varies considerably. The content of a program should ideally be tailored to maximize the chances that a patient's individual goals and the therapeutic goals of the rehabilitation interdisciplinary team should be met. Both patient-individual and team goals are based on a comprehensive baseline assessment at the beginning of pulmonary rehabilitation.[4]

In this article, 3 practical and related questions are discussed: (1) who should be referred for pulmonary rehabilitation? (2) Where should rehabilitation take place? (3) How long should rehabilitation last? Across the globe there is a large heterogeneity in these organizational components of rehabilitation.[5] Although seemingly simple, there is no

Supported by grant Flemish Research Foundation (gs1) FWO G.0871.13.
[a] Respiratory Rehabilitation and Respiratory Division, University Hospital Leuven, Leuven, Belgium; [b] KU Leuven, Department of Rehabilitation Sciences, Faculty of Kinesiology and Rehabilitation Sciences, 3000 Leuven, Belgium
* Corresponding author. Respiratory Division, University Hospital Gasthuisberg, Herestraat 49, 3000 Leuven, Belgium.
E-mail address: thierry.troosters@med.kuleuven.be

Clin Chest Med 35 (2014) 303–311
http://dx.doi.org/10.1016/j.ccm.2014.02.002

chestmed.theclinics.com

straightforward and fully evidence-based answer available to these questions. Several options are available for each. Based on the phenotype of an individual patient and on the characteristics of the rehabilitation team, the patient should be referred to the most suitable program. However, in practice decisions are often influenced by limited availability of programs and limited reimbursement options.

Who Should Be Referred?

Most research on the effects of pulmonary rehabilitation is performed in patients known to respiratory specialists and studies have consistently shown wide variability in outcomes of rehabilitation in virtually all outcome measures studied. Only a few studies have attempted to identify the best responders to rehabilitation programs. All these studies have defined responders in a particular dimension of outcome, and being a responder in that particular dimension does not automatically imply being a responder on other dimensions. Because rehabilitation requires substantial effort and investment on both the patient and the rehabilitation team, the targeted outcome or outcomes of the program need to be identified and there should be reasonable expectation that the patient can significantly improve in these outcomes. Adherence with programs is crucial if they are to result in benefits,[6] and several factors have been (weakly) associated with nonadherence to pulmonary rehabilitation. These include lower levels of social support,[7] active smoking,[7-9] extremes of age,[8,9] long-term oxygen use,[8] forced expiratory volume in 1 second,[8] a lower health-related quality of life score,[8,9] and longer traveling distance to the rehabilitation center.[8] A systematic review identified travel and transport issues and a lack of perceived benefit as barriers to both uptake and completion of programs. The only demographic features that consistently predicted noncompletion were being a current smoker and depression.[10] Apart from these quantifiable factors there are several personal and system factors that influence uptake and adherence. Qualitative studies identified that the service that is introduced and the capacity of the service to meet the patient's lifestyle needs are determinants of the willingness of patients to undertake the treatment. Themes that determined the decision not to start rehabilitation or to interrupt a program were difficulties with accessing the program (geography and timing); difficulties in prioritizing the treatment; contrary beliefs about the role and safety of exercise, and fears about criticism (being unable to cope with exercise, or smoking status).

These factors are only seldom recognized when the lack of uptake of rehabilitation is discussed. A patient who does not start a rehabilitation program clearly cannot become a responder.

A few studies have attempted to identify the best responders to exercise training. Prediction models are generally poor, but may give insight into the benefits that can be expected in individual patients. Patients with poor functional exercise capacity, more muscle dysfunction,[11,12] and better preserved ventilatory capacity[13] seem to respond slightly better to exercise training. Two studies found that patients with skeletal muscle fatigue after exercise[14] or an exercise training program[15] are more likely to experience physiologic benefits of a training program. Thus, those patients with poor skeletal muscle function at the beginning of pulmonary rehabilitation are more likely to benefit from the exercise stimulus. Although one study suggested that younger patients are more likely to respond favorably to exercise training,[16] age is generally not though to be an important discriminator between responders and nonresponders.[17-19] Gender and lung function also do not predict success of rehabilitation.

Responders are typically defined in just 1 dimension, such as exercise capacity or quality of life. However, as shown in **Fig. 1**, improvement in one outcome area, such as exercise capacity, is not necessarily related to improvement in another area, such as quality of life. Furthermore, for most end points, benefits can only be expected if there is a baseline abnormality. This rule also applies for less conventional end points, such as maintenance of postural control and balance or psychological abnormalities: benefits can only be attained if deficiencies in these dimensions are present at baseline, which reiterates the importance of comprehensive baseline screening and the identification of patient-specific goals for the rehabilitation program.

For people outside pulmonary rehabilitation (chest physicians, internal medicine, or general practitioners), there is no clear guidance on which patients should be referred for pulmonary rehabilitation. The most recent Global Initiative for Obstructive Lung Disease (GOLD) strategy document advocates pulmonary rehabilitation of GOLD category B, which means that virtually any symptomatic patient with COPD should be considered for this intervention.[20] A pragmatic approach is to refer any patient with persistent respiratory symptoms (dyspnea, fatigue) and/or functional status limitations despite otherwise optimal therapy.[4] The British Thoracic Society guidelines give more practical guidance as to who should be referred to rehabilitation, based on the Medical

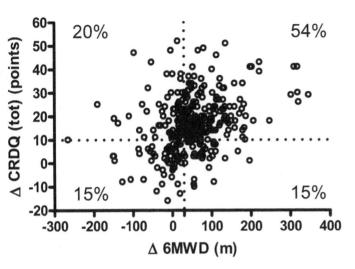

Fig. 1. Effects of 3 months' (3 week^{-1}) outpatient rehabilitation on functional exercise capacity and on health-related quality of life in 352 consecutive patients with COPD referred for pulmonary rehabilitation. Approximately 35% of patients had less than 30 meters improvement in 6-minute walk distance (6MWD), and approximately 26% of patients had less than 10 points' improvement in health-related quality of life. Only 15% of patients did not meet both criteria, whereas 54% did meet both criteria. CRDQ, Chronic Respiratory Disease Questionnaire; tot, total.

Research Council (MRC) dyspnea scale of the patients (**Box 1**).[21]

Complementing these general recommendations, there are some patients in whom rehabilitation should be prescribed without hesitation. These patients include (1) those with COPD who were recently admitted to the hospital with an acute exacerbation; they should be offered a plan for rehabilitation by the time they get discharged. In these patients rehabilitation could be initiated during the hospital admission (discussed later). The rehabilitation intervention in this setting also stresses self-management training in order to prevent subsequent hospital admissions.[22,23] (2) Patients with MRC dyspnea ratings of 3 or greater

---

Box 1
British Thoracic Society referral to pulmonary rehabilitation based on MRC dyspnea scale

- Patients with a MRC dyspnea score of 3 to 5 who are functionally limited by breathlessness should be referred for outpatient pulmonary rehabilitation (grade A).

- Patients with an MRC dyspnea score of 2 who are functionally limited by breathlessness should be referred for pulmonary rehabilitation (grade D).

- Patients with an MRC dyspnea score of 5 who are housebound should not routinely be offered supervised pulmonary rehabilitation within their homes (grade B).

- Flexible and pragmatic approaches should be considered to facilitate exercise training in patients who have less severe COPD and who are less breathless (expert consensus).

(ie, patients who walk slower than most people on level ground) in whom all pharmacologic options have been exhausted. According to the British Thoracic Society recommendations these patients should be referred to pulmonary rehabilitation regardless of their lung function impairment. However, patients with lower MRC dyspnea scores (eg, patients who get short of breath when hurrying or walking up a slight hill) may also benefit from pulmonary rehabilitation in terms of exercise capacity, symptoms of anxiety and depression, and symptoms of dyspnea.[24,25]

It is likely that, in the future, physical activity assessment will become an important criterion to select patients for pulmonary rehabilitation. Rehabilitation should be geared to reactivate patients with low physical activity levels, because low function in this area is an important factor in the systemic consequences of COPD, which are amenable to pulmonary rehabilitation. If a patient with severe lung function or exercise impairment is still active, it may be questionable that rehabilitation will lead to major benefits in this individual. However, although this reasoning seems intuitive, it still needs prospective validation. Valid activity monitors with patient-friendly and investigator-friendly user interfaces have recently become available[26]; in the future these tools will likely become important in the selection of appropriate candidates.

Besides identifying the best possible candidates for rehabilitation, consideration of those who should not be referred is also important. There are few absolute contraindications to pulmonary rehabilitation, apart from a complete lack of motivation. If exercise would be painful (severe arthritis) or potentially dangerous (uncontrolled cardiovascular disease), the indication for rehabilitation needs to be carefully considered, and risks and potential benefits must be carefully weighed. Comorbidities are often thought of as contraindications for referral to pulmonary rehabilitation. However, for many of the common comorbidities of COPD (diabetes, obesity, cardiovascular disease, cognitive problems, depression, and osteoporosis), rehabilitation, including adapted exercise training, is a recommended treatment. Programs need to be adapted to the problems of these patients such that the patients benefit from the program both in terms of their COPD-related problems and in terms of their comorbidity.[27]

Where Should Rehabilitation Take Place?

Pulmonary rehabilitation can be provided in several settings (**Table 1**). Programs were conventionally developed as outpatient programs in which patients visited clinical facilities on a regular basis, typically 2 to 3 times per week. Pulmonary rehabilitation also initially proved to be effective in the inpatient setting. More recently, pulmonary rehabilitation has been delivered successfully in alternative settings such as primary care (ie, in the home of the patient, or in a primary care health care provider's office, typically a physiotherapy office), in secondary care (ie, regional hospitals), in the community, or in nursing homes.[28] Even more recently, telehealth applications started to be made in rehabilitation in order to ensure proper follow-up of patients.[29]

Few studies have directly compared different settings. Two studies compared home-based with outpatient rehabilitation and found largely equivalent effects.[30,31] A third large study is currently underway.[32] A nonrandomized study in Denmark also confirmed comparable effects of rehabilitation in primary and secondary care.[33] Another study compared community-based with hospital outpatient-based rehabilitation, again without clear benefits of either program.[34] In a Brazilian study, unsupervised home-based rehabilitation showed significant benefits that were not different from outpatient rehabilitation in

Table 1
An overview of possible locations for rehabilitation programs

Type Program	Location	Typical Duration	Multidiscipline	Suitable Patients
Inpatient	Dedicated rehabilitation center	4 wk	++++	Complex patients with limited mobility or poor social support After ICU
Outpatient	Dedicated rehabilitation center	6 wk to 6 mo	+++	Complex patients with sufficient social support After exacerbation
	Second-line hospital	6–12 wk	++	Less complex patient
Community based	Fitness center, gym	8–12 wk or maintenance	+/−	Patients who need exercise only
	Nursing home	Maintenance exercise	+	Institutionalized patients
Primary care based	Physiotherapy practice	8–12 wk	+/−	Mobile patients who need exercise only and/or respiratory physiotherapy (mucus problems)
Home based	With physiotherapy supervision	12 wk	−	Less mobile patients who need exercise only and/or respiratory physiotherapy (mucus problems)
	Without supervision	NA	−	Patients who need only physical activity and mild exercises with proper self-management
Home based and telemonitored	—	Maintenance or primary	++ (educ.)	Patients who need mostly exercise and can manage technology

Abbreviations: educ., education; ICU, intensive care unit; NA, not applicable.

improvements on the 6-minute walking test. However, a study that used a similar comparison, which focused on more physiologic outcomes, showed superiority of a supervised outpatient program.[35,36] In a systematic review the effects of home-based rehabilitation were confirmed.[37] Even in the home setting several types of exercise training (strength or endurance) can be successfully applied.[38] However, home-based programs for the most severely disabled patients may not be suitable.[38,39]

The effectiveness of outpatient rehabilitation for patients with COPD has been confirmed outside the context of clinical trials.[40,41] To the best of our knowledge, the effectiveness of home-based programs has only been shown in the context of formal clinical trials, administered by experts. Such expertise may not be present when a trial is initiated in primary care practices.

Outpatient programs in specialized centers
Outpatient hospital-based programs have been successfully used to offer pulmonary rehabilitation to patients with COPD, and most of the data showing successful outcomes comes from this setting. Outpatient programs have an advantage in that they can rely on existing multidisciplinary expertise to assess each patient and to individually tailor the rehabilitation program to the patient's needs. Programs are typically run by dedicated and skilled staff. These programs allow for inclusion of complex patients and those with rare diseases or conditions such as restrictive lung disease, pulmonary hypertension, or patients before or after lung transplantation. Because of the available multidisciplinary staff, programs can easily be adapted to the specific needs of patients. Disciplines that can be involved in the rehabilitation process of a patient are the medical doctor (chest physician, specialized in rehabilitation), physiotherapist, specialized nurse, occupational therapist, nutritional specialist, psychologist, a social worker, and the patient's general practitioner. Although the benefits of exercise training are clear at a group level, other disciplines may contribute with targeted intervention to selected patients.

Patient mobility and transportation issues are major problems in adherence to outpatient problems, and are probably the most common reason why patients opt out of participation. Another issue is the limited number of programs available. In Belgium, only 4 centers are currently allowed to run highly specialized rehabilitation that is properly reimbursed for its complexity. These programs have a total capacity of about 300 patients per year, which is insufficient to serve all potential candidates. In addition, outpatient hospital-based programs are generally more expensive than programs offered in primary care or in the community. However, the expense should be given less weight because, even in a more expensive rehabilitation center setting, a rehabilitation program is affordable and effects at the patient level are largely clinically relevant.

Inpatient rehabilitation
Pulmonary rehabilitation provided in the inpatient setting generally has the same benefits as programs provided in outpatient hospital-based settings. An additional benefit to an inpatient program is the full-time availability of the patient to the rehabilitation team, allowing even more multidisciplinary work. In such programs other rehabilitation modules can be easily implemented. An example is the implementation of a balance training program that successfully improved patients' balance and confidence of balance.[42] Transportation is not an issue, but patients have to agree to be taken out of their daily routines for extended periods of time. Programs are typically shorter than outpatient programs, lasting around 4 weeks.

The major disadvantage of inpatient programs is their increased cost and (although not much studied) the potential risk of being institutionalized. In addition, most health care systems only have a limited number of rehabilitation beds (if any), limiting the number of potential beneficiaries of these programs, regardless of the cost.

The short-term effectiveness of inpatient programs has been well established.[43] Such programs may be of particular importance for patients with end-stage lung disease, those awaiting lung transplantation,[44] or in patients with acute exacerbations. For patients with acute exacerbations, programs can be short with the aim of preventing exacerbation-related deterioration in functional performance and muscle strength.[45] Such short programs need to be followed up by subsequent longer-term outpatient-based rehabilitation. In one study a follow-up home-based rehabilitation program was successful in maintaining the benefits of the initial hospital-based program.[46] When programs are initiated during admissions for COPD exacerbations, elements of multidisciplinary geriatric rehabilitation may also be beneficial as components of the inpatient program.[47] In addition, special attention should be paid to the mental health of patients in this setting. Depression and anxiety are independent risk factors for adverse outcomes of hospital admissions related to exacerbations.[48] The rehabilitation team is well placed to identify and tackle these problems.

Rehabilitation in primary care

Pulmonary rehabilitation can also be conducted successfully in the primary care setting. The major advantage for this venue is that the program is conducted in the patient's locale, thus facilitating easier access and perhaps a greater likelihood of initiating the intervention. A less explored potential advantage is that, because participation takes place in more familiar settings, the translation of benefits into enhanced physical activity in the home and community settings might be enhanced.[49] Studies performed in primary care have shown that exercise training can be successfully executed. Programs can be conducted in the physiotherapy office where equipment for exercise training is typically available.[50,51] As an alternative, the pulmonary rehabilitation may be conducted in the patient's home[39,52]; this may only be feasible if the proper exercise equipment is placed in the home[30] and proper instruction and monitoring is provided. Furthermore, an obstacle to delivery of rehabilitation in the primary care or home setting is the unavailability of a multidisciplinary team to assess the patient and direct the complex intervention in multimorbid patients. When these programs can make use of a network that embeds a specialized center where the assessment can take place and a proposal for a program can be made, these hurdles can be overcome. Home exercises are sometimes prescribed without supervision. Although these may improve patient-centered outcomes and functional exercise capacity,[31] their effectiveness on physiologic outcomes has not been shown.

Community centers

The use of community centers for pulmonary rehabilitation may also alleviate the travel burden for patients, but may allow group training supervised by physical therapists in a location that has appropriate equipment for exercise training in elderly or frail subjects. Community-centered pulmonary rehabilitation has been deployed successfully in stable respiratory patients in the form of maintenance programs,[53,54] or as primary programs.[55] The expertise for these programs is typically offered through an affiliated center of excellence. A community-based program was recently combined with telehealth support from a specialized center to deploy rehabilitation and education in the remote community.[29] These new and creative solutions may offer new opportunities to respiratory health care providers living remote from a rehabilitation center.

Telehealth

A more recent development in broadening the applicability of pulmonary rehabilitation is the initiation of telehealth applications.[56] This development allows remote monitoring by dedicated health care providers operating from specialized centers of the patients' training progress and of potential problems occurring during the training. Internet-based programs enable the rehabilitation team to have a presence in the patient's house through educational programs, videoconferencing, or telemonitoring. Although theoretically possible, feasible, and effective,[57] there are still several barriers to the adoption of telehealth. These barriers include the requirement for technical competence, the potential experience of disrupted services, and the possibility that opting into these services would cause disruptive changes to existing services.[58] It has yet to be determined from large multicenter studies whether telerehabilitation is a feasible option in patients with respiratory disease, including whether telehealth solutions can have a role in the maintenance of physical activity levels and whether it can be useful for monitoring and early detection of symptoms from exacerbations.

Duration of Rehabilitation

The duration of the pulmonary rehabilitation program remains a debated topic, and to date no consensus has been reached as to how long the intervention should last. In most guidelines a minimal duration of 6 to 8 weeks is mentioned,[4] but it is clear that longer programs may potentially render larger and more comprehensive benefits. The rehabilitation intervention should ideally last as long as gains are being made. However, the duration of programs is practically defined by the available health care (reimbursement) system rather than by the individual patient need. The impact of varying duration of programs has been studied only at a group level rather than at the individual patient level. At a group level, longer programs may be beneficial, but rehabilitation is unlikely to provide optimal results after a given number of weeks in every patient and for every desired outcome. One study suggested that, although benefits of a program in functional exercise tolerance were observed after 3 months, benefits in terms of enhanced physical activity levels were only observed after 6 months of rehabilitation.[59]

Duration and setting cannot be seen independently. Inpatient programs for patients experiencing exacerbations of COPD typically are short in duration, often lasting days or a few weeks. Even for respiratory patients who are clinically stable, it is generally economically unfeasible to make inpatient programs longer than few weeks. In contrast, outpatient programs can extend to 3 to 6 months. In addition, community programs may be set up as permanent maintenance programs.[54] Flexibility among settings may be a way forward in rehabilitation of patients with respiratory diseases. Rehabilitation may be seen more as a flexible plan of care not specifically tied to a single institution, rather than a specific package in 1 center and lasting just a few weeks. Few studies have explored this concept of using home-based rehabilitation to sustain benefits of an inpatient program started in patients with exacerbations[46] or exploring community-based rehabilitation following inpatient rehabilitation.[60]

SUMMARY

From a group perspective, pulmonary rehabilitation has produced positive and clinically meaningful effects across multiple outcome areas in patients with chronic respiratory diseases. This finding has increased enthusiasm for pulmonary rehabilitation among clinicians and third-party payers, and has ensured its status as a gold standard of treatment of patients with chronic respiratory disease such as COPD GOLD category B. However, the decision of whether a patient is a good candidate for rehabilitation, the place of the rehabilitation program, and the duration of this intervention are not straightforward. Rather than basing the type, location, and duration of the therapy on the unique needs of the patient, regional health care restrictions may limit referral to programs and may fix their duration and location. Flexibility should ideally be available, which reflects the medical and the patient needs (in terms of complexity and desired goals) and, importantly, the patient preferences in terms of location and duration of programs. This article stresses the desirability for personalized, flexible approaches to pulmonary rehabilitation in terms of referral, location, and duration. However, more research is needed to see whether these approaches have the anticipated benefits. In the absence of research that proves that such personalized, flexible programs lead to better outcomes, render more cost-effective results, and have improved uptake and adherence, clinicians must rely on conventional wisdom. In general, programs should last at least 8 weeks. Indications for referral include those patients recovering from severe exacerbations of their respiratory disease and those patients who walk slower than people of their age because of breathlessness or other exercise-related symptoms. In addition, patients with less severe symptoms may also benefit from rehabilitation, and likely programs for these patients can be set up in less costly settings, such as primary care or community locations.

ACKNOWLEDGMENTS

The authors acknowledge Drs Nici and ZuWallack for their editorial suggestions.

REFERENCES

1. Troosters T, van der Molen T, Polkey M, et al. Improving physical activity in COPD: towards a new paradigm. Respir Res 2013;14:115.
2. Troosters T, Gosselink R, Janssens W, et al. Exercise training and pulmonary rehabilitation: new insights and remaining challenges. Eur Respir Rev 2010;19:24–9.
3. Casaburi R, ZuWallack R. Pulmonary rehabilitation for management of chronic obstructive pulmonary disease. N Engl J Med 2009;360:1329–35.
4. Spruit MA, Singh SJ, Garvey C, et al. An official American Thoracic Society/European Respiratory Society statement: key concepts and advances in pulmonary rehabilitation. Am J Respir Crit Care Med 2013;188:e13–64.
5. Spruit MA, Pitta F, Garvey C, et al. Differences in content and organizational aspects of pulmonary rehabilitation programs. Eur Respir J 2013. [Epub ahead of print].
6. Scott AS, Baltzan MA, Fox J, et al. Success in pulmonary rehabilitation in patients with chronic obstructive pulmonary disease. Can Respir J 2010;17:219–23.
7. Young P, Dewse M, Fergusson W, et al. Respiratory rehabilitation in chronic obstructive pulmonary disease: predictors of nonadherence. Eur Respir J 1999;13:855–9.
8. Hayton C, Clark A, Olive S, et al. Barriers to pulmonary rehabilitation: characteristics that predict patient attendance and adherence. Respir Med 2013;107:401–7.
9. Selzler AM, Simmonds L, Rodgers WM, et al. Pulmonary rehabilitation in chronic obstructive pulmonary disease: predictors of program completion and success. COPD 2012;9:538–45.
10. Keating A, Lee AL, Holland AE. Lack of perceived benefit and inadequate transport influence uptake and completion of pulmonary rehabilitation in people with chronic obstructive pulmonary disease: a qualitative study. J Physiother 2011;57:183–90.
11. Troosters T, Gosselink R, Decramer M. Exercise training in COPD; how to distinguish responders from nonresponders. J Cardiopulm Rehabil 2001; 21:10–7.
12. Garrod R, Marshall J, Barley E, et al. Predictors of success and failure in pulmonary rehabilitation. Eur Respir J 2006;27:788–94.

13. Plankeel JF, McMullen B, MacIntyre NR. Exercise outcomes after pulmonary rehabilitation depend on the initial mechanism of exercise limitation among non-oxygen-dependent COPD patients. Chest 2005;127:110–6.

14. Mador MJ, Mogri M, Patel A. Contractile fatigue of the quadriceps muscle predicts improvement in exercise performance after pulmonary rehabilitation. J Cardiopulm Rehabil Prev 2014;34:54–61.

15. Burtin C, Saey D, Saglam M, et al. Effectiveness of exercise training in patients with COPD: the role of muscle fatigue. Eur Respir J 2012;40:338–44.

16. Walsh JR, McKeough ZJ, Morris NR, et al. Metabolic disease and participant age are independent predictors of response to pulmonary rehabilitation. J Cardiopulm Rehabil Prev 2013;33:249–56.

17. Di MF, Pedone C, Lubich S, et al. Age does not hamper the response to pulmonary rehabilitation of COPD patients. Age Ageing 2008;37:530–5.

18. Couser JI, Guthmann R, Hamadeh MA, et al. Pulmonary rehabilitation improves exercise capacity in older elderly patients with COPD. Chest 1995; 107:730–4.

19. Baltzan MA, Kamel H, Alter A, et al. Pulmonary rehabilitation improves functional capacity in patients 80 years of age or older. Can Respir J 2004;11:407–13.

20. Global strategy for diagnosis, management, and prevention of COPD. 2013. Available at: www.goldcopd. com. Accessed December 13, 2013.

21. Bolton CE, Bevan-Smith EF, Blakey JD, et al. British Thoracic Society guideline on pulmonary rehabilitation in adults. Thorax 2013;68(Suppl 2):ii1–30.

22. Casas A, Troosters T, Garcia-Aymerich J, et al. Integrated care prevents hospitalizations for exacerbations in COPD patients. Eur Respir J 2006;28: 123–30.

23. Bourbeau J, Julien M, Maltais F, et al. Reduction of hospital utilization in patients with chronic obstructive pulmonary disease: a disease-specific self-management intervention. Arch Intern Med 2003; 163:585–91.

24. Man WD, Grant A, Hogg L, et al. Pulmonary rehabilitation in patients with MRC Dyspnoea Scale 2. Thorax 2011;66:263.

25. Evans RA, Singh SJ, Collier R, et al. Pulmonary rehabilitation is successful for COPD irrespective of MRC dyspnoea grade. Respir Med 2009;103: 1070–5.

26. Rabinovich RA, Louvaris Z, Raste Y, et al. Validity of physical activity monitors during daily life in patients with COPD. Eur Respir J 2013;42:1205–15.

27. Hornikx M, Van Remoortel H, Demeyer H, et al. The influence of comorbidities on the outcomes of pulmonary rehabilitation programs in patients with COPD; a systematic review. Biomed Res Int 2013; 2013:146148.

28. van Dam van Isselt EF, Groenewegen-Sipkema KH, Spruit-van EM, et al. Geriatric rehabilitation for patients with advanced COPD: programme characteristics and case studies. Int J Palliat Nurs 2013; 19:141–6.

29. Stickland M, Jourdain T, Wong EY, et al. Using Tele-health technology to deliver pulmonary rehabilitation in chronic obstructive pulmonary disease patients. Can Respir J 2011;18:216–20.

30. Maltais F, Bourbeau J, Shapiro S, et al. Effects of home-based pulmonary rehabilitation in patients with chronic obstructive pulmonary disease: a randomized trial. Ann Intern Med 2008;149: 869–78.

31. Mendes de Oliveira JC, Studart Leitao Filho FS, Malosa Sampaio LM, et al. Outpatient vs. home-based pulmonary rehabilitation in COPD: a randomized controlled trial. Multidiscip Respir Med 2010;5:401–8.

32. Holland AE, Mahal A, Hill CJ, et al. Benefits and costs of home-based pulmonary rehabilitation in chronic obstructive pulmonary disease – a multi-centre randomised controlled equivalence trial. BMC Pulm Med 2013;13:57.

33. Vest S, Moll L, Petersen M, et al. Results of an outpatient multidisciplinary COPD rehabilitation programme obtained in two settings: primary and secondary health care. Clin Respir J 2011;5:84–91.

34. Waterhouse JC, Walters SJ, Oluboyede Y, et al. A randomised 2 × 2 trial of community versus hospital pulmonary rehabilitation, followed by telephone or conventional follow-up. Health Technol Assess 2010;14:i–xi, 1.

35. Puente-Maestu L, Sanz ML, Sanz P, et al. Effects of two types of training on pulmonary and cardiac responses to moderate exercise in patients with COPD. Eur Respir J 2000;15:1026–32.

36. Puente-Maestu L, Sanz ML, Sanz P, et al. Comparison of effects of supervised versus self-monitored training programmes in patients with chronic obstructive pulmonary disease. Eur Respir J 2000;15:517–25.

37. Liu XL, Tan JY, Wang T, et al. Effectiveness of home-based pulmonary rehabilitation for patients with chronic obstructive pulmonary disease: a meta-analysis of randomized controlled trials. Rehabil Nurs 2013;39:36–59.

38. McFarland C, Willson D, Sloan J, et al. A randomized trial comparing 2 types of in-home rehabilitation for chronic obstructive pulmonary disease: a pilot study. J Geriatr Phys Ther 2012; 35:132–9.

39. Wedzicha JA, Bestall JC, Garrod R, et al. Randomized controlled trial of pulmonary rehabilitation in severe chronic obstructive pulmonary disease patients, stratified with the MRC dyspnoea scale. Eur Respir J 1998;12:363–9.

40. Young P, Dewse M, Fergusson W, et al. Improvements in outcomes for chronic obstructive pulmonary disease (COPD) attributable to a hospital-based respiratory rehabilitation programme. Aust N Z J Med 1999;29:59–65.

41. Salhi B, Troosters T, Behaegel M, et al. Effects of pulmonary rehabilitation in patients with restrictive lung diseases. Chest 2010;137:273–9.

42. Beauchamp MK, Janaudis-Ferreira T, Parreira V, et al. A randomized controlled trial of balance training during pulmonary rehabilitation for individuals with COPD. Chest 2013;144:1803–10.

43. Goldstein RS, Gort EH, Stubbing D, et al. Randomised controlled trial of respiratory rehabilitation. Lancet 1994;344:1394–7.

44. Gloeckl R, Halle M, Kenn K. Interval versus continuous training in lung transplant candidates: a randomized trial. J Heart Lung Transplant 2012;31: 934–41.

45. Troosters T, Probst VS, Crul T, et al. Resistance training prevents deterioration in quadriceps muscle function during acute exacerbations of chronic obstructive pulmonary disease. Am J Respir Crit Care Med 2010;181:1072–7.

46. Behnke M, Taube C, Kirsten D, et al. Home-based exercise is capable of preserving hospital-based improvements in severe chronic obstructive pulmonary disease. Respir Med 2000;94:1184–91.

47. Ammenwerth W, Nosul M, Berliner M, et al. Implementation of an early geriatric rehabilitation in acute inpatient pneumology. Pneumologie 2012; 66:235–9 [in German].

48. Laurin C, Moullec G, Bacon SL, et al. Impact of anxiety and depression on chronic obstructive pulmonary disease exacerbation risk. Am J Respir Crit Care Med 2012;185:918–23.

49. Effing T, Zielhuis G, Kerstjens H, et al. Community based physiotherapeutic exercise in COPD self-management: a randomised controlled trial. Respir Med 2011;105:418–26.

50. Wijkstra PJ, Ten Vergert EM, van Altena R, et al. Long term benefits of rehabilitation at home on quality of life and exercise tolerance in patients with chronic obstructive pulmonary disease. Thorax 1995;50:824–8.

51. van Wetering CR, Hoogendoorn M, Mol SM, et al. Short- and long-term efficacy of a community-based COPD management program in less advanced COPD: a randomized controlled trial. Thorax 2009;65:7–13.

52. Strijbos JH, Postma DS, van Altena R, et al. A comparison between an outpatient hospital-based pulmonary rehabilitation program and a home-care pulmonary rehabilitation program in patients with COPD. A follow-up of 18 months. Chest 1996;109:366–72.

53. Beauchamp MK, Francella S, Romano JM, et al. A novel approach to long-term respiratory care: results of a community-based post-rehabilitation maintenance program in COPD. Respir Med 2013;107:1210–6.

54. Moullec G, Ninot G. An integrated programme after pulmonary rehabilitation in patients with chronic obstructive pulmonary disease: effect on emotional and functional dimensions of quality of life. Clin Rehabil 2010;24:122–36.

55. Golmohammadi K, Jacobs P, Sin DD. Economic evaluation of a community-based pulmonary rehabilitation program for chronic obstructive pulmonary disease. Lung 2004;182:187–96.

56. Tabak M, Vollenbroek-Hutten MM, van der Valk PD, et al. A telerehabilitation intervention for patients with Chronic Obstructive Pulmonary Disease: a randomized controlled pilot trial. Clin Rehabil 2013. [Epub ahead of print].

57. Zanaboni P, Lien LA, Hjalmarsen A, et al. Long-term telerehabilitation of COPD patients in their homes: interim results from a pilot study in northern Norway. J Telemed Telecare 2013;19:425–9.

58. Sanders C, Rogers A, Bowen R, et al. Exploring barriers to participation and adoption of telehealth and telecare within the Whole System Demonstrator trial: a qualitative study. BMC Health Serv Res 2012;12:220.

59. Pitta F, Troosters T, Probst V, et al. Are patients with COPD more active after pulmonary rehabilitation? Chest 2008;134:273–80.

60. Moullec G, Ninot G, Varray A, et al. An innovative maintenance follow-up program after a first inpatient pulmonary rehabilitation. Respir Med 2008; 102:556–66.

Exercise Training in Pulmonary Rehabilitation

Vasileios Andrianopoulos, MSc[a],*, Peter Klijn, PhD[b], Frits M.E. Franssen, PhD, MD[a], Martijn A. Spruit, PhD[a,c]

KEYWORDS

- Exercise • Rehabilitation • Pulmonary • Lungs • Intervention • Physical activity

KEY POINTS

- Exercise training remains a cornerstone of pulmonary rehabilitation (PR) in patients with chronic respiratory disease.
- The choice of type of exercise training depends on the physiologic requirements and goals of the individual patient as well as the available equipment at the PR center.
- Current evidence suggests that, ground walking exercise training, Nordic walking exercise training, resistance training, water-based exercise training, tai chi, and nonlinear periodized exercise are all feasible and effective in (subgroups) of patients with chronic obstructive pulmonary disease.

Pulmonary rehabilitation (PR) is defined as a comprehensive intervention based on a thorough patient assessment followed by patient-tailored therapies that include, but are not limited to, exercise training, education, and behavior change. PR programs are designed to improve the physical and psychological condition of people with chronic respiratory disease and to promote the long-term adherence to health-enhancing behaviors.[1] Therefore, exercise training is a core component of PR in patients with chronic respiratory disease.[1–6] This article provides an overview of various types of exercise training, including endurance exercise training, interval exercise training, ground walking exercise training, Nordic walking exercise training, resistance training, water-based (or aquatic) exercise training, tai chi, and nonlinear periodized exercise training (NLPE) (**Fig. 1**).

ENDURANCE EXERCISE TRAINING

Endurance training can be defined as an activity in which large muscle groups are used continuously.[7]

In the past, PR has focused primarily on aerobic endurance training (such as walking, cycling, stair climbing[8]), a training frequency of 3 to 4 days per week, with an initial work-phase duration of 10 to 15 minutes, progressively increasing up to 30 to 40 minutes.[9,10] Between 6 and 8 weeks of endurance exercise training is thought to be the minimum time frame needed to achieve substantial effects.[11,12] However, longer PR programs generally lead to more favorable results.[11]

The main aim of endurance training in patients with chronic obstructive pulmonary disease (COPD) is to improve aerobic capacity and augment the ability to perform daily activities.[10] Previous studies have shown that endurance exercise training also has beneficial effects on peripheral muscle force, functional exercise capacity, peak work rate, and health-related quality of life.[13–16] Increased exercise capacity following PR can be attributed, in part, to centrally mediated improvements, such as reduced ventilatory requirement for a given task and increased peak aerobic capacity.[8] There is also evidence that endurance exercise

[a] Department of Research & Education, CIRO+, Centre of Expertise for Chronic Organ Failure, Hornerheide 1, Horn 6085 NM, The Netherlands; [b] Department of Pulmonology, Merem Asthma Center Heideheuvel, Soestdijkerstraatweg 129, 1213 VX Hilversum, The Netherlands; [c] Faculty of Medicine and Life Sciences, REVAL-Rehabilitation Research Center, BIOMED-Biomedical Research Institute, Hasselt University, Agoralaan gebouw A, 3590, Diepenbeek, Belgium
* Corresponding author.
E-mail address: vasilisandrianopoulos@ciro-horn.nl

Clin Chest Med 35 (2014) 313–322
http://dx.doi.org/10.1016/j.ccm.2014.02.013
0272-5231/14/$ – see front matter © 2014 Elsevier Inc. All rights reserved.

Types of exercise in COPD

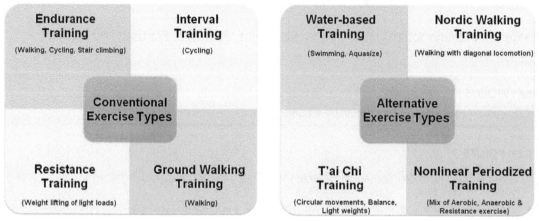

Fig. 1. Types of exercise in chronic obstructive pulmonary disease (COPD).

training elicits improvements in aerobic function and structure of the lower-limb muscles. The latter include increased muscle fiber capillarization, increased mitochondrial density, increased oxidative capacity of muscle fibers, and a delayed onset of the anaerobic metabolism.[8,17] Endurance exercise training also seems to improve arterial stiffness in patients with COPD,[18] but these results need to be verified in larger studies. Aortic pulse wave velocity did not change following a state-of-the-art PR program in patients with COPD, including endurance exercise training, interval exercise training, and strengthening exercises.[19] A lower BODE index (a composite COPD rating, including measures of body mass index, airway obstruction, dyspnea, and 6-minute walk distance) has also been observed after endurance exercise training.[20] Because higher (worse) BODE scores predict mortality in COPD,[21] this type of exercise intervention may improve mortality.[22] However, this finding has never been confirmed prospectively.

Endurance training, under the supervision of a health care professional such as a physiotherapist or exercise physiologist, is highly recommended for patients with COPD who are able to perform continuous training of at least moderate intensity.[23] In PR exercise training, the target training intensity is usually monitored by work rate and perceived exertion.

Exercise training at 60% to 90% of peak work rate is usually defined as high-intensity exercise,[5] and is thought to be superior to lower intensity training in achieving physiologic improvements in aerobic exercise capacity.[11,24–27] An intensity greater than 60% of the peak work rate can usually be sustained for short periods only, ranging from 4 to 10 minutes in patients with moderate to severe

COPD. Less than 20% of patients may be able to sustain this continuous high-intensity exercise throughout the PR program.[28] Although higher intensity of training generally leads to greater increases in exercise capacity, this is not always the case.[4,29] Low-intensity to moderate-intensity continuous training (50% to 60% of peak work rate or a score of 5 to 6 points on the modified Borg scale) can also lead to gains in exercise endurance, even in patients with advanced disease.[8,30]

INTERVAL EXERCISE TRAINING

Interval training can be defined as repeated short periods of exercise alternated with rest. The duration of the work interval and the recovery interval can vary greatly and depend on the duration of the work phase.[31,32] In healthy individuals the metabolic changes, including cardiorespiratory responses and low muscle lactate concentrations, during interval exercise are similar to those of continuous moderate exercise.[33]

Emerging research indicates that interval training is an attractive alternative to continuous training, especially in those patients with COPD who develop severe dyspnea during exercise[34–36]; these patients are often unable to sustain continuous exercise intensities sufficiently long enough to obtain physiologic training adaptations.[23,37] The intermittent recovery periods during interval training facilitate a decrease in end-expiratory lung volume and prevent high lactate accumulation, which results in lower ventilation and less dyspnea.[37–43]

Compared with continuous high-intensity training, interval training results in fewer unintended breaks, probably reflecting the decreased ventilatory requirement of continuous training.[37,38] Interval training can deliver an adequate load to the exercising muscles, resulting in the desired peripheral adaptations[44,45] with less dyspnea burden.

Studies in patients with COPD indicate that interval training has beneficial effects that are equivalent to those of continuous training in terms of exercise capacity and health-related quality of life.[34,42,46–49] Several interval protocols with varying work phases, and passive or active recovery, have been used in COPD exercise research with significant training effects.[31,34,42,46–48]

GROUND WALKING EXERCISE TRAINING

Treadmill walking and stationary cycle training have traditionally been the prominent exercise training modalities in comprehensive PR.[6,50] However, ground walking exercise training in COPD can also make oxygen more efficient.[51] A home-based unsupervised walking program, 6 days per week for 12 weeks, in patients with COPD almost doubled endurance walk time compared with a control group.[52] A study that compared ground walking with stationary cycle training in patients with COPD showed that ground walking improved endurance walking capacity to a greater degree, and was as effective in improving peak walking capacity, peak and endurance cycle capacity, and quality of life.[53]

The recommended ground walking intensity is 80% of the average speed on the 6-minute walk test, or 75% of peak speed attained with moderate dyspnea sensation (3 on the modified Borg scale) during the incremental shuttle walking test.[6,54] Ground-based walking exercise training is not the same as physical activity counseling: the former is performed at a higher intensity, whereas the latter is less rigorous and often uses feedback from activity monitors.[55,56]

NORDIC WALKING EXERCISE TRAINING

Nordic walking was developed as an off-season training method for competitive cross-country skiers and it is reputed to be Europe's fastest growing form of exercise.[57] It is an exercise technique characterized by diagonal locomotion using longer steps compared with regular walking,[58] and requires coordinated movements for balance and stability, strength and endurance, varied cardiovascular efforts, agility, and visual acuity.[59] In the last decade, Nordic walking has been promoted by the International Nordic Walking Association and has become increasingly popular as an endurance activity in the general population.[60–62]

In healthy individuals, Nordic walking is a more intense workout than normal walking at the same speed,[63] causing higher peak heart rate and oxygen consumption, even compared with jogging.[64] In general, Nordic walking is recommended as an effective and efficient mode of exercise to improve overall functional fitness in elderly people.[61] It may provide additional benefits in functional capacity and muscular strength compared with regular walking, and is suitable for improving endurance in elderly adults.[61,65] Nordic walking exercise also elicits several positive effects in people with chronic diseases, such as improved mobility in patients with Parkinson disease, increased exercise capacity in men after acute coronary syndrome, and enhanced quality of life in overweight individuals with diabetes.[66–68]

Nordic walking is safe, feasible, and effective in patients with COPD. Compared with usual care, a supervised, 3-month, outdoor Nordic walking exercise program at 75% of initial maximum heart rate, 3 times per week for 1 hour per session, increased exercise tolerance and daily physical activity (walking time and intensity).[69] The observed improvements in exercise capacity and physical activity remained up to 6 months after completion of the intervention.

RESISTANCE TRAINING

Muscle strength is important for optimal health, functional performance, and quality of life.[70,71] The expected loss of muscle mass and strength with age can progress more slowly when elderly individuals participate in resistance exercise training programs.[72] Resistance training is an intervention that can enhance or maintain muscle function (eg, maximal strength, muscle endurance and/or muscle mass).[73] The fundamental principles of resistance training are progressive overload, variation, and specificity. The intervention must be tailored to the specific needs of the individual to maximize outcomes.[73] The complex process of resistance training is accomplished by the incorporation and manipulation of the following variables: intensity, volume (ie, number of sets and repetitions), training frequency, rest interval between sets, sequence of exercises, and movement velocity.[73,74] Intensity is considered the most important variable, and is inversely related to the training volume.[74]

In addition to improvements in muscle mass and strength, studies in healthy elderly subjects show that resistance training also improves skeletal muscle oxidative capacity and endurance,[75] and increases capillarization and oxygen flux through the skeletal muscle.[76,77] Substantial increases in muscle strength and in power (standardized for body weight) occur in healthy women more than 75 years of age.[78] Furthermore, resistance training can increase leg strength and walking distance in healthy elderly people regardless of gender.[79]

Before 1990, resistance training was not recommended for rehabilitative exercise. Nowadays resistance training is recognized as being beneficial in people with chronic diseases.[50,80–83] In COPD, resistance training is an ideal intervention for those patients who have peripheral muscle weakness and intensive symptoms of dyspnea during physical activity or exercise.[84] In the course of daily activities, basic strength-related tasks such as maintaining balance while standing, rising from a chair, or lifting objects constitute a challenge.[12,85–87] It is assumed that resistance exercise training can partially reverse peripheral muscle weakness and thus reduce this aspect of the systemic burden of COPD.[11] In a recent study, upper and lower extremity resistance training added to aerobic training resulted in improvements in strength, lean body mass, functional exercise capacity, and in 3 of 8 simulated activity of daily living tasks compared with aerobic training alone.[88] In addition, patients with COPD who underwent resistance exercise training program showed increased improvements in quality of life.[89]

According to current American Thoracic Society/European Respiratory Society statement on PR,[1] resistance training should be performed at moderate intensity (50%–85% of the single-repetition maximum) and include 2 to 4 sets of 6 to 12 repetitions. Several exercise studies in patients with COPD, using similar approaches to resistance training,[13–16] showed increased peripheral muscle strength. Although increases in peripheral muscle strength can improve endurance measures, improvement is neither consistent nor optimal.[14,15,90]

WATER-BASED (OR AQUATIC) EXERCISE TRAINING

Water-based (or aquatic) exercise training is a lower extremity exercise in a low-impact, resistance-based environment, and uses similar training principles to land-based training. Water-based programs allow people to gain all the advantages of land-based exercise, but the buoyancy of water facilitates balance and gait without overt stress or strain on arthritic joints.[91] Several exercises, such as walking, cycling, and lifting weight, can be performed in a swimming pool.[92] Suggested water temperatures vary from 29°C to 38°C.[93,94] Water-based exercise training programs confer improvements

in exercise performance, muscle strength, and balance in the elderly with and without chronic conditions.[95–99]

Aquatic exercise training has also been suggested as a new therapeutic training modality in patients with COPD.[94,100–102] It shows promise in improving exercise capacity and quality of life in this patient population and can be an alternative training approach to traditional land-based exercise programs. Land-based programs can be difficult for patients who have coexisting obesity, musculoskeletal, or neurologic limitations.[102] However, water-based exercise training requires adequate duration and frequency in order to provide important benefits to patients with COPD. A recent study found that a single, weekly maintenance water-based exercise session program did not maintain the improvements in physical activity and quality of life that had resulted from 3 sessions per week on a high-intensity, 3-month water-based training program.[103]

In patients with COPD, exercise in the swimming pool can have an additional beneficial physiologic effect caused by the hydrostatic pressure. The hydrostatic pressure exerted during immersion can facilitate expiration and thereby reduce the degree of air trapping.[104–107] For example, vital capacity decreases up to 10%,[107,108] functional residual capacity reduces to about 54%, and expiratory reserve volume decreases by 75% with partial immersion.[109,110]

TAI CHI

Tai chi is a thirteenth century Chinese martial art rooted in Taoist philosophy and Chinese philosophic principles, and it includes gentle circular movements, balance exercise, weight lifting, breathing techniques, and mental concentration.[111–116] Traditional tai chi includes various movements that are performed in a slow, relaxed manner for 30 minutes.[115] There are many styles of tai chi and each style has its own form. The most popular and widely practiced style of tai chi is the Yang style, which includes 24 movements in its simple form and 108 movements in its traditional form.[112,117] The frequency and duration of tai chi that may result in beneficial effects varies from 1 to 3 times per week for 4 to 16 weeks, with individual sessions lasting 45 to 60 minutes.[118–124] The exercise intensity of tai chi depends on its training style and different skill levels.[125] However, the recommended intensity is 50% to 58% of heart rate reserve for people from 25 to 80 years old.[126,127]

Long-term regular tai chi exercise training has beneficial effects on balance, flexibility, muscular strength, cardiovascular fitness, cognition, sleep quality, and emotional functioning in elderly adults.[128–134] Furthermore, Tai chi also has beneficial effects in individuals with mild hypertension,[135] stroke,[136] fibromyalgia,[137,138] rheumatoid arthritis,[139] knee osteoarthritis,[140] diabetes,[141] Parkinson disease,[142] and other chronic diseases.[117,127]

Limited data suggest that tai chi may be beneficial in patients with COPD.[6,143,144] A recent study that investigated a 12-week program of short-form sun-style tai chi of moderate intensity, found that this form of exercise increased endurance shuttle walk time, reduced medial-lateral body sway in semitandem stand, and increased total score on the Chronic Respiratory Questionnaire.[145,146] In a meta-analysis of 8 randomized controlled trials, tai chi improved exercise capacity, dyspnea, quality of life, and lung function compared with general exercise or usual care in COPD.[147]

NLPE

Traditional exercise training during PR uses a non-varied, linear-progressive protocol.[31] With this type of protocol an orderly increase in exercise stress (eg, intensity and duration) is placed on the body. A traditional session usually consists of a combination of endurance and resistance training with both the aerobic and anaerobic systems providing the necessary energy for muscular contractions. However, this mix-type protocol may compromise adaptations.[31]

Athletes use sophisticated nonlinear training methods directed to specific individual training goals. NLPE is a training strategy that is designed to maximize individual adaptation, prevent overtraining, and attain an optimal training effect[31,73] by frequent variation in number of exercises, training intensity, exercise duration, and resting periods.[31] To optimize physiologic adaptation, the aerobic and anaerobic energy systems are preferentially stimulated and matched during endurance and resistance exercise within 1 training session. Moreover, variation in low-intensity and high-intensity exercise interspersed with adequate recovery has been shown to be important for healthy adults and is suggested to result in a more fatigue-resistant fiber type.[31]

Applying principles of nonlinear exercise training in athletes to patients with severe to very severe COPD is feasible and worthwhile. Klijn and colleagues[31] showed that a 10-week NLPE program (3 sessions per week) was superior in improving cycle endurance and health-related quality of life compared with traditional nonvaried

exercise training. These promising results need to be corroborated by others, and should also focus on long-term outcomes.

SUMMARY

Exercise training remains a cornerstone of PR in patients with chronic respiratory disease. Although treadmill walking and stationary cycle ergometry training constitute the most common forms of exercise training in PR[50] and have been shown to improve muscle function, exercise performance, and health status, other types of exercise training may also be beneficial. The choice of type of exercise training depends on the physiologic requirements and goals of the individual patient as well as the available equipment at the PR center. Current evidence suggests that, at ground walking exercise training, Nordic walking exercise training, resistance training, water-based exercise training, tai chi, and NLPE are all feasible and effective in (subgroups) of patients with COPD. In turn, these exercise training modalities can be considered as part of a comprehensive, interdisciplinary PR program.

REFERENCES

1. Spruit MA, Singh SJ, Garvey C, et al. An official American Thoracic Society/European Respiratory Society statement: key concepts and advances in pulmonary rehabilitation. Am J Respir Crit Care Med 2013;188(8):e13–64.
2. Lacasse Y, Goldstein R, Lasserson TJ, et al. Pulmonary rehabilitation for chronic obstructive pulmonary disease. Cochrane Database Syst Rev 2006;(4):CD003793.
3. Sillen MJ, Speksnijder CM, Eterman RM, et al. Effects of neuromuscular electrical stimulation of muscles of ambulation in patients with chronic heart failure or COPD: a systematic review of the English-language literature. Chest 2009;136(1):44–61.
4. Zainuldin R, Mackey MG, Alison JA. Optimal intensity and type of leg exercise training for people with chronic obstructive pulmonary disease. Cochrane Database Syst Rev 2011;(11):CD008008.
5. Puhan MA, Schunemann HJ, Frey M, et al. How should COPD patients exercise during respiratory rehabilitation? Comparison of exercise modalities and intensities to treat skeletal muscle dysfunction. Thorax 2005;60(5):367–75.
6. Spruit MA, Wouters EF. New modalities of pulmonary rehabilitation in patients with chronic obstructive pulmonary disease. Sports Med 2007;37(6):501–18.

7. Mazzeo RS, Cavanagh P, Evans WJ, et al. ACSM position stand: Exercise and physical activity for older adults. Med Sci Sports Exerc 1998;30(6): 992–1008.

8. Rochester CL. Exercise training in chronic obstructive pulmonary disease. J Rehabil Res Dev 2003; 40(5 Suppl 2):59–80.

9. Lacasse Y, Martin S, Lasserson TJ, et al. Meta-analysis of respiratory rehabilitation in chronic obstructive pulmonary disease. A Cochrane Systematic Review. Eura Medicophys 2007;43(4): 475–85.

10. Gloeckl R, Marinov B, Pitta F. Practical recommendations for exercise training in patients with COPD. Eur Respir Rev 2013;22(128):178–86.

11. Troosters T, Casaburi R, Gosselink R, et al. Pulmonary rehabilitation in chronic obstructive pulmonary disease. Am J Respir Crit Care Med 2005;172(1): 19–38.

12. Ries AL, Bauldoff GS, Carlin BW, et al. Pulmonary rehabilitation: joint ACCP/AACVPR evidence-based clinical practice guidelines. Chest 2007; 131(Suppl 5):4S–42S.

13. Bernard S, Whittom F, Leblanc P, et al. Aerobic and strength training in patients with chronic obstructive pulmonary disease. Am J Respir Crit Care Med 1999;159(3):896–901.

14. Ortega F, Toral J, Cejudo P, et al. Comparison of effects of strength and endurance training in patients with chronic obstructive pulmonary disease. Am J Respir Crit Care Med 2002;166(5):669–74.

15. Spruit MA, Gosselink R, Troosters T, et al. Resistance versus endurance training in patients with COPD and peripheral muscle weakness. Eur Respir J 2002;19(6):1072–8.

16. Mador MJ, Bozkanat E, Aggarwal A, et al. Endurance and strength training in patients with COPD. Chest 2004;125(6):2036–45.

17. Vogiatzis I, Terzis G, Nanas S, et al. Skeletal muscle adaptations to interval training in patients with advanced COPD. Chest 2005;128(6):3838–45.

18. Vivodtzev I, Minet C, Wuyam B, et al. Significant improvement in arterial stiffness after endurance training in patients with COPD. Chest 2010; 137(3):585–92.

19. Vanfleteren LE, Spruit MA, Groenen MT, et al. Arterial stiffness in patients with COPD: the role of systemic inflammation and the effects of pulmonary rehabilitation. Eur Respir J 2013. [Epub ahead of print].

20. Cote CG, Celli BR. Pulmonary rehabilitation and the BODE index in COPD. Eur Respir J 2005;26(4): 630–6.

21. Celli BR, Cote CG, Marin JM, et al. The body-mass index, airflow obstruction, dyspnea, and exercise capacity index in chronic obstructive pulmonary disease. N Engl J Med 2004;350(10):1005–12.

22. Nasis IG, Vogiatzis I, Stratakos G, et al. Effects of interval-load versus constant-load training on the BODE index in COPD patients. Respir Med 2009; 103(9):1392–8.

23. Langer D, Hendriks E, Burtin C, et al. A clinical practice guideline for physiotherapists treating patients with chronic obstructive pulmonary disease based on a systematic review of available evidence. Clin Rehabil 2009;23(5):445–62.

24. Casaburi R, Patessio A, Ioli F, et al. Reductions in exercise lactic acidosis and ventilation as a result of exercise training in patients with obstructive lung disease. Am Rev Respir Dis 1991;143(1): 9–18.

25. Maltais F, LeBlanc P, Simard C, et al. Skeletal muscle adaptation to endurance training in patients with chronic obstructive pulmonary disease. Am J Respir Crit Care Med 1996;154(2 Pt 1):442–7.

26. Gimenez M, Servera E, Vergara P, et al. Endurance training in patients with chronic obstructive pulmonary disease: a comparison of high versus moderate intensity. Arch Phys Med Rehabil 2000;81(1): 102–9.

27. Puente-Maestu L, Sanz ML, Sanz P, et al. Effects of two types of training on pulmonary and cardiac responses to moderate exercise in patients with COPD. Eur Respir J 2000;15(6):1026–32.

28. Maltais F, LeBlanc P, Jobin J, et al. Intensity of training and physiologic adaptation in patients with chronic obstructive pulmonary disease. Am J Respir Crit Care Med 1997;155(2):555–61.

29. Goldstein RS, Hill K, Brooks D, et al. Pulmonary rehabilitation: a review of the recent literature. Chest 2012;142(3):738–49.

30. Puente-Maestu L, Sanz ML, Sanz P, et al. Comparison of effects of supervised versus self-monitored training programmes in patients with chronic obstructive pulmonary disease. Eur Respir J 2000;15(3):517–25.

31. Klijn P, van Keimpema A, Legemaat M, et al. Nonlinear exercise training in advanced chronic obstructive pulmonary disease is superior to traditional exercise training. A randomized trial. Am J Respir Crit Care Med 2013;188(2):193–200.

32. Laursen PB, Jenkins DG. The scientific basis for high-intensity interval training: optimising training programmes and maximising performance in highly trained endurance athletes. Sports Med 2002;32(1):53–73.

33. Astrand P, Rodahl K. Textbook of work physiology. New York: McGraw-Hill; 1986.

34. Vogiatzis I, Nanas S, Roussos C. Interval training as an alternative modality to continuous exercise in patients with COPD. Eur Respir J 2002;20(1): 12–9.

35. Elkins MR, Dwyer TJ. Interval and continuous training are similarly effective in chronic obstructive

pulmonary disease. Br J Sports Med 2011;45(2): 155–6.

36. Beauchamp MK, Nonoyama M, Goldstein RS, et al. Interval versus continuous training in individuals with chronic obstructive pulmonary disease–a systematic review. Thorax 2010;65(2):157–64.

37. Sabapathy S, Kingsley RA, Schneider DA, et al. Continuous and intermittent exercise responses in individuals with chronic obstructive pulmonary disease. Thorax 2004;59(12):1026–31.

38. Vogiatzis I, Nanas S, Kastanakis E, et al. Dynamic hyperinflation and tolerance to interval exercise in patients with advanced COPD. Eur Respir J 2004;24(3):385–90.

39. Gosselink R, Troosters T, Decramer M. Exercise training in COPD patients: the basic questions. Eur Respir J 1997;10(12):2884–91.

40. Spruit MA, Troosters T, Trappenburg JC, et al. Exercise training during rehabilitation of patients with COPD: a current perspective. Patient Educ Couns 2004;52(3):243–8.

41. Meyer K, Samek L, Schwaibold M, et al. Physical responses to different modes of interval exercise in patients with chronic heart failure–application to exercise training. Eur Heart J 1996;17(7):1040–7.

42. Puhan MA, Busching G, Schunemann HJ, et al. Interval versus continuous high-intensity exercise in chronic obstructive pulmonary disease: a randomized trial. Ann Intern Med 2006;145(11):816–25.

43. Gloeckl R, Halle M, Kenn K. Interval versus continuous training in lung transplant candidates: a randomized trial. J Heart Lung Transplant 2012; 31(9):934–41.

44. Vogiatzis I, Athanasopoulos D, Habazettl H, et al. Intercostal muscle blood flow limitation during exercise in chronic obstructive pulmonary disease. Am J Respir Crit Care Med 2010;182(9):1105–13.

45. Vogiatzis I, Terzis G, Stratakos G, et al. Effect of pulmonary rehabilitation on peripheral muscle fiber remodeling in patients with COPD in GOLD stages II to IV. Chest 2011;140(3):744–52.

46. Arnardottir RH, Boman G, Larsson K, et al. Interval training compared with continuous training in patients with COPD. Respir Med 2007;101(6): 1196–204.

47. Coppoolse R, Schols AM, Baarends EM, et al. Interval versus continuous training in patients with severe COPD: a randomized clinical trial. Eur Respir J 1999;14(2):258–63.

48. Mador MJ, Krawza M, Alhajhusian A, et al. Interval training versus continuous training in patients with chronic obstructive pulmonary disease. J Cardiopulm Rehabil Prev 2009;29(2):126–32.

49. Varga J, Porszasz J, Boda K, et al. Supervised high intensity continuous and interval training vs. self-paced training in COPD. Respir Med 2007; 101(11):2297–304.

50. Spruit MA, Pitta F, Garvey C, et al. Differences in content and organizational aspects of pulmonary rehabilitation programs. Eur Respir J 2013. [Epub ahead of print].

51. Leader D. The benefits of walking for people with COPD. 2009. Available at: http://copd.about.com/od/livingwithcopd/tp/Exercise.htm. Accessed January 20, 2014.

52. Hernandez MT, Rubio TM, Ruiz FO, et al. Results of a home-based training program for patients with COPD. Chest 2000;118(1):106–14.

53. Leung RW, Alison JA, McKeough ZJ, et al. Ground walk training improves functional exercise capacity more than cycle training in people with chronic obstructive pulmonary disease (COPD): a randomised trial. J Physiother 2010;56(2):105–12.

54. The Australian Lung Foundation and Australian Physiotherapy Association. Pulmonary rehabilitation toolkit: exercise prescription table. 2011. Available at: http://www.pulmonaryrehab.com.au/index.asp?page598. Accessed January 20, 2014.

55. Moy ML, Weston NA, Wilson EJ, et al. A pilot study of an Internet walking program and pedometer in COPD. Respir Med 2012;106(9):1342–50.

56. Vaes AW, Cheung A, Atakhorrami M, et al. Effect of 'activity monitor-based' counseling on physical activity and health-related outcomes in patients with chronic diseases: a systematic review and meta-analysis. Ann Med 2013;45(5–6):397–412.

57. Pantzar M, Shove E. Understanding innovation in practice: a discussion of the production and reproduction of Nordic walking. Technol Anal Strateg 2010;22(4):447–61.

58. Hansen L, Henriksen M, Larsen P, et al. Nordic walking does not reduce the loading of the knee joint. Scand J Med Sci Sports 2008;18(4):436–41.

59. Nottingham S, Jurasin A. Nordic walking for total fitness. Champaign-Illinois, USA: Human Kinetics; 2010.

60. Schiffer T, Knicker A, Dannohl R, et al. Energy cost and pole forces during Nordic walking under different surface conditions. Med Sci Sports Exerc 2009;41(3):663–8.

61. Takeshima N, Islam M, Rogers M, et al. Effects of Nordic walking compared to conventional walking and band-based resistance exercise on fitness in older adults. J Sports Sci Med 2013;2013(12):422–30.

62. Tschentscher M, Niederseer D, Niebauer J. Health benefits of Nordic walking: a systematic review. Am J Prev Med 2013;44(1):76–84.

63. Kukkonen-Harjula K, Hiilloskorpi H, Manttari A, et al. Self-guided brisk walking training with or without poles: a randomized-controlled trial in middle-aged women. Scand J Med Sci Sports 2007;17(4):316–23.

64. Schiffer T, Knicker A, Hoffman U, et al. Physiological responses to Nordic walking, walking and jogging. Eur J Appl Physiol 2006;98(1):56–61.

65. Parkatti T, Perttunen J, Wacker P. Improvements in functional capacity from Nordic walking: a randomized-controlled trial among elderly people. J Aging Phys Act 2012;20(1):93–105.

66. van Eijkeren FJ, Reijmers RS, Kleinveld MJ, et al. Nordic walking improves mobility in Parkinson's disease. Mov Disord 2008;23(15):2239–43.

67. Kocur P, Deskur-Smielecka E, Wilk M, et al. Effects of Nordic walking training on exercise capacity and fitness in men participating in early, short-term inpatient cardiac rehabilitation after an acute coronary syndrome–a controlled trial. Clin Rehabil 2009;23(11):995–1004.

68. Fritz T, Caidahl K, Osler M, et al. Effects of Nordic walking on health-related quality of life in overweight individuals with type 2 diabetes mellitus, impaired or normal glucose tolerance. Diabet Med 2011;28(11):1362–72.

69. Breyer MK, Breyer-Kohansal R, Funk GC, et al. Nordic walking improves daily physical activities in COPD: a randomised controlled trial. Respir Res 2010;11:112.

70. Seymour JM, Spruit MA, Hopkinson NS, et al. The prevalence of quadriceps weakness in COPD and the relationship with disease severity. Eur Respir J 2010;36(1):81–8.

71. Bird SP, Tarpenning KM, Marino FE. Designing resistance training programmes to enhance muscular fitness: a review of the acute programme variables. Sports Med 2005;35(10):841–51.

72. Seguin R, Nelson ME. The benefits of strength training for older adults. Am J Prev Med 2003; 25(3 Suppl 2):141–9.

73. American College of Sports Medicine. American College of Sports Medicine position stand. Progression models in resistance training for healthy adults. Med Sci Sports Exerc 2009; 41(3):687–708.

74. Kraemer WJ, Ratamess NA. Fundamentals of resistance training: progression and exercise prescription. Med Sci Sports Exerc 2004;36(4): 674–88.

75. Jubrias SA, Esselman PC, Price LB, et al. Large energetic adaptations of elderly muscle to resistance and endurance training. J Appl Physiol (1985) 2001;90(5):1663–70.

76. Hepple RT, Mackinnon SL, Goodman JM, et al. Resistance and aerobic training in older men: effects on VO2peak and the capillary supply to skeletal muscle. J Appl Physiol (1985) 1997;82(4): 1305–10.

77. McGuigan MR, Bronks R, Newton RU, et al. Resistance training in patients with peripheral arterial disease: effects on myosin isoforms, fiber type distribution, and capillary supply to skeletal muscle. J Gerontol A Biol Sci Med Sci 2001; 56(7):B302–10.

78. Skelton DA, Young A, Greig CA, et al. Effects of resistance training on strength, power, and selected functional abilities of women aged 75 and older. J Am Geriatr Soc 1995;43(10):1081–7.

79. Ades PA, Ballor DL, Ashikaga T, et al. Weight training improves walking endurance in healthy elderly persons. Ann Intern Med 1996;124(6):568–72.

80. Nici L, ZuWallack R, Wouters E, et al. On pulmonary rehabilitation and the flight of the bumblebee: the ATS/ERS statement on pulmonary rehabilitation. Eur Respir J 2006;28(3):461–2.

81. Feigenbaum MS, Pollock ML. Prescription of resistance training for health and disease. Med Sci Sports Exerc 1999;31(1):38–45.

82. Pollock ML, Evans WJ. Resistance training for health and disease: introduction. Med Sci Sports Exerc 1999;31(1):10–1.

83. Spruit MA, Eterman RM, Hellwig VA, et al. Effects of moderate-to-high intensity resistance training in patients with chronic heart failure. Heart 2009; 95(17):1399–408.

84. O'Shea SD, Taylor NF, Paratz J. Peripheral muscle strength training in COPD: a systematic review. Chest 2004;126(3):903–14.

85. Annegarn J, Meijer K, Passos VL, et al. Problematic activities of daily life are weakly associated with clinical characteristics in COPD. J Am Med Dir Assoc 2012;13(3):284–90.

86. Annegarn J, Spruit MA, Savelberg HH, et al. Differences in walking pattern during 6-min walk test between patients with COPD and healthy subjects. PLoS One 2012;7(5):e37329.

87. Mesquita R, Janssen DJ, Wouters EF, et al. Within-day test-retest reliability of the timed up & go test in patients with advanced chronic organ failure. Arch Phys Med Rehabil 2013;94(11):2131–8.

88. Panton LB, Golden J, Broeder CE, et al. The effects of resistance training on functional outcomes in patients with chronic obstructive pulmonary disease. Eur J Appl Physiol 2004;91(4):443–9.

89. Benton MJ, Wagner CL. Effect of single-set resistance training on quality of life in COPD patients enrolled in pulmonary rehabilitation. Respir Care 2013;58(3):487–93.

90. Casaburi R, Bhasin S, Cosentino L, et al. Effects of testosterone and resistance training in men with chronic obstructive pulmonary disease. Am J Respir Crit Care Med 2004;170(8):870–8.

91. Grosse SJ. Aquatic progressions. The buoyancy of water facilitates balance and gait. Rehab Manag 2009;22(3):25–7.

92. Geytenbeek J. Aquatic physiotherapy evidence-based practice guide. Sydney (Australia): National Aquatic Physiotherapy Group: Australian Physiotherapy Association; 2008.

93. Kurabayashi H, Machida I, Tamura K, et al. Breathing out into water during subtotal immersion: a

therapy for chronic pulmonary emphysema. Am J Phys Med Rehabil 2000;79(2):150–3.

94. Wadell K, Sundelin G, Henriksson-Larsen K, et al. High intensity physical group training in water–an effective training modality for patients with COPD. Respir Med 2004;98(5):428–38.

95. Rica RL, Carneiro RM, Serra AJ, et al. Effects of water-based exercise in obese older women: impact of short-term follow-up study on anthropometric, functional fitness and quality of life parameters. Geriatr Gerontol Int 2013;13(1):209–14.

96. Fernandez-Lao C, Cantarero-Villanueva I, Ariza-Garcia A, et al. Water versus land-based multimodal exercise program effects on body composition in breast cancer survivors: a controlled clinical trial. Support Care Cancer 2013;21(2):521–30.

97. Bergamin M, Ermolao A, Tolomio S, et al. Water- versus land-based exercise in elderly subjects: effects on physical performance and body composition. Clin Interv Aging 2013;8:1109–17.

98. Hale LA, Waters D, Herbison P. A randomized controlled trial to investigate the effects of water-based exercise to improve falls risk and physical function in older adults with lower-extremity osteoarthritis. Arch Phys Med Rehabil 2012;93(1):27–34.

99. Bento PC, Pereira G, Ugrinowitsch C, et al. The effects of a water-based exercise program on strength and functionality of older adults. J Aging Phys Act 2012;20(4):469–83.

100. de Souto Araujo ZT, de Miranda Silva Nogueira PA, Cabral EE, et al. Effectiveness of low-intensity aquatic exercise on COPD: a randomized clinical trial. Respir Med 2012;106(11):1535–43.

101. Lotshaw AM, Thompson M, Sadowsky HS, et al. Quality of life and physical performance in land- and water-based pulmonary rehabilitation. J Cardiopulm Rehabil 2007;27(4):247–51.

102. McNamara RJ, McKeough ZJ, McKenzie DK, et al. Water-based exercise in COPD with physical co-morbidities: a randomised controlled trial. Eur Respir J 2013;41(6):1284–91.

103. Wadell K, Henriksson-Larsen K, Lundgren R, et al. Group training in patients with COPD - long-term effects after decreased training frequency. Disabil Rehabil 2005;27(10):571–81.

104. Dahlback GO, Jonsson E, Liner MH. Influence of hydrostatic compression of the chest and intrathoracic blood pooling on static lung mechanics during head-out immersion. Undersea Biomed Res 1978;5(1):71–85.

105. Schoenhofer B, Koehler D, Polkey MI. Influence of immersion in water on muscle function and breathing pattern in patients with severe diaphragm weakness. Chest 2004;125(6):2069–74.

106. DeLisa J, Gans B, Walsh L. Physical medicine and rehabilitation: principles and practice. Philadelphia: Lippincott Williams & Wilkins; 2004.

107. Hall J, Bisson D, O'Hare P. The physiology of immersion. J Appl Physiol 1990;76:517–21.

108. Anste K, Roskell C. Hydrotherapy. Detrimental or beneficial to the respiratory system? Physiotherapy 2000;86:5–13.

109. Agostoni E, Gurtner G, Torri G, et al. Respiratory mechanics during submersion and negative-pressure breathing. J Appl Physiol 1966;21(1):251–8.

110. Hong SK, Cerretelli P, Cruz JC, et al. Mechanics of respiration during submersion in water. J Appl Physiol 1969;27(4):535–8.

111. Cheng M. Master Cheng's thirteen chapters on T'ai Chi Chuan. New York: Sweet Chi Press; 1982.

112. Frantzis B. Tai Chi: health for life. Berkeley (CA): Energy Arts; 2006.

113. Helm B. Gateways to health: Taijiquan and traditional Chinese medicine. Taijiquan J 2002;2002:8–12.

114. Klein PJ, Adams WD. Comprehensive therapeutic benefits of Taiji: a critical review. Am J Phys Med Rehabil 2004;83(9):735–45.

115. Koh TC. Tai Chi Chuan. Am J Chin Med 1981;9(1):15–22.

116. Gong LS, Qian JA, Zhang JS, et al. Changes in heart rate and electrocardiogram during taijiquan exercise: analysis by telemetry in 100 subjects. Chin Med J (Engl) 1981;94(9):589–92.

117. Wang C, Collet JP, Lau J. The effect of Tai Chi on health outcomes in patients with chronic conditions: a systematic review. Arch Intern Med 2004;164(5):493–501.

118. Wolf SL, Barnhart HX, Ellison GL, et al. The effect of Tai Chi Quan and computerized balance training on postural stability in older subjects. Atlanta FICSIT Group. Frailty and Injuries: cooperative studies on intervention techniques. Phys Ther 1997;77(4):371–81 [discussion: 82–4].

119. Wolf SL, Barnhart HX, Kutner NG, et al. Reducing frailty and falls in older persons: an investigation of Tai Chi and computerized balance training. Atlanta FICSIT Group. Frailty and Injuries: cooperative studies of intervention techniques. J Am Geriatr Soc 1996;44(5):489–97.

120. Tsang WW, Hui-Chan CW. Effect of 4- and 8-wk intensive Tai Chi training on balance control in the elderly. Med Sci Sports Exerc 2004;36(4):648–57.

121. Hartman CA, Manos TM, Winter C, et al. Effects of T'ai Chi training on function and quality of life indicators in older adults with osteoarthritis. J Am Geriatr Soc 2000;48(12):1553–9.

122. Kirsteins AE, Dietz F, Hwang SM. Evaluating the safety and potential use of a weight-bearing exercise, Tai-Chi Chuan, for rheumatoid arthritis patients. Am J Phys Med Rehabil 1991;70(3):136–41.

123. Lan C, Lai JS, Chen SY, et al. Tai Chi Chuan to improve muscular strength and endurance in

elderly individuals: a pilot study. Arch Phys Med Rehabil 2000;81(5):604–7.

124. Lan C, Lai JS, Wong MK, et al. Cardiorespiratory function, flexibility, and body composition among geriatric Tai Chi Chuan practitioners. Arch Phys Med Rehabil 1996;77(6):612–6.

125. Xiong KY, He H, Ni GX. Effect of skill level on cardiorespiratory and metabolic responses during Tai Chi training. Eur J Sport Sci 2013;13(4):386–91.

126. Lan C, Chen SY, Lai JS. Relative exercise intensity of Tai Chi Chuan is similar in different ages and gender. Am J Chin Med 2004;32(1):151–60.

127. Lan C, Chen SY, Lai JS, et al. Tai Chi Chuan in medicine and health promotion. Evid Based Complement Alternat Med 2013;2013:1–17.

128. Hong Y, Li JX, Robinson PD. Balance control, flexibility, and cardiorespiratory fitness among older Tai Chi practitioners. Br J Sports Med 2000;34(1):29–34.

129. Blake H, Hawley H. Effects of Tai Chi exercise on physical and psychological health of older people. Curr Aging Sci 2012;5(1):19–27.

130. Taylor-Piliae RE, Haskell WL, Stotts NA, et al. Improvement in balance, strength, and flexibility after 12 weeks of Tai chi exercise in ethnic Chinese adults with cardiovascular disease risk factors. Altern Ther Health Med 2006;12(2):50–8.

131. Li F, Fisher KJ, Harmer P, et al. Tai chi and self-rated quality of sleep and daytime sleepiness in older adults: a randomized controlled trial. J Am Geriatr Soc 2004;52(6):892–900.

132. Li F, Harmer P, Fisher KJ, et al. Tai Chi and fall reductions in older adults: a randomized controlled trial. J Gerontol A Biol Sci Med Sci 2005;60(2):187–94.

133. Taylor-Piliae RE, Haskell WL, Froelicher ES. Hemodynamic responses to a community-based Tai Chi exercise intervention in ethnic Chinese adults with cardiovascular disease risk factors. Eur J Cardiovasc Nurs 2006;5(2):165–74.

134. Mortimer JA, Ding D, Borenstein AR, et al. Changes in brain volume and cognition in a randomized trial of exercise and social interaction in a community-based sample of non-demented Chinese elders. J Alzheimers Dis 2012;30(4):757–66.

135. Tsai JC, Wang WH, Chan P, et al. The beneficial effects of Tai Chi Chuan on blood pressure and lipid profile and anxiety status in a randomized

controlled trial. J Altern Complement Med 2003;9(5):747–54.

136. Hart J, Kanner H, Gilboa-Mayo R, et al. Tai Chi Chuan practice in community-dwelling persons after stroke. Int J Rehabil Res 2004;27(4):303–4.

137. Wang C, Schmid CH, Rones R, et al. A randomized trial of tai chi for fibromyalgia. N Engl J Med 2010;363(8):743–54.

138. Jones KD, Sherman CA, Mist SD, et al. A randomized controlled trial of 8-form Tai chi improves symptoms and functional mobility in fibromyalgia patients. Clin Rheumatol 2012;31(8):1205–14.

139. Wang C. Tai Chi improves pain and functional status in adults with rheumatoid arthritis: results of a pilot single-blinded randomized controlled trial. Med Sport Sci 2008;52:218–29.

140. Hochberg MC, Altman RD, April KT, et al. American College of Rheumatology 2012 recommendations for the use of nonpharmacologic and pharmacologic therapies in osteoarthritis of the hand, hip, and knee. Arthritis Care Res (Hoboken) 2012;64(4):465–74.

141. Wang JH. Effects of Tai Chi exercise on patients with type 2 diabetes. Med Sport Sci 2008;52:230–8.

142. Li F, Harmer P, Fitzgerald K, et al. Tai chi and postural stability in patients with Parkinson's disease. N Engl J Med 2012;366(6):511–9.

143. Sharma M, Haider T. Tai Chi as an alternative and complementary therapy for patients with asthma and chronic obstructive pulmonary disease. J Evid Based Complementary Altern Med 2013;18(3):209–15.

144. Chan AW, Lee A, Suen LK, et al. Tai chi Qigong improves lung functions and activity tolerance in COPD clients: a single blind, randomized controlled trial. Complement Ther Med 2011;19(1):3–11.

145. Leung RW, McKeough ZJ, Peters MJ, et al. Short-form Sun-style t'ai chi as an exercise training modality in people with COPD. Eur Respir J 2013;41(5):1051–7.

146. Spruit MA, Polkey MI. T'ai chi for individuals with COPD: an ancient wisdom for a 21st century disease? Eur Respir J 2013;41(5):1005–7.

147. Yan JH, Guo YZ, Yao HM, et al. Effects of Tai Chi in patients with chronic obstructive pulmonary disease: preliminary evidence. PLoS One 2013;8(4):e61806.

Strategies to Enhance the Benefits of Exercise Training in the Respiratory Patient

Kylie Hill, PhD[a,b,c],*, Anne E. Holland, PhD[d,e,f]

KEYWORDS

- Chronic obstructive pulmonary disease • Exercise training • Heliox
- Neuromuscular electrical stimulation • Noninvasive ventilation • Rollators • Supplemental oxygen

KEY POINTS

- In people with chronic obstructive pulmonary disease, exercise training offered as part of pulmonary rehabilitation has strong evidence for increasing exercise capacity, reducing symptoms of dyspnea and fatigue, and improving health-related quality of life.
- Nevertheless, there is a proportion of people referred to pulmonary rehabilitation who achieve minimal gains, most likely because of profound ventilatory limitation during exercise or the presence of comorbid conditions that limit participation in exercise training.
- Several adjuncts or strategies have been explored to optimize the proportion of people referred to pulmonary rehabilitation who achieve significant and meaningful gains on program completion.

INTRODUCTION

Pulmonary rehabilitation has been defined as a comprehensive intervention that follows a thorough patient assessment and includes therapies such as exercise training and education.[1] The aim of pulmonary rehabilitation is to improve the physical and psychological condition of people with chronic respiratory disease as well as promote long-term adherence to health-enhancing behaviors.[1] Exercise training is the cornerstone of an effective pulmonary rehabilitation program. Most studies examining the effect of pulmonary rehabilitation have been conducted in people with chronic obstructive pulmonary disease (COPD).[2] In this population, there is strong

Disclosure and Conflict of Interest Statement: Neither author has any conflict of interest with the content of this article.

[a] School of Physiotherapy and Exercise Science, Faculty of Health Science, Curtin University, GPO Box U1987, Perth, Western Australia 6845, Australia; [b] Lung Institute of Western Australia, Centre for Asthma, Allergy and Respiratory Research, University of Western Australia, Hospital Avenue, Nedlands, Western Australia 6009, Australia; [c] Physiotherapy Department, Royal Perth Hospital, Wellington Street, Perth, Western Australia 6000, Australia; [d] Department of Physiotherapy, La Trobe University, Level 4, The Alfred Centre, 99 Commercial Road, Melbourne, Victoria 3004, Australia; [e] Department of Physiotherapy, Alfred Health, Commercial Road, Melbourne, Victoria 3004, Australia; [f] Institute for Breathing and Sleep, Studley Road, Heidelberg, Victoria 3084, Australia
* Corresponding author. School of Physiotherapy and Exercise Science, Faculty of Health Science, Curtin University, GPO Box U1987, Perth, Western Australia 6845, Australia.
E-mail address: k.hill@curtin.edu.au

Clin Chest Med 35 (2014) 323–336
http://dx.doi.org/10.1016/j.ccm.2014.02.003

evidence that pulmonary rehabilitation, which includes exercise training, confers significant and important improvements in exercise capacity, symptoms such as dyspnea and fatigue, and health-related quality of life as well as reductions in health care use.[2-4] These effects are seen in people with stable disease as well as during or immediately after an acute exacerbation of their condition.[2,5] The mechanism of improvement relates largely to conditioning the muscles of locomotion, namely the quadriceps.[6,7] After rehabilitation, the changes in muscle morphology and biochemistry optimize the capacity of the quadriceps to meet the demands of exercise using aerobic energy systems.[6,7] This process in turn reduces the early reliance on anaerobic energy systems, delays the onset of blood lactate accumulation, and decreases the ventilatory load and sensation of dyspnea at submaximal exercise intensities.[6,7]

Although the evidence for pulmonary rehabilitation is strong, there are a proportion of people who do not achieve meaningful gains in exercise capacity.[8,9] These so called "nonresponders" seem to be characterized by more severe airflow obstruction and profound ventilatory limitation during exercise.[8,9] This situation may preclude the person from reaching an exercise intensity that constitutes an adequate stimulus to induce a training adaptation in the peripheral muscles. Furthermore, at least half of all people referred to pulmonary rehabilitation have 1 or more comorbid conditions, including musculoskeletal disorders, which compromise the training dose that can be achieved.[10] This situation has led to an interest in the role of adjuncts or alternative strategies, implemented during an exercise training program, to increase the load borne by the muscles of locomotion. Some of these strategies are commonplace and may be perceived by clinicians as easy to implement, such as the use of (1) supplemental oxygen, (2) rollators or wheeled walkers, (3) water-based exercise modalities, and (4) inspiratory muscle training (IMT). Others are less commonly used and may be perceived by clinicians as more difficult to implement, such as the use of (1) heliox (a helium-oxygen mixture), (2) noninvasive ventilation (NIV), (3) neuromuscular electrical stimulation (NMES), and (4) partitioning the exercising muscle mass. These approaches are described in this article.

SUPPLEMENTAL OXYGEN

Exercise-induced oxyhemoglobin desaturation is common in pulmonary rehabilitation participants. In 572 people with COPD undertaking a 6-minute walk test (6MWT), most of whom were entering a pulmonary rehabilitation program, desaturation of 4% or greater to less than 90% occurred in 47% of tests.[11] Although there are no strong data regarding the adverse effects of transient oxyhemoglobin desaturation during exercise, supplemental oxygen improves exercise performance and reduces dyspnea in people with COPD.[12] This finding is primarily related to a reduction in ventilation for a given exercise workload, leading to a delay in dynamic hyperinflation and prolonged exercise time.[13] These effects have been shown both in desaturators[13] and nondesaturators.[14] The reduction in ventilation at submaximal workloads may be associated with a slower increase in blood lactate as a result of better oxygen delivery to peripheral muscle[15] or direct chemoreceptor inhibition.[14] These acute effects of supplemental oxygen may facilitate training of the locomotor muscles at a higher intensity, or for a longer duration, to enhance training benefits.

There are now 7 randomized controlled trials (RCTs) that have evaluated the impact of supplemental oxygen during exercise training in COPD (Table 1). Despite the good physiologic rationale underpinning this intervention, 5 of the 7 trials found no beneficial effect on pulmonary rehabilitation outcomes.[16-20] Another trial measured exercise outcomes on the assigned gas, so it was unclear whether the benefits seen in the oxygen trained participants were related to the training program or the acute effects of the gas on exercise performance.[21] One well-designed trial that included participants who did not desaturate during exercise showed significantly increased endurance time during a constant power cycle ergometry test in the group who trained on supplemental oxygen compared with the air trained group after 7 weeks.[22] The oxygen group trained at a higher work rate, which progressed more rapidly over the course of the program, consistent with the hypothesis that the benefits of supplemental oxygen are attributable to a higher training intensity. It is unclear whether application of supplemental oxygen in previous trials had facilitated higher training workloads, which may explain the lack of positive findings in these studies. A Cochrane review[23] including 5 of these trials has concluded that there are small effects of supplemental oxygen during training on endurance time at the end of the program (mean improvement in exercise time compared with room air 2.69 minutes, 95% confidence interval 0.07–5.28 minutes, 2 trials with 53 participants) and Borg dyspnea score at the end of the endurance test (mean reduction in dyspnea 1.22 points, 95%

Table 1
Effect of supplemental oxygen during exercise training on exercise outcomes in COPD RCTs

Study	Included Participants	Exercise Program (wk, times/wk)	Treatment Group Sample Size	FEV$_1$ (% pred)	Oxygen	Control Group Sample Size	FEV$_1$ (% pred)	Comparator Treatment	Between Group Difference in Exercise Capacity After Training
Rooyackers, 1997	Desaturators	10, 5	12	29 ± 7	4 L/min	12	38 ± 11	Room air	No difference Wmax No difference 6MWD
Fichter, 1999	Moderate to severe COPD	4, 5	5	—	F$_{IO_2}$ 35%	5	—	Room air	No difference Wmax
Garrod, 2000	Desaturators	6, 3	12	35 ± 10	4 L/min	13	29 ± 10	Compressed air 4 L/min	No difference ISWT
Wadell, 2001	Desaturators	8, 3	10	39[a]	5 L/min	10	52[a]	Compressed air 5 L/min	No difference 6MWD
Emtner, 2003	Nondesaturators	7, 3	14	35 ± 10	3 L/min	15	38 ± 8	Compressed air 3 L/min	↑ endurance time in oxygen group
Scorsone, 2010	Desaturators	8, 3	10	47 ± 10	F$_{IO_2}$ 40%	10	50 ± 12	Room air	No difference Wmax No difference endurance time
Dyer, 2012	Desaturators, ↑ ESWT at least 10% on oxygen	6–7, 2	24	39 ± 16	2–6 L/min	23	44 ± 11	Room air	↑ ESWT in oxygen group Each group performed ESWT on allocated gas

Data are mean ± standard deviation, except [a]median.
Abbreviations: 6MWD, 6-minute walk distance; ESWT, endurance shuttle walk test; FEV$_1$ (% pred), forced expiratory volume in first second expressed as a percentage of the predicted value; F$_{IO_2}$, fraction of inspired oxygen; ISWT, incremental shuttle walk test; Wmax, maximum workload on cycle ergometer.

confidence interval 0.06–2.39 points, 2 trials with 53 participants). There were no data to support effects on health-related quality of life or longer-term clinical outcomes.

Recent guidelines for pulmonary rehabilitation reflect both the uncertainty arising from this body of literature and the common use of supplemental oxygen in clinical practice. The British Thoracic Society guidelines for pulmonary rehabilitation state that supplemental oxygen should not be used routinely, but should be offered to those who fulfill the criteria for long-term oxygen therapy or ambulatory oxygen therapy.[24] The American Thoracic Society/European Respiratory Society statement on pulmonary rehabilitation suggests that individualized oxygen titration trials should be used to identify those people with COPD who may respond to oxygen supplementation during exercise testing.[1] Given the potent effects of oxygen supplementation in reducing operating lung volumes and evidence of its usefulness to increase training intensity, a trial of supplemental oxygen may be justified in both desaturators and nondesaturators if dynamic hyperinflation or severe dyspnea limit the progression of exercise intensity or duration.

ROLLATORS (WHEELED WALKERS)

Most clinicians who work in the area of pulmonary rehabilitation have had their patients tell them they find it easier to walk in shopping centers where they can use a trolley or a cart. There are now data of people with COPD showing that the provision of a rollator (or wheeled walker) increases the distance achieved during the 6MWT and reduces dyspnea on test completion.[25,26] This effect was most evident in those with marked functional limitation (ie, 6-minute walk distance <300 m).[25] The mechanisms underpinning these improvements are likely to be multifactorial and include an increased capacity to use the accessory muscles of respiration when the arms are fixed, as well as the greater pressure-generating capacity of the inspiratory muscles in the forward lean position.[27,28] Further, it may relate to a reduction in the metabolic cost of walking.[29] Taken together, these factors serve to optimize the capacity of the respiratory system to meet the ventilatory demands imposed during walking-based exercise and offset the sensation of dyspnea.[30]

Despite these effects being shown on completion of walking tasks, no study has explored the effect of using a rollator to optimize walking-based exercise training in the context of pulmonary rehabilitation. The use of rollators as part of pulmonary rehabilitation is likely to increase given the predominance of comorbid conditions, including musculoskeletal disorders among people who are referred to pulmonary rehabilitation.[10] In contrast with many of the other approaches described in this article, there are data to show that rollators, when prescribed for use by an appropriately trained health care professional, are used frequently in the home environment, and people report a high level of satisfaction with them.[31] Specifically, rollators seem to promote walking outdoors[31] and may therefore increase participation in physical activity on completion of pulmonary rehabilitation.

WATER-BASED EXERCISE

Given the high prevalence of comorbid conditions in people who have been referred to a pulmonary rehabilitation program,[10] studies have explored alternative training modalities to traditional land-based exercise, such as water-based exercise. Three RCTs have compared the effects of land-based exercise, water-based exercise, and a control group.[32–34] The first group comprised water-based or land-based training, performed 3 times per week, for 45 minutes per session, over 12 weeks. Compared with both the control group and the group who underwent land-based exercise, those who completed the water-based training achieved greater gains in endurance walking capacity measured via the endurance shuttle walk test.[32] The second study included participants with 1 or more physical comorbidities, defined as obesity, musculoskeletal disorders, peripheral vascular disease, or neurologic conditions. Compared with a group who received usual care, or land-based exercise, those who underwent water-based training 3 times a week, for 60 minutes per session, over 8 weeks achieved greater gains in exercise capacity, measured via the incremental and endurance shuttle walk tests. Similar results were shown for the fatigue domain of a health-related quality-of-life questionnaire.[34] The results of a third RCT[33] also showed gains in exercise capacity, measured via the 6MWT on completion of a water-based training program, conducted 3 times a week, for 90 minutes per session, over 8 weeks. However, these gains were not of greater magnitude than those seen in a group that completed land-based training.

Studies in this area have reported no serious adverse events and high levels of acceptability of water-based exercise as an alternative training modality.[32–35] In addition to the effect that buoyancy has on unloading of peripheral and spinal joints, the hydrostatic force on the chest wall associated with water immersion may assist in reducing lung volumes during exercise[36]; an effect similar to that reported in obese people with COPD.[37] In turn, these effects may serve to increase the training dose that can be tolerated and thus optimize the magnitude of any physiologic training adaptation. Therefore, for people with COPD, especially those who have difficulty participating in land-based exercise because of comorbid conditions, consideration should be given to implementing a water-based exercise training program.

INSPIRATORY MUSCLE TRAINING

In people with COPD, pulmonary hyperinflation serves to shorten and flatten the diaphragm, reducing its mechanical advantage and pressure-generating capacity.[38] This reduction in pressure-generating capacity has been associated with the severity of dyspnea and also with impairments in exercise capacity.[39,40] Traditional exercise training, such as walking and cycling, does not impose sufficient load on the inspiratory muscles to induce a training adaptation. This situation has led to an interest in the role of specifically loading the inspiratory muscles, with the goal of improving their function as a way to ameliorate dyspnea and optimize exercise tolerance. The results of early studies in this area were confounded by limitations of resistive loading devices.[41] Studies that used a resistive device to load the inspiratory muscles without constraining the breathing pattern were unlikely to have imposed a load that was of sufficient magnitude to induce a training adaptation.[42] However, since that time, several robust RCTs have examined the effects of IMT applied in isolation and combined with exercise training. Meta-analyses of these trials provide strong evidence that IMT improves inspiratory muscle function (strength and endurance) and reduces dyspnea.[43] There is some evidence that IMT improves exercise capacity and health-related quality of life.[43] However, the effects are less convincing when the meta-analyses were restricted to those RCTs that specifically explored the role of IMT as an adjunct to a program of exercise training. In these studies, gains were reported in inspiratory muscle strength, but not exercise tolerance, symptoms, or health-related quality of life.[43,44]

The role of IMT in the rehabilitation of people with COPD is often debated.[45,46] Proponents of this approach support its use in those people with marked inspiratory muscle weakness.[47] Further, there is evidence that as little as 5 weeks of high-intensity IMT is capable of inducing changes in respiratory muscle morphology.[48] Based on current evidence, it seems reasonable to offer IMT to those people who continue to experience intractable dyspnea despite completion of a comprehensive pulmonary rehabilitation program.

NON-INVASIVE VENTILATION

The use of NIV during exercise is an alternative strategy to counter the deleterious effects of dynamic hyperinflation on respiratory muscle function. Whereas IMT aims to strengthen the respiratory muscles, the aim of NIV during exercise is to unload the respiratory muscles, thus reducing the oxygen cost of breathing and delaying the onset of intolerable dyspnea. Within a single exercise session, NIV has been shown to decrease inspiratory muscle effort, increase inspiratory and expiratory flows, increase minute ventilation, and improve gas exchange compared with exercise without ventilatory support.[49–51] There is a significant reduction in dyspnea at equivalent exercise workloads, the extent of which is proportional to degree of respiratory muscle unloading achieved with NIV.[49] As a result of these acute changes in physiology and symptoms, exercise tolerance is increased. A systematic review and meta-analysis including 7 trials of NIV versus unassisted breathing during cycling or walking in COPD found that NIV increased endurance time by an average of 3.3 minutes (55%).[52] Similarly, NIV during lower limb resistance exercise has been shown to delay the onset of quadriceps fatigue.[53] An increase in blood flow to the locomotor muscles may contribute to these findings, possibly as a result of redirection of the available cardiac output from respiratory muscles that are unloaded under NIV.[54]

Use of NIV during an entire 6-week to 8-week exercise training program has consistently been associated with improved exercise outcomes in people with advanced COPD. Compared with training on room air or oxygen, NIV-assisted training confers greater gains in maximum exercise performance,[55,56] functional exercise capacity,[57] and endurance exercise capacity.[56] These benefits are likely related to training at a higher intensity.[55,56,58] No studies have evaluated whether these benefits persist over the longer-term. Whether the increase in exercise capacity with NIV can be translated into greater improvements in symptoms and health-related quality of life when compared with unassisted training is not yet clear, because studies have not been powered to assess these outcomes.[57] No additional benefits of NIV were seen in an RCT in which participants had less severe disease.[59]

Current evidence indicates that NIV may be a useful adjunct to exercise training in carefully selected individuals. As well as potential application during outpatient pulmonary rehabilitation, consideration should be given to use of NIV to facilitate early exercise training in hospitalized patients recovering from acute exacerbations of COPD, in whom it has been shown to increase walking time, improve oxyhemoglobin saturation, and reduce dyspnea.[60] However, only a few people are suitable, and it may not be an acceptable treatment to those who are not using NIV.[61]

Use of NIV during training requires consideration of equipment and technique. Acute improvements in exercise endurance are more consistent when using inspiratory pressure support than other ventilatory modes.[52] This evidence, together with its ready availability and ease of use, suggests that inspiratory pressure support is the first choice for NIV-assisted training. Higher levels of inspiratory pressure support, in the region of 8 to 12 cm H_2O, give rise to better training outcomes than lower pressure levels.[62] A systematic review showed that positive effects of NIV-assisted training are seen in RCTs in which the mean FEV_1 (forced expiratory volume in 1 second) was less than 40% predicted, confirming that this technique is useful only in advanced disease.[62] Some studies have shown significant dropout rates during NIV-assisted training, with several citing discomfort related to the mask or ventilator.[62] For people to successfully use NIV during exercise, rehabilitation clinicians must have sufficient time and expertise in its implementation and titration, which is likely to limit this adjunct to a few centers.

HELIOX/HELIUM-HYPEROXIA

Heliox is formed when the nitrogen in air is replaced by helium, resulting in a gas that is 79% helium and 21% oxygen. Because helium has a lower density than nitrogen, heliox has a density nearly 3 times lower than air. As a result, the inhalation of heliox results in significantly lower turbulence and a greater tendency toward laminar flow, with an overall decrease in airway resistance. The beneficial effects of inhaling heliox during a single session of submaximal exercise in COPD have been well described, including reduced dynamic hyperinflation,[63–65] reduced respiratory muscle loading,[66,67] increased exercise endurance time,[63,64] less dyspnea,[63,66] and less leg fatigue.[66] Increasing the concentration of oxygen in the inhaled gas (eg, 40% oxygen, 70% helium), known as helium-hyperoxia, may have even greater effects on dynamic hyperinflation and exercise endurance than either normoxic helium or hyperoxia alone, with additive and independent effects of each gas on the work of breathing.[68–70] Physiologic benefits of inhaling helium gas mixtures are most evident in those with more severe airflow obstruction.[68]

Recent studies have shown that heliox results in increased locomotor muscle oxygen delivery in people with moderate to severe COPD,[64,66,67] as a result of improvements in both systemic oxygen delivery and locomotor muscle blood flow.[66] This finding suggests a potential role for helium gas mixtures in optimizing the effects of exercise training on locomotor muscles during pulmonary rehabilitation. Three RCTs have investigated the effects of heliox during exercise training in COPD (**Table 2**), with conflicting results. A single study showed a greater increase in endurance time in participants trained on helium-hyperoxia compared with training on room air,[71] whereas 2 others have shown no benefits of either heliox[72] or helium-hyperoxia.[20] These disparate results are likely a result of the training stimulus applied. The first study commenced training at a higher absolute workload in the helium-hyperoxia group than the air group, with regular increments thereafter.[71] In the other 2 studies,[20,72] the training intensity achieved with helium gas mixtures did not exceed the training intensity achieved in the control groups. This finding suggests that the benefits of breathing helium gas mixtures during exercise training may be apparent only if this intervention allows a higher training load to be applied. No studies have directly assessed the effects of exercise training using helium gas mixtures on adaptations in the muscles of locomotion.

The complex nature of applying helium gas mixtures during exercise training, together with the added expense and lack of conclusive clinical benefits, suggests that this therapy does not have a routine role in pulmonary rehabilitation for COPD. Further studies are required to establish whether heliox or helium-hyperoxia can augment the effects of exercise training in selected people with COPD, with sustained benefits after the training period.

Table 2
RCTs that have investigated the effects of heliox or helium-hyperoxia during exercise training in COPD

Study	Program Details	Treatment Group			Control Groups			Between Group Differences After Exercise Training
		Sample Size	FEV$_1$ (% pred)	Intervention	Sample Size	FEV$_1$ (% pred)	Comparators	
Johnson, 2002	6 wk, twice weekly, 20 min treadmill training and education	11	34 ± 13	Heliox	13 / 15	31 ± 11 / 32 ± 9	Humidified air NIV during training, EPAP 2 cm H$_2$O, IPAP 8–12 cm H$_2$O	No difference in total exercise time on treadmill between groups
Eves, 2009	6 wk, thrice weekly, 30 min exercise and education	19	47 ± 19	HH 60% helium, 40% oxygen	19	46 ± 14	Air	Greater change in constant load exercise time in HH group Greater change in SGRQ total score in HH group but no difference in domain scores
Scorsone, 2010	8 wk, thrice weekly, 30 min cycle ergometer	10	49 ± 12	HH 60% helium, 40% oxygen	10 / 10	47 ± 10 / 50 ± 12	Supplemental oxygen 40% Humidified air	No difference in constant load exercise time between groups

Data are mean ± standard deviation.
Abbreviations: EPAP, expiratory positive airway pressure; FEV$_1$ (% pred), forced expiratory volume in first second expressed as a percentage of the predicted value; HH, helium-hyperoxia; IPAP, inspiratory positive airway pressure; SGRQ, St George's Respiratory Questionnaire.

NEUROMUSCULAR ELECTRICAL STIMULATION

NMES involves applying an intermittent electrical current to a superficial peripheral muscle using electrodes and a stimulator.[73] The electrical current serves to trigger an action potential and depolarize the motor nerve to elicit an involuntary muscle contraction.[74] Although any superficial peripheral muscle can be stimulated to contract in this way, most studies have focused on stimulating the quadriceps femoris. The stimulator can be programmed to elicit contractions that are more likely to favor gains in strength or endurance. Strength protocols involve relatively few contractions, using high-frequency stimulation, at the highest current that can be tolerated.[73] A short duty cycle, characterized by a long contraction period followed by an even longer rest period, may be advantageous.[75] In contrast, endurance protocols involve multiple contractions over prolonged periods (often hours), using low-frequency stimulation and a moderate current with relatively short contractions followed by short rest periods.[76] Electrical stimulation is an attractive option to train the peripheral muscles in people characterized by profound ventilatory limitation, because it evokes minimal ventilatory response and therefore minimal experience of dyspnea.[77] This situation is true for high-frequency and low-frequency stimulation parameters.[77]

The RCTs that have investigated NMES, in isolation from other therapies, in people with COPD are summarized in **Table 3**.[78–82] All have reported consistent changes in muscle function, including gains in force-generating capacity, endurance, cross-sectional area, and upregulation of pathways involved in muscle anabolism. Most have also reported gains in exercise capacity. These studies were conducted in participants characterized by moderate to severe disease, and 2 were conducted in participants who were hospitalized with an acute exacerbation. In contrast to these RCTs, 2 randomized crossover studies of NMES applied in isolation from exercise training have failed to show any gains in muscle force-generating capacity or exercise capacity.[83,84] Both of these studies recruited participants with less severe lung disease ($FEV_1 \sim 50\%$ predicted), which may have contributed to the lack of effect. Earlier work[82,84] has reported that the capacity of the person to tolerate a progressive increase in current is a consistent predictor of response to NMES. Higher currents are associated with greater gains in muscle function,[81,82] and men may be more likely to tolerate the sensation associated with high currents.[81]

Two RCTs have investigated the effects of adding NMES to a program of exercise.[85,86] Both were conducted among inpatients, characterized by severe functional limitation and muscle atrophy, who were receiving rehabilitation after a period of serious illness. Many participants in these studies were essentially bedbound, and exercise training comprised active or active-assisted limb movements and treadmill walking when able. Compared with the group who underwent exercise training alone, the grouped who received NMES in addition to exercise training achieved benefits in muscle force-generating capacity, measures of dyspnea during activities of daily living, and the capacity to undertake functional tasks. Further work is needed to determine whether offering NMES confers additional benefits among those people who are referred to outpatient pulmonary rehabilitation.

PARTITIONING EXERCISING MUSCLE MASS

The ventilatory load imposed during exercise is related to the intensity and duration of exercise as well as the volume of exercising muscle mass. During pulmonary rehabilitation, for those people who are unable to cope with high-intensity exercise, the ventilatory load is often reduced by reducing exercise intensity.[87] Such an approach may compromise the effectiveness of the training program and reduce the likelihood of any physiologic adaptation in the exercising muscles.[6] In 1999, Richardson and colleagues[88] reported that partitioning the exercise muscle mass served to reduce the ventilatory load associated with exercise and, in turn, optimize the muscle-specific work rate. This concept was suggested as a training strategy by Dolmage and colleagues,[89] who reported that, compared with cycling using both legs, cycling at the same relevant intensity using only 1 leg increased constant power exercise time by a factor of 3.6. Since this time, there have been 2 studies that have compared the effect of completing a cycle-based exercise training program, using 2 legs simultaneously versus training each leg independently.[90,91] These studies are summarized in **Table 4**. Both studies have shown that a protocol of 1-leg versus 2-leg cycling conferred greater gains in the peak power and peak rate of oxygen uptake measured on completion of the training program. This approach seems to be readily translated into clinical practice.[92]

Table 3
RCTs that have investigated the effects of NMES in patients with COPD

Study	Treatment Group							Control Group			Between Group Differences After Intervention
	Setting	Sample Size	FEV$_1$ (% pred)	Muscles Stimulated	Stimulation Frequency (Hz)	Initial Duty Cycle	Program Details	Sample Size	FEV$_1$ (% pred)	Sham Protocol	
Bourjeily-Habr, 2002	Outpatient training	9	36 ± 4	Quadriceps, hamstrings and calves	50	200 ms on: 1500 ms off	20 min, 3 × per wk, 6 wk	9	41 ± 4	Yes	↑ quadriceps and hamstring strength, ↑ exercise capacity
Neder, 2002	Home-based training	9	38 ± 10	Quadriceps	50	2 s on: 18 s off	15 min increased to 30 min after first wk, 5 × per wk, 6 wk	6	40 ± 13	No	↑ V$_{O2peak}$, ↑ exercise time, ↑ quadriceps strength, ↓ quadriceps fatigue
Abdellaoui, 2011	Inpatient	9	15 [17]	Quadriceps and hamstrings	35	Not stated	60 min, 5 × per wk, 6 wk	6	25 [24]	Yes	↑ quadriceps strength, ↑ exercise capacity, change in proportion of muscle fibers
Giavendoni, 2012	Inpatient	11	41 ± 6	Quadriceps (dominant leg only)	50	8 s on: 20 s off	30 min daily sessions for 14 d	11	41 ± 6	No stimulation of nondominant leg	↑ quadriceps strength
Vivodtzev, 2012	Home-based training	12	30 ± 4	Quadriceps and calves	50	6 s on: 16 s off	5 × per wk, 60 min per session, for 6 wk	12	34 ± 3	Yes	↑ muscle CSA, ↑ quadriceps strength and endurance, ↑ muscle signaling pathways favoring anabolism

Data are mean ± standard deviation or median [interquartile range].
Abbreviations: CSA, cross-sectional area; FEV$_1$ (% pred), forced expiratory volume in first second expressed as a percentage of the predicted value; V$_{O2peak}$, peak rate of oxygen consumption.

Table 4
RCTs that have investigated the effects of 1-leg cycling in patients with COPD

Study	Program Details	Treatment Group Sample Size	Treatment Group FEV_1 (% pred)	Treatment Group Training Intensity	Control Group Sample Size	Control Group FEV_1 (% pred)	Control Group Training Intensity	Between Group Differences After Training
Dolmage, 2008	Supervised 30 min sessions, 3 × a wk, 7 wk	9	37 ± 8	50% of peak power achieved during CPET	9	40 ± 23	70% of peak power achieved during CPET	↑Vo_{2peak}, ↑ peak power, ↑Vco_{2peak}, ↑V_{Epeak}, ↓ minute ventilation and heart rate at submaximal Vo_2
Bjorgen, 2009	Supervised, 16 min, 3 × a wk, 8 wk	12	41 ± 10	Interval training: 4 × 4 min exercise at 85%–95% HRmax (measured during 1-leg CPET) Each 4 min exercise period alternated between the 2 legs, giving a total of 8 intervals	7	45 ± 8	Interval training: 4 × 4 min exercise at 85%–95% HRmax (measured during 2-leg CPET), interspersed with 3 min active rest (60%–70% HRmax)	↑Vo_{2peak}, ↑ peak power, ↑Vco_{2peak} and ↑V_{Epeak}

Data are mean ± standard deviation.

Abbreviations: CPET, cardiopulmonary exercise test; FEV_1 (% pred), forced expiratory volume in first second expressed as a percentage of the predicted value; HRmax, maximum heart rate; Vco_{2peak}, peak rate of carbon dioxide production; V_{Epeak}, peak rate of minute ventilation; Vo_{2peak}, peak rate of oxygen consumption.

SUMMARY

Several exercise training adjuncts can be used to maximize benefit through increasing the load on the locomotor muscles during pulmonary rehabilitation programs. This article has presented several strategies for which there is a strong physiologic rationale for their use in patients with COPD. However, most are suitable for only a carefully selected subgroup of individuals attending pulmonary rehabilitation, and in many cases, their long-term effects have not been examined. Clinicians should consider the judicious use of training adjuncts such as these to optimize training intensity and maximize the number of people who achieve meaningful improvements in outcomes that are important to patients after pulmonary rehabilitation.

REFERENCES

1. Spruit MA, Singh S, Garvey C, et al. An official American Thoracic Society/European Respiratory Society statement: key concepts and advances in pulmonary rehabilitation–an executive summary. Am J Respir Crit Care Med 2013;188(8):e13–64.

2. Lacasse Y, Goldstein R, Lasserson TJ, et al. Pulmonary rehabilitation for chronic obstructive pulmonary disease. Cochrane Database Syst Rev 2006;(4):CD003793.

3. Raskin J, Spiegler P, McCusker C, et al. The effect of pulmonary rehabilitation on healthcare utilization in chronic obstructive pulmonary disease: the Northeast Pulmonary Rehabilitation Consortium. J Cardiopulm Rehabil 2006;26(4):231–6.

4. Cecins N, Geelhoed E, Jenkins SC. Reduction in hospitalisation following pulmonary rehabilitation in patients with COPD. Aust Health Rev 2008; 32(3):415–22.

5. Puhan MA, Gimeno-Santos E, Scharplatz M, et al. Pulmonary rehabilitation following exacerbations of chronic obstructive pulmonary disease. Cochrane Database Syst Rev 2011;(10):CD005305.

6. Casaburi R, Patessio A, Ioli F, et al. Reductions in exercise lactic acidosis and ventilation as a result of exercise training in patients with obstructive lung disease. Am Rev Respir Dis 1991;143(1): 9–18.

7. Maltais F, LeBlanc P, Simard C, et al. Skeletal muscle adaptation to endurance training in patients with chronic obstructive pulmonary disease. Am J Respir Crit Care Med 1996;154(2 Pt 1):442–7.

8. Troosters T, Gosselink R, Decramer M. Exercise training in COPD: how to distinguish responders from nonresponders. J Cardiopulm Rehabil 2001; 21(1):10–7.

9. Scott AS, Baltzan MA, Fox J, et al. Success in pulmonary rehabilitation in patients with chronic obstructive pulmonary disease. Can Respir J 2010;17(5):219–23.

10. Crisafulli E, Costi S, Luppi F, et al. Role of comorbidities in a cohort of patients with COPD undergoing pulmonary rehabilitation. Thorax 2008;63(6): 487–92.

11. Jenkins S, Cecins N. Six-minute walk test: observed adverse events and oxygen desaturation in a large cohort of patients with chronic lung disease. Intern Med J 2011;41(5):416–22.

12. Dean NC, Brown JK, Himelman RB, et al. Oxygen may improve dyspnea and endurance in patients with chronic obstructive pulmonary disease and only mild hypoxemia. Am Rev Respir Dis 1992; 146(4):941–5.

13. O'Donnell DE, D'Arsigny C, Webb KA. Effects of hyperoxia on ventilatory limitation during exercise in advanced chronic obstructive pulmonary disease. Am J Respir Crit Care Med 2001;163(4): 892–8.

14. Somfay A, Porszasz J, Lee SM, et al. Dose-response effect of oxygen on hyperinflation and exercise endurance in nonhypoxaemic COPD patients. Eur Respir J 2001;18(1):77–84.

15. O'Donnell DE, Bain DJ, Webb KA. Factors contributing to relief of exertional breathlessness during hyperoxia in chronic airflow limitation. Am J Respir Crit Care Med 1997;155(2):530–5.

16. Rooyackers JM, Dekhuijzen PN, Van Herwaarden CL, et al. Training with supplemental oxygen in patients with COPD and hypoxaemia at peak exercise. Eur Respir J 1997;10(6): 1278–84.

17. Fichter J, Fleckenstein J, Stahl C, et al. Effect of oxygen (FIO2: 0.35) on the aerobic capacity in patients with COPD. Pneumologie 1999;53(3): 121–6 [in German].

18. Garrod R, Paul EA, Wedzicha JA. Supplemental oxygen during pulmonary rehabilitation in patients with COPD with exercise hypoxaemia. Thorax 2000;55(7):539–43.

19. Wadell K, Henriksson-Larsen K, Lundgren R. Physical training with and without oxygen in patients with chronic obstructive pulmonary disease and exercise-induced hypoxaemia. J Rehabil Med 2001;33(5):200–5.

20. Scorsone D, Bartolini S, Saporiti R, et al. Does a low-density gas mixture or oxygen supplementation improve exercise training in COPD? Chest 2010;138(5):1133–9.

21. Dyer F, Callaghan J, Cheema K, et al. Ambulatory oxygen improves the effectiveness of pulmonary rehabilitation in selected patients with chronic obstructive pulmonary disease. Chron Respir Dis 2012;9(2):83–91.

22. Emtner M, Porszasz J, Burns M, et al. Benefits of supplemental oxygen in exercise training in nonhypoxemic chronic obstructive pulmonary disease patients. Am J Respir Crit Care Med 2003;168(9): 1034–42.

23. Nonoyama ML, Brooks D, Lacasse Y, et al. Oxygen therapy during exercise training in chronic obstructive pulmonary disease. Cochrane Database Syst Rev 2007;(2):CD005372.

24. Bolton CE, Bevan-Smith EF, Blakey JD, et al. British Thoracic Society guideline on pulmonary rehabilitation in adults. Thorax 2013;68(Suppl 2):ii1–30.

25. Solway S, Brooks D, Lau L, et al. The short-term effect of a rollator on functional exercise capacity among individuals with severe COPD. Chest 2002;122(1):56–65.

26. Probst VS, Troosters T, Coosemans I, et al. Mechanisms of improvement in exercise capacity using a rollator in patients with COPD. Chest 2004;126(4): 1102–7.

27. O'Neill S, McCarthy DS. Postural relief of dyspnoea in severe chronic airflow limitation: relationship to respiratory muscle strength. Thorax 1983;38(8): 595–600.

28. Cavalheri V, Camillo CA, Brunetto AF, et al. Effects of arm bracing posture on respiratory muscle strength and pulmonary function in patients with chronic obstructive pulmonary disease. Rev Port Pneumol 2010;16(6):887–91.

29. Hill K, Dolmage TE, Woon LJ, et al. Rollator use does not consistently change the metabolic cost of walking in people with chronic obstructive pulmonary disease. Arch Phys Med Rehabil 2012; 93(6):1077–80.

30. Parshall MB, Schwartzstein RM, Adams L, et al. An official American Thoracic Society statement: update on the mechanisms, assessment, and management of dyspnea. Am J Respir Crit Care Med 2012;185(4):435–52.

31. Hill K, Goldstein R, Gartner EJ, et al. Daily utility and satisfaction with rollators among persons with chronic obstructive pulmonary disease. Arch Phys Med Rehabil 2008;89(6):1108–13.

32. Wadell K, Sundelin G, Henriksson-Larsen K, et al. High intensity physical group training in water–an effective training modality for patients with COPD. Respir Med 2004;98(5):428–38.

33. de Souto Araujo ZT, de Miranda Silva Nogueira PA, Cabral EE, et al. Effectiveness of low-intensity aquatic exercise on COPD: a randomized clinical trial. Respir Med 2012;106(11):1535–43.

34. McNamara RJ, McKeough ZJ, McKenzie DK, et al. Water-based exercise in COPD with physical comorbidities: a randomised controlled trial. Eur Respir J 2013;41(6):1284–91.

35. Rae S, White P. Swimming pool-based exercise as pulmonary rehabilitation for COPD patients in primary care: feasibility and acceptability. Prim Care Respir J 2009;18(2):90–4.

36. Girandola RN, Wiswell RA, Mohler JG, et al. Effects of water immersion on lung volumes: implications for body composition analysis. J Appl Physiol Respir Environ Exerc Physiol 1977;43(2):276–9.

37. Ora J, Laveneziana P, Wadell K, et al. Effect of obesity on respiratory mechanics during rest and exercise in COPD. J Appl Physiol (1985) 2011; 111(1):10–9.

38. Smith J, Bellemare F. Effect of lung volume on in vivo contraction characteristics of human diaphragm. J Appl Physiol (1985) 1987;62(5): 1893–900.

39. Hamilton AL, Killian KJ, Summers E, et al. Symptom intensity and subjective limitation to exercise in patients with cardiorespiratory disorders. Chest 1996; 110(5):1255–63.

40. Gosselink R, Troosters T, Decramer M. Peripheral muscle weakness contributes to exercise limitation in COPD. Am J Respir Crit Care Med 1996;153(3): 976–80.

41. Smith K, Cook D, Guyatt GH, et al. Respiratory muscle training in chronic airflow limitation: a meta-analysis. Am Rev Respir Dis 1992;145(3): 533–9.

42. Belman MJ, Thomas SG, Lewis MI. Resistive breathing training in patients with chronic obstructive pulmonary disease. Chest 1986;90(5): 662–9.

43. Gosselink R, De Vos J, van den Heuvel SP, et al. Impact of inspiratory muscle training in patients with COPD: what is the evidence? Eur Respir J 2011;37(2):416–25.

44. O'Brien K, Geddes EL, Reid WD, et al. Inspiratory muscle training compared with other rehabilitation interventions in chronic obstructive pulmonary disease: a systematic review update. J Cardiopulm Rehabil Prev 2008;28(2):128–41.

45. Ambrosino N. The case for inspiratory muscle training in COPD. For. Eur Respir J 2011;37(2): 233–5.

46. Polkey MI, Moxham J, Green M. The case against inspiratory muscle training in COPD. Against. Eur Respir J 2011;37(2):236–7.

47. Charususin N, Gosselink R, Decramer M, et al. Inspiratory muscle training protocol for patients with chronic obstructive pulmonary disease (IMTCO study): a multicentre randomised controlled trial. BMJ Open 2013;3(8).

48. Ramirez-Sarmiento A, Orozco-Levi M, Guell R, et al. Inspiratory muscle training in patients with chronic obstructive pulmonary disease: structural adaptation and physiologic outcomes. Am J Respir Crit Care Med 2002;166(11):1491–7.

49. Maltais F, Reissmann H, Gottfried SB. Pressure support reduces inspiratory effort and dyspnea

during exercise in chronic airflow obstruction. Am J Respir Crit Care Med 1995;151(4):1027–33.

50. Kyroussis D, Polkey MI, Hamnegard CH, et al. Respiratory muscle activity in patients with COPD walking to exhaustion with and without pressure support. Eur Respir J 2000;15(4):649–55.

51. Dreher M, Storre JH, Windisch W. Noninvasive ventilation during walking in patients with severe COPD: a randomised cross-over trial. Eur Respir J 2007;29(5):930–6.

52. van 't Hul A, Kwakkel G, Gosselink R. The acute effects of noninvasive ventilatory support during exercise on exercise endurance and dyspnea in patients with chronic obstructive pulmonary disease: a systematic review. J Cardiopulm Rehabil 2002;22(4):290–7.

53. Borghi-Silva A, Di Thommazo L, Pantoni CB, et al. Non-invasive ventilation improves peripheral oxygen saturation and reduces fatigability of quadriceps in patients with COPD. Respirology 2009; 14(4):537–44.

54. Borghi-Silva A, Oliveira CC, Carrascosa C, et al. Respiratory muscle unloading improves leg muscle oxygenation during exercise in patients with COPD. Thorax 2008;63(10):910–5.

55. Reuveny R, Ben-Dov I, Gaides M, et al. Ventilatory support during training improves training benefit in severe chronic airway obstruction. Isr Med Assoc J 2005;7(3):151–5.

56. van 't Hul A, Gosselink R, Hollander P, et al. Training with inspiratory pressure support in patients with severe COPD. Eur Respir J 2006;27(1):65–72.

57. Borghi-Silva A, Mendes RG, Toledo AC, et al. Adjuncts to physical training of patients with severe COPD: oxygen or noninvasive ventilation? Respir Care 2010;55(7):885–94.

58. Hawkins P, Johnson LC, Nikoletou D, et al. Proportional assist ventilation as an aid to exercise training in severe chronic obstructive pulmonary disease. Thorax 2002;57(10):853–9.

59. Bianchi L, Foglio K, Porta R, et al. Lack of additional effect of adjunct of assisted ventilation to pulmonary rehabilitation in mild COPD patients. Respir Med 2002;96(5):359–67.

60. Menadue C, Alison JA, Piper AJ, et al. Bilevel ventilation during exercise in acute on chronic respiratory failure: a preliminary study. Respir Med 2010; 104(2):219–27.

61. Dyer F, Flude L, Bazari F, et al. Non-invasive ventilation (NIV) as an aid to rehabilitation in acute respiratory disease. BMC Pulm Med 2011;11:58.

62. Corner E, Garrod R. Does the addition of non-invasive ventilation during pulmonary rehabilitation in patients with chronic obstructive pulmonary disease augment patient outcome in exercise tolerance? A literature review. Physiother Res Int 2010;15(1):5–15.

63. Palange P, Valli G, Onorati P, et al. Effect of heliox on lung dynamic hyperinflation, dyspnea, and exercise endurance capacity in COPD patients. J Appl Physiol (1985) 2004;97(5):1637–42.

64. Chiappa GR, Queiroga F Jr, Meda E, et al. Heliox improves oxygen delivery and utilization during dynamic exercise in patients with chronic obstructive pulmonary disease. Am J Respir Crit Care Med 2009;179(11):1004–10.

65. Laveneziana P, Valli G, Onorati P, et al. Effect of heliox on heart rate kinetics and dynamic hyperinflation during high-intensity exercise in COPD. Eur J Appl Physiol 2011;111(2):225–34.

66. Vogiatzis I, Habazettl H, Aliverti A, et al. Effect of helium breathing on intercostal and quadriceps muscle blood flow during exercise in COPD patients. Am J Physiol Regul Integr Comp Physiol 2011;300(6):R1549–59.

67. Louvaris Z, Zakynthinos S, Aliverti A, et al. Heliox increases quadriceps muscle oxygen delivery during exercise in COPD patients with and without dynamic hyperinflation. J Appl Physiol (1985) 2012; 113(7):1012–23.

68. Laude EA, Duffy NC, Baveystock C, et al. The effect of helium and oxygen on exercise performance in chronic obstructive pulmonary disease: a randomized crossover trial. Am J Respir Crit Care Med 2006;173(8):865–70.

69. Eves ND, Petersen SR, Haykowsky MJ, et al. Helium-hyperoxia, exercise, and respiratory mechanics in chronic obstructive pulmonary disease. Am J Respir Crit Care Med 2006;174(7):763–71.

70. Queiroga F Jr, Nunes M, Meda E, et al. Exercise tolerance with helium-hyperoxia versus hyperoxia in hypoxaemic patients with COPD. Eur Respir J 2013;42(2):362–70.

71. Eves ND, Sandmeyer LC, Wong EY, et al. Helium-hyperoxia: a novel intervention to improve the benefits of pulmonary rehabilitation for patients with COPD. Chest 2009;135(3):609–18.

72. Johnson JE, Gavin DJ, Adams-Dramiga S. Effects of training with heliox and noninvasive positive pressure ventilation on exercise ability in patients with severe COPD. Chest 2002; 122(2):464–72.

73. Maffiuletti NA. Physiological and methodological considerations for the use of neuromuscular electrical stimulation. Eur J Appl Physiol 2010;110(2): 223–34.

74. Vivodtzev I, Lacasse Y, Maltais F. Neuromuscular electrical stimulation of the lower limbs in patients with chronic obstructive pulmonary disease. J Cardiopulm Rehabil Prev 2008;28(2): 79–91.

75. Filipovic A, Kleinoder H, Dormann U, et al. Electromyostimulation–a systematic review of the influence of training regimens and stimulation

parameters on effectiveness in electromyostimulation training of selected strength parameters. J Strength Cond Res 2011;25(11):3218–38.

76. Nuhr MJ, Pette D, Berger R, et al. Beneficial effects of chronic low-frequency stimulation of thigh muscles in patients with advanced chronic heart failure. Eur Heart J 2004;25(2):136–43.

77. Sillen MJ, Wouters EF, Franssen FM, et al. Oxygen uptake, ventilation, and symptoms during low-frequency versus high-frequency NMES in COPD: a pilot study. Lung 2011;189(1):21–6.

78. Bourjeily-Habr G, Rochester CL, Palermo F, et al. Randomised controlled trial of transcutaneous electrical muscle stimulation of the lower extremities in patients with chronic obstructive pulmonary disease. Thorax 2002;57(12):1045–9.

79. Neder JA, Sword D, Ward SA, et al. Home based neuromuscular electrical stimulation as a new rehabilitative strategy for severely disabled patients with chronic obstructive pulmonary disease (COPD). Thorax 2002;57(4):333–7.

80. Abdellaoui A, Prefaut C, Gouzi F, et al. Skeletal muscle effects of electrostimulation after COPD exacerbation: a pilot study. Eur Respir J 2011;38(4):781–8.

81. Giavedoni S, Deans A, McCaughey P, et al. Neuromuscular electrical stimulation prevents muscle function deterioration in exacerbated COPD: a pilot study. Respir Med 2012;106(10):1429–34.

82. Vivodtzev I, Debigare R, Gagnon P, et al. Functional and muscular effects of neuromuscular electrical stimulation in patients with severe COPD: a randomized clinical trial. Chest 2012;141(3):716–25.

83. Dal Corso S, Napolis L, Malaguti C, et al. Skeletal muscle structure and function in response to electrical stimulation in moderately impaired COPD patients. Respir Med 2007;101(6):1236–43.

84. Napolis LM, Dal Corso S, Neder JA, et al. Neuromuscular electrical stimulation improves exercise tolerance in chronic obstructive pulmonary disease patients with better preserved fat-free mass. Clinics (Sao Paulo) 2011;66(3):401–6.

85. Zanotti E, Felicetti G, Maini M, et al. Peripheral muscle strength training in bed-bound patients with COPD receiving mechanical ventilation: effect of electrical stimulation. Chest 2003;124(1):292–6.

86. Vivodtzev I, Pepin JL, Vottero G, et al. Improvement in quadriceps strength and dyspnea in daily tasks after 1 month of electrical stimulation in severely deconditioned and malnourished COPD. Chest 2006;129(6):1540–8.

87. Maltais F, LeBlanc P, Jobin J, et al. Intensity of training and physiologic adaptation in patients with chronic obstructive pulmonary disease. Am J Respir Crit Care Med 1997;155(2):555–61.

88. Richardson RS, Sheldon J, Poole DC, et al. Evidence of skeletal muscle metabolic reserve during whole body exercise in patients with chronic obstructive pulmonary disease. Am J Respir Crit Care Med 1999;159(3):881–5.

89. Dolmage TE, Goldstein RS. Response to one-legged cycling in patients with COPD. Chest 2006;129(2):325–32.

90. Dolmage TE, Goldstein RS. Effects of one-legged exercise training of patients with COPD. Chest 2008;133(2):370–6.

91. Bjorgen S, Hoff J, Husby VS, et al. Aerobic high intensity one and two legs interval cycling in chronic obstructive pulmonary disease: the sum of the parts is greater than the whole. Eur J Appl Physiol 2009;106(4):501–7.

92. Evans RA, Dolmage TE, Mangovski-Alzamora S, et al. One-legged cycling for chronic obstructive pulmonary disease (COPD): knowledge translation to pulmonary rehabilitation. Am J Respir Crit Care Med 2013;A2574.

Collaborative Self-Management and Behavioral Change

Kathryn Rice, MD[a],*, Jean Bourbeau[b],
Roderick MacDonald, MS[a], Timothy J. Wilt, MD, MPH[a]

KEYWORDS

- Chronic obstructive pulmonary disease • Collaborative self-management • Behavioral change
- Pulmonary rehabilitation

KEY POINTS

- Behavioral change is critical for improving health outcomes in patients with chronic obstructive pulmonary disease.
- An educational approach alone is insufficient; effective collaborative self-management (CSM) to promote adaptive behaviors is necessary.
- CSM should be integrated with pulmonary rehabilitation programs, one of the main goals of which is to induce long-term changes in behavior.
- More research is needed to evaluate the effectiveness of assimilating CSM into primary care, patient-centered medical homes, and palliative care teams.

INTRODUCTION

According to the World Health Organization (WHO), chronic noncommunicable medical conditions, including chronic obstructive pulmonary disease (COPD), comprise more than half of the total global burden of disease. People who suffer from chronic diseases have complex medical, emotional, and social needs during the changing trajectory of their illnesses. These needs cannot be met by education alone; changes in behavior, especially the acquisition of self-care skills, are also required.[1] Chronic disease management, also termed collaborative self-management (CSM), is defined by the Disease Management Association of America as "a system of coordinated health care interventions and communications for populations with conditions in which patient self-care efforts are significant."[2] There is mounting evidence that embedding CSM within existing health care systems provides an effective model to meet these needs. The Joint Commission on Patient Safety and Quality in the United States has recently set out an evidence-based framework to improve self-management support for people with chronic conditions.[3] For people suffering from COPD, CSM is a multicomponent model of health care delivery that guides self-management behaviors to help patients lead lives that are as healthy and functional as possible.

Regarding COPD, the first Cochrane review in 2003 found insufficient evidence to demonstrate the effectiveness of CSM.[4] The next Cochrane review of 14 randomized controlled trials (RCTs) reported that COPD CSM improved dyspnea scores and reduced respiratory-related hospitalizations.[5] In 2013, a new Cochrane review of 26 RCTs found that COPD CSM not only improved disease-specific health status and exercise capacity but also reduced hospital admissions and hospital days per person.[6] This meta-analysis found no difference in mortality, although more

[a] Minneapolis VA Health Care System, One Veterans Drive, Minneapolis, MN 55417, USA; [b] Montreal Chest Institute, McGill University Health Centre, Montréal, Québec, Canada
* Corresponding author.
E-mail address: kathryn.rice@va.gov

Clin Chest Med 35 (2014) 337–351
http://dx.doi.org/10.1016/j.ccm.2014.02.004
0272-5231/14/$ – see front matter Published by Elsevier Inc.

recent studies were not included. There was insufficient evidence to either refute or confirm the long-term effectiveness of COPD CSM.

CHALLENGES TO PROVIDING HIGH-QUALITY COPD CARE

Health care systems face major challenges in reducing the burden of illness and improving the functional status of people with chronic health problems.[7] Challenges for patients include the complexity of behavioral changes they are asked to make, communication problems, such as the fear of asking questions or "white-coat silence,"[8] a lack understanding of the disease and the severity of its symptoms, and nonadherence to medication.[9] Provider challenges include knowledge deficits and pessimism about COPD,[9-14] and acquiring the skills needed to guide behavioral changes. Challenges to health care systems are the availability of resources, including sufficient provider time to elicit and answer questions and ensure understanding[8]; role clarity for members of the health care team[15]; and systematic evaluation of the effectiveness of interventions.

Team-based models of care such as COPD CSM provide a framework for overcoming many of these challenges. The theoretical frameworks for these systems have been previously described in some detail.[16] CSM is based on Wagner's Chronic Care Model as shown in **Fig. 1**,[17] which emphasizes patient self-efficacy and behavior change. An additional framework for behavioral change is provided by the precede-proceed model.[18] According to this model, it is important to identify participants' learning needs based on the evaluation of factors that can influence their behavior, as follows. (1) The predisposing factors that refer to existing health-related knowledge, beliefs, attitudes, and values, and expected changes in behavior; in addition, the level of self-efficacy is an important predisposing factor to behavioral change. (2) The facilitating factors or barriers that are based on patients' past life experiences, knowledge, and skills already acquired, and the accessibility to services and financial resources. (3) The reinforcing factors that depend on patients' social support network and their successful past life experiences. Behavioral interventions must be planned in relation to identified learning needs that are meaningful for the patient and applied through methods enhancing self-efficacy to achieve the expected behavioral changes and outcomes.

Evidence supports the integration of CSM into routine health care for several chronic diseases,

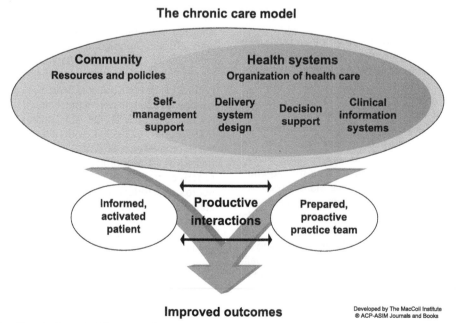

The chronic care model

Community
Resources and policies

Health systems
Organization of health care

Self-management support

Delivery system design

Decision support

Clinical information systems

Informed, activated patient

Productive interactions

Prepared, proactive practice team

Improved outcomes

Developed by The MacColl Institute
® ACP-ASIM Journals and Books

Fig. 1. The Chronic Care Model. Notes: The Improving Chronic Illness Care Program is supported by The Robert Wood Johnson Foundation, with direction and technical assistance provided by Group Health Cooperative of Puget Sound's MacColl Institute for Healthcare Innovation, and its relationship to the Patient-Centered Medical Home. (*From* Wagner EH. Chronic disease management: what will it take to improve care for chronic illness? Eff Clin Pract 1998;1(1):2–4; with permission.)

including congestive heart failure (CHF),[19,20] diabetes,[21] depression[22] and asthma.[23] In a systematic review of CSM for patients with COPD, a multicomponent, as opposed to single-component, CSM intervention was required for success.[24] Specifically, the inclusion of 2 or more of the following components were associated with better clinical outcomes: (1) self-management, (2) advanced access care delivery, (3) decision support, and (4) clinical information systems. Categories of these components and specific examples of the types of care in COPD CSM are shown in **Tables 1** and **2**. Support for multicomponent COPD CSM was also provided in another systematic review, which found that successful interventions included all of the following dimensions: patient-related, professional-directed, and organizational.[23]

The primary aim of COPD CSM is to help patients deal with the spectrum of their condition, including both the "good days" and the "bad days"; that is, acute exacerbation of COPD (AECOPD). This goal is accomplished by providing careful and continuous communication with a case manager, fostering disease-specific knowledge and skills guided by a mutually understood care plan, and encouraging patient self-efficacy behaviors.

COPD CSM FOR THE "GOOD DAYS"

Behavioral change and psychological components of COPD CSM are aimed at helping patients lead as functional and as healthy a life (with as many "good days") as possible throughout the course of their condition. CSM enhances patients' knowledge and understanding of the disease, and, more importantly, encourages self-efficacious behavioral lifestyle changes. This self-management includes goal-setting, increased physical activity, adherence to exercise programs after completion of pulmonary rehabilitation, and coping with breathlessness, anxiety, and depression. Preventive behaviors include vaccination, smoking cessation, diet, good hand hygiene, and adherence to respiratory medication.

Knowledge and Understanding

Although education alone in COPD CSM is insufficient to accomplish the myriad goals of managing this chronic condition throughout its course, it does provide an informational framework for shared decision making and correcting common misperceptions.[25] For example, a lack of understanding by patients and providers about correct inhalational techniques and the benefits of controller medications[11,12,14] can result in poor adherence. Likewise, because adherence to long-term oxygen treatment (LTOT) is often suboptimal,[26] patients should understand that improved survival, not merely immediate symptom relief, is the ultimate goal of LTOT.[27] There are many educational resource materials for COPD CSM, such as "Living Well with COPD" by the American College of Chest Physicians (2012), and the Canadian program for patients "Living Well with COPD" (www.livingwellwithcopd.com) and health professional guide "Krames On-Demand" (www.kramesstaywell.com).[28] Evidence that COPD CSM improves patient understanding of the disease is compelling. Knowledge informs the patient of the probable consequences and outcomes of their choices. Six of 7 RCTs that have reported this outcome have found a benefit.[29–35] Although new knowledge inspires individuals to consider changes in behavior, empirical evidence has shown that it is insufficient for generating sustained behavioral change.

Table 1
COPD CSM structure and examples

Categories of Care	Examples
Self-management	Ongoing education behavioral support Prevention (vaccination, smoking) Motivation, self-efficacy, and goal-setting Physical activity programs Disease exacerbation action plans Team training in cognitive behavior change
Advanced access care delivery	24/7 plan for care accessibility Shared/group appointments Nonappointment care/telephone follow-up Home tele-care
Decision support	Integration of guidelines Specialty expertise and ongoing input Barrier identification Performance review
Clinical information system	Disease registries Provider reminders Provider feedback Quality improvement Risk management/resource utilization

Adapted from Adams SG, Smith PK, Allan PF, et al. Systematic review of the chronic care model in chronic obstructive pulmonary disease prevention and management. Arch Intern Med 2007;167(6):551–61.

Table 2
Self-management skills and healthy behaviors for self-management of COPD

Healthy Behavior	Self-Management Skill (Strategy)
Live in a smoke-free environment	Quit smoking and remain nonsmoker, and avoid secondhand smoke
Comply with your medication	Take medication as prescribed on a regular basis and use proper inhalation techniques
Manage your breathing	Use according to directives: • The pursed-lip breathing technique • The forward body positions • The coughing techniques
Conserve your energy	Prioritize your activities, plan your schedule, and pace yourself
Manage your stress and anxiety	Use your relaxation and breathing techniques, try to solve one problem at a time, talk about your problems, and do not hesitate to ask for help and maintain a positive attitude
Prevent and manage aggravations of your symptoms (exacerbations)	Get your flu shot every year and your vaccine for pneumonia Identify and avoid factors that can make your symptoms worse Use your Plan of Action according to the directives (recognition of symptoms deterioration and actions to perform) Contact your resource person when needed
Maintain an active life	Maintain physical activities (activities of daily living, walking, climbing stairs, etc) Exercise regularly (according to a prescribed home exercise program)
Keep a healthy diet	Maintain a healthy weight, eat food high in protein, and eat smaller meals more often (5–6 meals/day)
Have good sleep habits	Maintain a routine, avoid heavy meals and stimulants before bedtime, and relax before bedtime
Maintain a satisfying sex life	Use positions that require less energy Share your feelings with your partner Do not limit yourself to intercourse, create a romantic atmosphere Use your breathing, relaxation, and coughing techniques
Get involved in leisure activities	Choose leisure activities that you enjoy Choose environments where your symptoms will not be aggravated Pace yourself through the activities while using your breathing techniques Respect your strengths and limitations

Adapted from Bourbeau J, Nault D. Self-management strategies in chronic obstructive pulmonary disease. Clin Chest Med 2007;28(3):617–28; with permission.

Self-Efficacy Behaviors for Healthy Living

Few trials have reported on the direct effect of COPD CSM on measures of self-efficacy: whereas self-efficacy scores improved in one study,[36] another found no impact of COPD CSM on self-efficacy overall, although a post hoc analysis did find a reduction in COPD admissions and deaths in the subset of successful self-managers, who also had had lower baseline self-efficacy scores.[37] A qualitative analysis embedded in another RCT showed that 59% of the CSM patients felt more self-confident and more secure.[38] Self-efficacy is lower in patients with low compliance to a maintenance exercise program than in patients with high compliance to maintenance exercise,[29,30] a finding that concurs with health behavior theory.[39] Specific disease-related self-efficacy goals for healthy living are discussed in subsequent sections.

Physical activity

Lower levels of physical activity in COPD are linked to a vicious circle of exertional dyspnea causing avoidance of activity, resulting in deconditioning, thereby exacerbating exertional dyspnea and ultimately leading to a loss of self-confidence about the ability to perform activities of daily living.[40] Although COPD CSM differs somewhat from pulmonary rehabilitation in emphasis and approach, guiding patient behavior to increase regular physical activity is a core component of both.[25,41] Clinical trials of COPD CSM have mainly focused on exercise and physical capacity and not on physical activity.

Earlier trials that did not include a structured or supervised exercise program found no significant effect on exercise capacity.[5,42–46] An a posteriori qualitative study[38] of a small sample of patients who received CSM showed an increase in activities of daily living and regular exercise. Although the results of this qualitative study may have relevance, further quantitative studies are needed.

Health status, psychological well-being, and dyspnea

Several recent studies of COPD CSM have found significant and clinically meaningful improvements in health status, as measured by the St George's Respiratory Questionnaire (SGRQ)[47] or the Chronic Respiratory Questionnaire (CRQ).[31,48–51] Other studies have reported no overall difference in health status,[29,34,36,44,45,52–56] but several of them reported improvements in selected domains, including the symptom and impact subscales of the SGRQ,[33,37,42] and the fatigue and mastery components of the CRQ.[46] The 2007 Cochrane analysis found a statistically significant difference in overall SGRQ scores, but it did not achieve the accepted minimal clinically important difference (MCID).[5] The most recent Cochrane update found a pooled mean difference on the SGRQ total score of −3.71 in favor of CSM that approached the MCID of −4 points.[6]

Psychological components of well-being are strong determinants of health status. Studies of the effect of COPD CSM on anxiety and depression are mixed, whereas the impact on subjective dyspnea scales has been generally positive. A study that compared cognitive-behavioral therapy for depression/anxiety with self-efficacy behavior education in COPD patients found that both interventions sustainably improved depression and health status.[50] By contrast, 2 RCTs of CSM found no differences in anxiety or depression scores.[36,37]

By providing ongoing team support, promoting self-efficacy, and teaching breathing-related behavioral skills, CSM can help break the vicious cycle of dyspnea, inactivity, deconditioning, and resulting worsening dyspnea. The 2007 Cochrane analysis of CSM in COPD found significant improvements in dyspnea scores,[5] and 3 of the 4 RCTs since 2006 that reported dyspnea scores also reported improvement.[57–60]

Preventive behaviors

Advice and assistance on smoking cessation is a standard component of COPD CSM,[5] although the few studies that examined its effect on smoking status reported mixed results.[31,33,43,46] Vaccination for respiratory infection is also a component of COPD CSM, although information

is lacking about its efficacy of COPD CSM in increasing respiratory vaccination rates and health outcomes.[61–63] Good hand hygiene behavior, which reduces respiratory infections in patients at risk for influenza,[64] is also recommended in COPD CSM,[61] and was a core component in at least one successful trial.[51] Optimal nutrition is important for everyone's health, including those with COPD. An abnormally low body mass index is associated with increased mortality in patients with COPD,[65] and increased fruit intake in COPD patients is associated with decreased mortality.[66] A dietary intervention for patients with COPD improved exercise capacity in one study.[67] As a component of COPD CSM,[61] patients are encouraged to eat a healthy, balanced diet and are taught potentially beneficial eating techniques including multiple small meals, adequate fluid intake, and eating slowly. There is a dedicated diet module in the Canadian CSM Living Well with COPD[61] that has recently been developed by a team of dietitians. Despite the importance of this topic, information is lacking on the effect of COPD CSM on improving dietary habits.

Adherence to inhaled controller medications can maximize the number of "good days" for COPD patients by reducing dyspnea and by decreasing the frequency of exacerbations.[68,69] Studies that have measured the impact of COPD CSM on adherence to maintenance medications have generally been positive,[33,51,70] with the exceptions of 2 smaller trials.[46,71]

Change in Provider Behavior

The ultimate success in dealing with the current primary care crisis in providing chronic care hinges on establishing trust between providers and patients, developing team relationships, and promoting essential skills, including active listening and motivational interviewing.[72] However, there is a paucity of information about the effect of CSM on provider behavior. Successful implementation of the Chronic Care Model may provide a surrogate measure in this regard. The establishment of team-based medical homes has been shown to reduce physician burnout and improve patient experience ratings without increasing costs.[73] More specific insight about the effect on providers is provided by a study which found that health care workers who participated in COPD CSM developed a new sense of cooperation, and began to enjoy working with their patients.[58]

COPD CSM FOR THE "BAD DAYS"
Action Plans for AECOPD

AECOPD is a major negative determinant of health status: health status is worse in frequent exacerbators and contributes to the decline in pulmonary function.[74,75] Early recognition and treatment of AECOPD is associated with more rapid recovery, and failure to treat is associated with worse health status and increased emergency hospitalizations.[76] Reliance on traditional models of health care delivery to identify and treat AECOPD is suboptimal: half of all episodes go unreported to health care providers, and both reported and unreported exacerbations are associated with declines in health status.[77]

Most COPD CSM programs have included action plans for self-management of AECOPD, and adherence to written action plans for prompt treatment of AECOPD is associated with more rapid recovery times.[78] A retrospective study of a relatively small cohort of 89 patients found that action plans increased the use of prednisone and antibiotics without decreasing unplanned visits.[79] A systematic review of 5 RCTs that compared the provision of action plans for AECOPD (with minimal or no self-management education) versus usual care found that the former improved patients' ability to respond appropriately to COPD exacerbation symptoms but had no effect on health care utilization.[80] These results suggest that action plans should generally be used in the setting of a more comprehensive intervention, such as COPD CSM. Individually tailored action plans provide instructions on what the exacerbation is and what to do about it. This approach typically includes refillable prescriptions for antibiotics and short courses of oral corticosteroids to be initiated at onset of exacerbation symptoms, and emergency and follow-up information. Close follow-up, including regular communication with a case manager, is important. Action plans should also include instructions for patients to report exacerbations requiring prednisone or antibiotics to the CSM team, as well as any exacerbation not responding to action-plan medications. Patients must have a thorough understanding of the appropriate use of action plans so as to avoid delays or failure to initiate treatment, in addition to the potential dangers of excessive use of action plans, including adverse effects from frequent or prolonged systemic steroids, antibiotic resistance, and *Clostridium difficile* infections.[79] Another potential benefit of action plans may be to encourage patients to restrict oral corticosteroid exposure to short-term use only.[40] Patients must also learn how to recognize life-threatening symptoms that require prompt professional medical treatment. Even patients with a high burden of disease can achieve appropriate self-management behaviors in this setting, and this behavior may reduce health care utilization.[81]

In COPD, studies evaluating the effectiveness of action plans in exacerbation outcomes have had mixed results. In one study, adherence to action plans was strongly associated with a reduction in the number of days to total recovery from AECOPD.[36,52] Other studies reported that use of the action plan resulted in earlier identification and treatment of AECOPD.[44,70] However, a large Veterans Affairs (VA) Cooperative trial of CSM (centered on an action plan) versus usual care found no difference in self-reported exacerbations and no difference in the time from onset of symptoms to initiation of treatment.[36] Furthermore, although CSM patients were instructed to call the case manager in the event of an exacerbation, very few patients did indeed call. These data suggest that the CSM plan in this trial failed in its intent to provide timely care for patients with worsening symptoms of an exacerbation, and underlines the importance of following up and measuring the intended behavioral changes associated with COPD self-management.

Effect of CSM on Hospitalizations for AECOPD

Although hospitalizations for AECOPD are costly and burdensome to patients and society, there is a relative dearth of published information on CSM in this area.[82] One meta-analysis found that CSM decreased hospitalizations, but concluded that there was insufficient information about which components of CSM contribute the most benefit.[83] Although the most recent Cochrane review found reductions in respiratory-related hospital admissions over 12 months,[6] information is lacking on how to tailor this intervention to the heterogeneous population of patients with COPD; more specifically, it is not known why CSM reduces health care utilization in some patients and not in others.

COPD CSM RCTs that decreased hospitalizations

A relatively intense model of COPD CSM (education, 7–8 in-home sessions with nurses, respiratory therapists, or physiotherapists) in 191 patients previously hospitalized for AECOPD in Quebec, Canada, resulted in decreased respiratory-related hospitalizations (39.8%), and hospitalizations unrelated to COPD (57.1%).[42] A moderately intense COPD CSM intervention (tailored care plan including self-medication option, monthly nurse clinic visits, and general practice clinic visits every month for 1 year) in 135 outpatients in New Zealand with moderate to severe COPD decreased respiratory-related admissions, with an apparent reduction in all-cause admissions and a reduction in length of stay.[46] Another CSM study in Spain and Belgium (individually tailored care plans, a 2-hour education at discharge including strategies for future exacerbations, a home visit by a physician, nurse, and social worker, followed by telephone calls weekly for 1 month, 3 months, and 9 months) of 155 patients who were previously admitted for AECOPD resulted in a 45% reduction in hospitalizations.[43] The largest RCT to date (a single group session, customized action plans with refillable medication, and monthly phone contact with respiratory therapy disease managers) included 743 patients in the Midwest United States VA health care system at high risk for hospitalization for COPD.[51] Compared with usual care, CSM decreased respiratory-related hospitalizations by 30%, and all-cause hospitalizations or emergency department (ED) visits by 27%. Of note, cardiac and non-COPD hospitalizations also decreased by 32% in this study. One potential reason for this finding is that non-COPD cardiorespiratory admissions such as CHF are often preceded by pneumonia or another primary respiratory process.[84]

Other RCTs that have demonstrated reductions in hospitalizations include a study in 122 LTOT patients, which found that home-based visits every 3 months and monthly calls decreased hospital admissions by more than 50%[54]; a study of 50 patients in Germany with mild to very severe COPD that reported decreased hospitalizations[85]; a study of a relatively simplified model in 173 patients in Northern Ireland[33]; and an RCT of 85 patients in Japan of 6 months of tailored education with an action plan.[60] All the individual trials that have shown these benefits have in common a CSM intervention that included an AECOPD action plan embedded in an integrated health care system coordinated by a case manager, with regular communication (monthly visits or telephone calls) to reinforce patient empowerment.

COPD CSM RCTs that did not decrease hospitalizations

Several relatively large studies of COPD CSM have not demonstrated reductions in hospitalizations. One RCT of CSM (4 weekly group sessions for a total of 10 hours, a feedback session 3 months later, an action plan, a 2-year physical training program, and no scheduled follow-up calls or contacts) versus usual care in 248 outpatients with moderately severe COPD who were not otherwise at high risk for hospitalization[44] showed an apparent trend in decreased hospitalizations; however, in a subsequent economic analysis this was not considered cost-effective.[45] The VA Cooperative trial of CSM (the BREATH trial) (four 90-minute educational sessions, a group reinforcement session, action plans, and follow-up

phone calls once a month for 3 months, then every 3 months thereafter) versus usual care had to be prematurely discontinued for safety concerns (increased mortality in the treatment group) after enrollment of 426 patients out of an anticipated 960.[36] At the time of discontinuation, the investigators found no suggestion of a reduction in COPD-related hospitalizations or hospitalizations for any cause. In contrast to other studies, the intervention did not change patient behaviors related to AECOPD. The times between the onset of AECOPD symptoms and self-treatment did not differ between the groups (1 week), and the difference in the use of action-plan medications was much lower than that reported in the other VA study.[51] Finally, the Glasgow-supported self-management trial (GSuST) of 464 high-risk patients found no overall effect on hospitalizations, although a post hoc analysis found reduction in COPD hospitalizations and deaths in the 40% of patients who were successful self-managers.[37]

Why some RCTs may have been successful while others were not

Determining why some COPD CSM programs succeed while others fail is challenging, but of considerable importance. Possible reasons for negative studies include: (1) lack of statistical power, as many studies enrolled fewer than 200 patients[29,32,52,53,55,56,86]; (2) inclusion of patients who were not at high risk for hospitalization (ie, the ceiling effect)[34,44,52,53,55]; and (3) follow-up for less than 1 year.[32,49,53] In addition, failure to empower patients to appropriately manage AECOPDs by not providing an action plan with refillable home prescriptions[32,53,55,87] or insufficient ongoing communication to reinforce patients' empowerment to change behavior could explain negative results in some studies.[34,36]

The aforementioned large, apparently well-designed, but ultimately negative, VA and Glasgow trials merit further discussion.[36,37] Although both were based on a successful CSM model,[42] there may have been discrepancies between the intent of the CSM programs and their actual administration; that is, "the devil is in the details." Possible discrepancies might have been ensuring sufficient background and training for disease managers, or heterogeneity in the delivery of the educational content. The main focus may have been on education and not on promoting and supporting adaptive behaviors. Key messages about self-management might have been lost amid the complexity of the educational content, particularly among patients who were too recently ill to receive information and participate collaboratively. In addition, the educational content delivered might have made some patients overly confident about their ability to self-manage, and unable to recognize an urgent need for professional medical attention.

Mortality and safety concerns in COPD CSM

The benefits of COPD CSM must be carefully balanced against potential harms. Concerns about the safety of COPD CSM were recently raised when the BREATH study (see earlier discussion) had to be stopped prematurely because of increased all-cause and respiratory deaths in the CSM group in comparison with the usual care group (28 vs 10 deaths, $P = .003$).[36] In this study, the investigators made an extensive effort to collect and analyze complete information about the deaths, but could find no explanation for the excess mortality. Aside from the possibility of actual harm from COPD CSM, one potential explanation for the increased deaths is random chance, as discussed in the accompanying editorial.[88] Apparent, albeit small, imbalances in the distribution of baseline characteristics such as marital status, ethnicity, and cardiac comorbidities could conceivably have resulted in an imbalance in mortality.

Three meta-analyses of mortality from COPD CSM versus usual care are currently available.

Although the trials included in each analysis varied slightly, they all concluded that there was no statistically significant difference in mortality between groups, at both short-term and long-term follow-up,[6,89] and in patients who were enrolled after a COPD hospitalization and those who were not (**Table 3**). Despite these encouraging data, safety must never be underestimated. CSM programs should be properly adapted to respond to patient needs, taking into account disease severity and comorbidities. It may not be realistic or safe for some patients to make independent medical decisions without proper support and communication with a health care professional.

INTEGRATION OF COPD CSM AND PULMONARY REHABILITATION

Although studies with a primary focus on pulmonary rehabilitation were excluded from Cochrane reviews of COPD CSM, the integration of COPD CSM with pulmonary rehabilitation provides a natural, evidence-based health care delivery model for managing COPD patients of all degrees of severity. It allows the inclusion of patients with more severe disease, more comorbidities, inability to exercise, or limited ability to attend multiple

Table 3
All-cause mortality: randomized controlled trials for COPD CDM

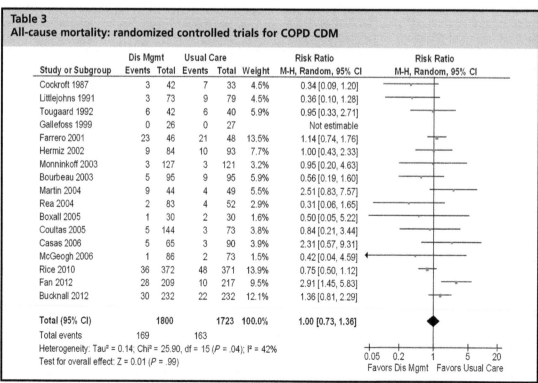

Study or Subgroup	Dis Mgmt Events	Total	Usual Care Events	Total	Weight	Risk Ratio M-H, Random, 95% CI
Cockroft 1987	3	42	7	33	4.5%	0.34 [0.09, 1.20]
Littlejohns 1991	3	73	9	79	4.5%	0.36 [0.10, 1.28]
Tougaard 1992	6	42	6	40	5.9%	0.95 [0.33, 2.71]
Gallefoss 1999	0	26	0	27		Not estimable
Farrero 2001	23	46	21	48	13.5%	1.14 [0.74, 1.76]
Hermiz 2002	9	84	10	93	7.7%	1.00 [0.43, 2.33]
Monninkoff 2003	3	127	3	121	3.2%	0.95 [0.20, 4.63]
Bourbeau 2003	5	95	9	95	5.9%	0.56 [0.19, 1.60]
Martin 2004	9	44	4	49	5.5%	2.51 [0.83, 7.57]
Rea 2004	2	83	4	52	2.9%	0.31 [0.06, 1.65]
Boxall 2005	1	30	2	30	1.6%	0.50 [0.05, 5.22]
Coultas 2005	5	144	3	73	3.8%	0.84 [0.21, 3.44]
Casas 2006	5	65	3	90	3.9%	2.31 [0.57, 9.31]
McGeogh 2006	1	86	2	73	1.5%	0.42 [0.04, 4.59]
Rice 2010	36	372	48	371	13.9%	0.75 [0.50, 1.12]
Fan 2012	28	209	10	217	9.5%	2.91 [1.45, 5.83]
Bucknall 2012	30	232	22	232	12.1%	1.36 [0.81, 2.29]
Total (95% CI)		1800		1723	100.0%	1.00 [0.73, 1.36]
Total events	169		163			

Heterogeneity: Tau² = 0.14; Chi² = 25.90, df = 15 (P = .04); I² = 42%
Test for overall effect: Z = 0.01 (P = .99)

Favors Dis Mgmt   Favors Usual Care

Courtesy of Roderick MacDonald, MS and Timothy Wilt, MD, Center for Chronic Disease Outcomes Research, Minneapolis Veterans Affairs Health Care System, Minneapolis, MN.

sessions.[41,81] Both COPD CSM and pulmonary rehabilitation share similar holistic and systematic approaches, and both can rapidly adapt their practices in the face of new evidence. Pulmonary rehabilitation, with its strong emphasis on formal exercise training, is the best intervention to improve exercise capacity, with a primary objective of relieving disability by decreasing dyspnea and improving the ability to perform activities of daily living.[90] However, improvements in exercise capacity do not automatically equate with increases in physical activity. In other words, pulmonary rehabilitation provides patients the "can do," whereas CSM provides patients the "will do." Pulmonary rehabilitation is too often restricted to an acute care time frame (6–12 weeks). Integrating pulmonary rehabilitation with ongoing CSM provides a longer-term, day-to-day approach to change and maintain behavior, including adherence to exercise programs and increases in day-to-day physical activity. In the most recent American Thoracic Society/European Respiratory Society Statement on Pulmonary Rehabilitation,[41] behavioral changes and CSM are emphasized as essential components of pulmonary rehabilitation: "Health behavior change is vital to optimization and maintenance of benefits from any intervention in chronic care, and pulmonary rehabilitation has taken a lead in implementing strategies to achieve this goal."

Several recent studies have successfully combined pulmonary rehabilitation with components of COPD CSM. A nurse-led study of home-based pulmonary rehabilitation combined with patient education in Turkey improved lung function, health status, dyspnea, and functional capacity.[91] An RCT of 4 months of multidisciplinary rehabilitation followed by 20 months of maintenance support with comprehensive COPD CSM education in the Netherlands improved health status and exercise capacity.[59] A study of personalized physical activity training, continuous self-management education including personal goal-setting, optimization of medications, action plans, and adherence monitoring in 2 towns in the Netherlands improved health status and dyspnea scores.[58] Another study of postpulmonary rehabilitation maintenance, education, and psychosocial support intervention embedded within a health care network in France improved health status and exercise capacity.[92] An RCT of home pulmonary rehabilitation, education, and promotion of healthy behaviors in Egypt improved exercise capacity and health status.[93] An RCT of pulmonary rehabilitation, self-management education, action plans, monthly telephone calls, and home visits in London reported improved self-management of AECOPD

and decreased mortality.[94] An RCT that combined hospital-based, supervised exercise sessions with self-management education in France improved the 6-minute walk distance by an average 50.5 m, improved health status, and decreased COPD medication costs.[95] A recent study with a rigorous process evaluation has demonstrated how CSM integrated into pulmonary rehabilitation can deliver high-quality, consistent, and equitable education sessions during hospital and community-based pulmonary rehabilitation.[96]

TRANSLATIONAL STUDIES OF COPD CSM

Although RCTs provide the strongest scientific evidence of the efficacy of an intervention such as COPD CSM, translational studies of comparative effectiveness provide real-world information for the betterment of health and cost-benefit analysis. A national audit in the United Kingdom of discharge programs for COPD embedded in the health care system found reductions in the length of stay in hospital without increases in mortality.[97] An analysis of a clinical cohort of COPD patients in Quebec, Canada found that participation in CSM was effective in reducing rehospitalization rates.[92] A pre-post evaluation of COPD CSM implementation in the Netherlands found improvements in self-care behaviors, adherence to medication, physical activity, and smoking cessation, and decreased hospitalization rates.[98] A large cohort of patients who participated in telephonic COPD CSM based in Denver, Colorado had decreased health care utilization and improved health status.[99] In Quebec, Canada, patients who returned to real-life clinical care for 2 years after ending their participation a CSM trial had sustained reductions in all-cause hospitalizations and ED visits.[42,100] The same group of investigators recently published another study of a cohort of patients with more severe COPD than patients in the original 2003 RCT.[81] In real-life practice, COPD CSM was effective in sustaining healthy self-management behavior and reducing health care utilization.

Costs

In addition to direct benefits to patient health, translating COPD CSM into practice has the potential to help control rising health care costs through reducing expensive health care utilization and promoting healthy behaviors. Reports of the impact of CSM in reducing medical expenditures are mixed. An early systematic review[101] and several other studies found no significant cost savings.[45,49,98,102] However, other trials have suggested that health service utilization and associated costs can be decreased.[54,86,103–106]

INTEGRATION OF COPD CSM INTO CLINICAL PRACTICE
Medical Home Model

The integration of COPD CSM into the patient-centered medical home (PCMH) model provides an opportunity to change the focus from a pessimistic, reactive, rescue approach to proactive, collaborative management. By teaching patients the behavioral skills required to implement disease-specific regimens, CSM can serve as a link between primary care and secondary care. Incorporating COPD CSM into the PCMH model can improve access to care, allow team members to practice at the "top of their license," establish continuity with other providers and community resources, and use health information technology to more efficiently manage care and assess quality improvement, risk-management performance, and resource utilization.[107]

Qualification and Training of COPD CSM Managers

The chronic disease manager is the linchpin of the CSM team, and the importance of his or her experience, training, and skills cannot be overemphasized.[81] CSM team members should have up-to-date training in cognitive-behavioral therapy (CBT) and motivational interviewing. CBT has proved to be effective in inducing behavioral change in patients with chronic respiratory disease such as COPD.[108] CBT offers relatively simple and structured techniques that can be incorporated by the members of a multidisciplinary team, for example in pulmonary rehabilitation. Successful implementation depends on interprofessional training and the development of team relationships and skills, such as active listening and motivational interviewing,[72] and adapting CSM to fit local health care delivery systems.[82]

The professional qualifications of successful COPD CSM managers vary according to the health care systems in which they are embedded. Successful trials have employed nurses,[42,109] respiratory therapists,[42,51] pharmacists,[110] and physiotherapists.[42] Employing lay community care guides as members of the CSM team is another recent innovation reported in a study of patients with the chronic metabolic syndrome.[111] As suggested in the accompanying editorial, the success of this strategy might be attributable to the concept that "knowing just the basics may have its advantages—what people don't know is less likely to distract them."[112]

The COPD CSM case manager should be a facilitator agent with skills in COPD content and CBT, and the ability to evaluate patients' learning outcomes, for example, patients' achievement of changes in behavior. The COPD CSM case manager should also be a resource person and, above all, he or she should have good communication skills and a nonjudgmental approach. Reference guides are available to help COPD CSM case managers implement programs (www.livingwell withcopd.com). However, studies are needed that better define the expertise and validate the training required by the COPD CSM managers.

Frequency and Intensity of Contacts

COPD CSM is founded on collaboration between patients and care team members, which, by definition, is ongoing. The amount of ongoing CSM contact has been correlated with positive outcomes.[51] Successful approaches have used 1-on-1 or group sessions, streamlined education and behavioral change sessions with follow-up telephone reinforcement,[33,51,58,59] or more numerous and comprehensive sessions.[42]

While effective CSM interventions do exist, the implementation rate of such interventions is lagging behind the increasing burden of chronic disease on an already strained health care system, with shortages in case managers who have the expertise to deliver such interventions. As a result, facets of communication, monitoring, reinforcement, and the intensity of the intervention for COPD CSM may vary among health care systems, although they ideally should be matched to patients' needs. Health information technology is another approach to provide effective, timely, and sustained patient support. Home tele-care presents an innovative tool for CSM that provides targeted "automated hovering."[113] An automated tele-care platform has been reported to help patients successfully identify AECOPDs.[57] Combining education with home tele-care can reduce ED visits and hospitalizations, improve health status, increase exercise capacity and BODE (Body mass index, airflow Obstruction, Dyspnea, Exercise capacity) index, and reduce smoking rates.[114] A recent Cochrane review of 10 RCTs of tele-care for COPD confirmed reductions in health care utilization, but noted that more research is needed to determine how this fits into more complex CSM delivery models.[115]

Patient Selection for COPD CSM

Uncertainty exists regarding which patients should be targeted for COPD CSM. To avoid a ceiling effect, many, but not all, successful COPD CSM interventions have focused on patients with advanced disease. A more proactive approach in patients who are less sick may be justified, however, if resources can be efficiently applied. Evidence for inclusion of patients with less severe COPD is suggested by the 2007 Cochrane review, which found reductions in hospitalizations in both low-risk and high-risk patients.[5] Whether to include or exclude patients with various comorbidities is also unclear. Patients with severe comorbidities, especially CHF,[43] have been excluded from some studies, presumably because of the difficulty in distinguishing the cause of symptoms. A recent study[36] suggests that CSM may increase mortality in patients with severe disease and cardiac comorbidities. Such patients, therefore, may not be good candidates for CSM that includes medical self-management.

Other studies, reflecting the real-world clinical setting, have not excluded these types of patients.[42,46,51] Targeting patients who are more likely to adopt successful behavioral change is also a consideration, as suggested by one study in which COPD admissions and deaths decreased in the subset of successful self-managers.[37] However, it is unclear how these patients might be identified in advance. Conversely, enrollment of patients with psychiatric disorders, a history of nonadherence, or other behavioral problems was actively encouraged in the Midwest VA study,[51] in reflection of real-world clinical needs.

THE CONTINUUM OF DISEASE: ADVANCE CARE PLANNING AND PALLIATIVE CARE

As COPD patients continue along the trajectory of their illness, strategies of care delivery must be adjusted to continue supporting the goal of providing the best possible quality of life, including relief of physical and psychological suffering. Achieving these goals requires coordination between primary care providers, the CSM team, and the palliative care team. COPD patients experience inadequacies in discussing details about the progression of illness, prognosis, and dying in traditional health care systems.[116] The inclusion of the palliative care team at earlier stages of any serious chronic illness not only addresses suffering but also assists patients in understanding the likely outcomes of their illness and in setting realistic goals.[117]

SUMMARY

Patients with COPD have complex medical, emotional, and social needs throughout the changing course of their disease. COPD CSM is based on the principle that guiding individual behavioral changes is the key to meeting these complex changing needs. Many models of

multicomponent, team-based COPD CSM have been shown to improve outcomes, such as health status and health care utilization, in rigorously designed RCTs. However, self-management may not suit all patients. Patient care and medical decisions may need to be assumed by health professionals at certain points in the disease trajectory that pose an unacceptable risk of mortality; that is, severe disease instability or comorbidities that interfere with decision-making capacity. Ideally, integrated systems of care such as CSM should adapt and adjust to these changing patient needs.

More importance must be lent to the training of the CSM team members in CBT and motivational interviewing. There is still a lot to learn, such as how to make sure that the CSM team members are qualified to properly guide the patients on their behavior-modification process; for example, helping them to set realistic goals and improve their motivation and self-efficacy. Furthermore, various evaluation methods need to be better defined and standardized so as to assess patients' readiness and progress at each intervention point. These issues will need to be incorporated into future trials, and adapted for use in clinical practice.

Larger, high-quality, longer-term studies using customized, well-described self-management interventions aimed at behavioral change are needed to evaluate real-world effectiveness, safety, and costs of integrating COPD CSM with pulmonary rehabilitation, the PCMH model, and palliative care teams. Finally, new technological communication interfaces are promising additions to the management of chronic diseases including COPD, and further studies that incorporate them with COPD CSM are needed.

ACKNOWLEDGMENTS

The authors would like to thank Louise Auclair and Esther Tomkee for their clerical work.

REFERENCES

1. Bourbeau J. Clinical decision processes and patient engagement in self-management. Dis Manag Health Outcome 2008;16(5):327–33.
2. Windham BG, Bennett RG, Gottlieb S. Care management interventions for older patients with congestive heart failure. Am J Manag Care 2003; 9(6):447–59.
3. Battersby M, Von KM, Schaefer J, et al. Twelve evidence-based principles for implementing self-management support in primary care. Jt Comm J Qual Patient Saf 2010;36(12):561–70.
4. Monninkhof E, van der Valk P, van der Palen J, et al. Self-management education for patients with

chronic obstructive pulmonary disease: a systematic review. Thorax 2003;58(5):394–8.

5. Effing T, Monninkhof E, van der Valk PD, et al. Self-management education for patients with chronic obstructive pulmonary disease. Cochrane Database Syst Rev 2007;(4):CD002990.

6. Kruis AL, Smidt N, Assendelft WJ, et al. Integrated disease management interventions for patients with chronic obstructive pulmonary disease. Cochrane Database Syst Rev 2013;(10):CD009437.

7. Schoen C, Osborn R, How SK, et al. In chronic condition: experiences of patients with complex health care needs, in eight countries, 2008. Health Aff (Millwood) 2009;28(1):w1–16.

8. Judson TJ, Detsky AS, Press MJ. Encouraging patients to ask questions: how to overcome "white-coat silence". JAMA 2013;309(22):2325–6.

9. Cooke CE, Sidel M, Belletti DA, et al. Review: clinical inertia in the management of chronic obstructive pulmonary disease. COPD 2012; 9(1):73–80.

10. Johnson DR, Nichol KL, Lipczynski K. Barriers to adult immunization. Am J Med 2008;121(7 Suppl 2):S28–35.

11. Melani AS, Canessa P, Coloretti I, et al. Inhaler mishandling is very common in patients with chronic airflow obstruction and long-term home nebuliser use. Respir Med 2012;106(5):668–76.

12. Mularski RA, Asch SM, Shrank WH, et al. The quality of obstructive lung disease care for adults in the United States as measured by adherence to recommended processes. Chest 2006;130(6):1844–50.

13. Rutschmann OT, Janssens JP, Vermeulen B, et al. Knowledge of guidelines for the management of COPD: a survey of primary care physicians. Respir Med 2004;98(10):932–7.

14. Solem CT, Lee TA, Joo MJ, et al. Complexity of medication use in newly diagnosed chronic obstructive pulmonary disease patients. Am J Geriatr Pharmacother 2012;10(2):110–22.

15. Johnston KN, Young M, Grimmer-Somers KA, et al. Why are some evidence-based care recommendations in chronic obstructive pulmonary disease better implemented than others? Perspectives of medical practitioners. Int J Chron Obstruct Pulmon Dis 2011;6:659–67.

16. Bourbeau J, Nault D. Self-management strategies in chronic obstructive pulmonary disease. Clin Chest Med 2007;28(3):617–28.

17. Wagner EH. Chronic disease management: what will it take to improve care for chronic illness? Eff Clin Pract 1998;1(1):2–4.

18. Green LW, Kreuter MW. Health promotion planning: an educational and environmental approach. 3rd edition. London: Mayfield Publishing Company; 1999.

19. McAlister FA, Lawson FM, Teo KK, et al. A systematic review of randomized trials of disease management programs in heart failure. Am J Med 2001;110(5):378–84.

20. Weintraub A, Gregory D, Patel AR, et al. A multicenter randomized controlled evaluation of automated home monitoring and telephonic disease management in patients recently hospitalized for congestive heart failure: the SPAN-CHF II trial. J Card Fail 2010;16(4):285–92.

21. Pimouguet C, Le GM, Thiebaut R, et al. Effectiveness of disease-management programs for improving diabetes care: a meta-analysis. CMAJ 2011;183(2):E115–27.

22. Kates N, Mach M. Chronic disease management for depression in primary care: a summary of the current literature and implications for practice. Can J Psychiatry 2007;52(2):77–85.

23. Lemmens KM, Nieboer AP, Huijsman R. A systematic review of integrated use of disease-management interventions in asthma and COPD. Respir Med 2009;103(5):670–91.

24. Adams SG, Smith PK, Allan PF, et al. Systematic review of the chronic care model in chronic obstructive pulmonary disease prevention and management. Arch Int Med 2007;167:551–61.

25. Nici L, Donner C, Wouters E, et al. American Thoracic Society/European Respiratory Society statement on pulmonary rehabilitation. Am J Respir Crit Care Med 2006;173(12):1390–413.

26. Lacasse Y, Lecours R, Pelletier C, et al. Randomised trial of ambulatory oxygen in oxygen-dependent COPD. Eur Respir J 2005;25(6):1032–8.

27. Stuart-Harris CH, Bishop JM, Clark TJ, et al. Long term domiciliary oxygen therapy in chronic hypoxic cor pulmonale complicating chronic bronchitis and emphysema: report of the Medical Research Council Working Party. Lancet 1981; 1(8222):681–6.

28. Huang L. Krames on-demand (KOD). J Med Libr Assoc 2006;94(2):234–5.

29. Cockcroft A, Bagnall P, Heslop A, et al. Controlled trial of respiratory health worker visiting patients with chronic respiratory disability. Br Med J (Clin Res Ed) 1987;294(6566):225–8.

30. Hill K, Mangovski-Alzamora S, Blouin M, et al. Disease-specific education in the primary care setting increases the knowledge of people with chronic obstructive pulmonary disease: a randomized controlled trial. Patient Educ Couns 2010; 81(1):14–8.

31. Efraimsson EO, Hillervik C, Ehrenberg A. Effects of COPD self-care management education at a nurse-led primary health care clinic. Scand J Caring Sci 2008;22(2):178–85.

32. Hermiz O, Comino E, Marks G, et al. Randomised controlled trial of home based care of patients with chronic obstructive pulmonary disease. BMJ 2002;325(7370):938–42.

33. Khdour MR, Kidney JC, Smyth BM, et al. Clinical pharmacy-led disease and medicine management programme for patients with COPD. Br J Clin Pharmacol 2009;68(4):588–98.

34. McGeoch GR, Willsman KJ, Dowson CA, et al. Self-management plans in the primary care of patients with chronic obstructive pulmonary disease. Respirology 2006;11(5):611–8.

35. Sashima S, Takahashi I, Nakazawa K. Identification and characterization of beta-D-galactosyl-transferase in chick corneas. Jpn J Ophthalmol 2002;46(6):607–15.

36. Fan VS, Gaziano JM, Lew R, et al. A comprehensive care management program to prevent chronic obstructive pulmonary disease hospitalizations: a randomized, controlled trial. Ann Intern Med 2012;156(10):673–83.

37. Bucknall CE, Miller G, Lloyd SM, et al. Glasgow supported self-management trial (GSuST) for patients with moderate to severe COPD: randomised controlled trial. BMJ 2012;344:e1060.

38. Bourbeau J, Nault D, Dang-Tan T. Self-management and behaviour modification in COPD. Patient Educ Couns 2004;52(3):271–7.

39. Bandura A. Social cognitive theory: an agentic perspective. Annu Rev Psychol 2001;52:1–26.

40. Tiep B. Disease management of COPD with pulmonary rehabilitation. Chest 1997;112(6):1630–56.

41. Spruit MA, Singh SJ, Garvey C, et al. An official American Thoracic Society/European Respiratory Society statement: key concepts and advances in pulmonary rehabilitation. Am J Respir Crit Care Med 2013;188(8):e13–64.

42. Bourbeau J, Julien M, Maltais F, et al. Reduction of hospital utilization in patients with chronic obstructive pulmonary disease: a disease-specific self-management intervention. Arch Intern Med 2003;163(5):585–91.

43. Casas A, Troosters T, Garcia-Aymerich J, et al. Integrated care prevents hospitalisations for exacerbations in COPD patients. Eur Respir J 2006;28(1):123–30.

44. Monninkhof E, van der Valk P, van der Palen J, et al. Effects of a comprehensive self-management programme in patients with chronic obstructive pulmonary disease. Eur Respir J 2003;22(5):815–20.

45. Monninkhof E, van der Valk P, Schermer T, et al. Economic evaluation of a comprehensive self-management programme in patients with moderate to severe chronic obstructive pulmonary disease. Chron Respir Dis 2004;1(1):7–16.

46. Rea H, McAuley S, Stewart A, et al. A chronic disease management programme can reduce days in hospital for patients with chronic obstructive pulmonary disease. Intern Med J 2004;34(11):608–14.

47. Jones PW, Quirk FH, Baveystock CM, et al. A self-complete measure of health status for chronic airflow limitation. The St. George's Respiratory Questionnaire. Am Rev Respir Dis 1992;145(6):1321–7.

48. Guyatt GH, Berman LB, Townsend M, et al. A measure of quality of life for clinical trials in chronic lung disease. Thorax 1987;42(10):773–8.

49. Koff PB, Jones RH, Cashman JM, et al. Proactive integrated care improves quality of life in patients with COPD. Eur Respir J 2009;33(5):1031–8.

50. Kunik ME, Veazey C, Cully JA, et al. COPD education and cognitive behavioral therapy group treatment for clinically significant symptoms of depression and anxiety in COPD patients: a randomized controlled trial. Psychol Med 2008;38(3):385–96.

51. Rice KL, Dewan N, Bloomfield HE, et al. Disease management program for chronic obstructive pulmonary disease: a randomized controlled trial. Am J Respir Crit Care Med 2010;182(7):890–6.

52. Bischoff EW, Akkermans R, Bourbeau J, et al. Comprehensive self management and routine monitoring in chronic obstructive pulmonary disease patients in general practice: randomised controlled trial. BMJ 2012;345:e7642.

53. Coultas D, Frederick J, Barnett B, et al. A randomized trial of two types of nurse-assisted home care for patients with COPD. Chest 2005;128(4):2017–24.

54. Farrero E, Escarrabill J, Prats E, et al. Impact of a hospital-based home-care program on the management of COPD patients receiving long-term oxygen therapy. Chest 2001;119(2):364–9.

55. Littlejohns P, Baveystock C, Parnell H, et al. Randomised controlled trial of the effectiveness of a respiratory health worker in reducing impairment, disability, and handicap due to chronic airflow limitation. Thorax 1991;46(8):559–64.

56. Martin IR, McNamara D, Sutherland FR, et al. Care plans for acutely deteriorating COPD: a randomized controlled trial. Chron Respir Dis 2004;1(4):191–5.

57. Bischoff EW, Boer LM, Molema J, et al. Validity of an automated telephonic system to assess COPD exacerbation rates. Eur Respir J 2012;39:1090–6.

58. Chavannes NH, Schermer TR, Wouters EF, et al. Predictive value and utility of oral steroid testing for treatment of COPD in primary care: the COOPT study. Int J Chron Obstruct Pulmon Dis 2009;4:431–6.

59. van Wetering CR, Hoogendoorn M, Mol SJ, et al. Short- and long-term efficacy of a community-based COPD management programme in less advanced COPD: a randomised controlled trial. Thorax 2010;65(1):7–13.

60. Wakabayashi R, Motegi T, Yamada K, et al. Efficient integrated education for older patients with chronic obstructive pulmonary disease using the Lung

Information Needs Questionnaire. Geriatr Gerontol Int 2011;11(4):422–30.

61. Living well with COPD. Available at: http://living wellwithcopd.com. 2013. Accessed March 17, 2014.

62. Nichol KL, Baken L, Nelson A. Relation between influenza vaccination and outpatient visits, hospitalization, and mortality in elderly persons with chronic lung disease. Ann Intern Med 1999; 130(5):397–403.

63. Nichol KL, Nordin JD, Nelson DB, et al. Effectiveness of influenza vaccine in the community-dwelling elderly. N Engl J Med 2007;357(14):1373–81.

64. Godoy P, Castilla J, Gado-Rodriguez M, et al. Effectiveness of hand hygiene and provision of information in preventing influenza cases requiring hospitalization. Prev Med 2012;54(6):434–9.

65. Landbo C, Prescott E, Lange P, et al. Prognostic value of nutritional status in chronic obstructive pulmonary disease. Am J Respir Crit Care Med 1999; 160(6):1856–61.

66. Walda IC, Tabak C, Smit HA, et al. Diet and 20-year chronic obstructive pulmonary disease mortality in middle-aged men from three European countries. Eur J Clin Nutr 2002;56(7):638–43.

67. Slinde F, Gronberg AM, Engstrom CR, et al. Individual dietary intervention in patients with COPD during multidisciplinary rehabilitation. Respir Med 2002;96(5):330–6.

68. Calverley PM, Anderson JA, Celli B, et al. Salmeterol and fluticasone propionate and survival in chronic obstructive pulmonary disease. N Engl J Med 2007;356(8):775–89.

69. Tashkin DP, Celli B, Senn S, et al. A 4-year trial of tiotropium in chronic obstructive pulmonary disease. N Engl J Med 2008;359(15):1543–54.

70. Garcia-Aymerich J, Hernandez C, Alonso A, et al. Effects of an integrated care intervention on risk factors of COPD readmission. Respir Med 2007; 101(7):1462–9.

71. Gallefoss F, Bakke PS. How does patient education and self-management among asthmatics and patients with chronic obstructive pulmonary disease affect medication? Am J Respir Crit Care Med 1999;160(6):2000–5.

72. Frolkis JP. A piece of my mind. The Columbo phenomenon. JAMA 2013;309(22):2333–4.

73. Reid RJ, Fishman PA, Yu O, et al. Patient-centered medical home demonstration: a prospective, quasi-experimental, before and after evaluation. Am J Manag Care 2009;15(9):e71–87.

74. Donaldson GC, Seemungal TA, Bhowmik A, et al. Relationship between exacerbation frequency and lung function decline in chronic obstructive pulmonary disease. Thorax 2002;57(10):847–52.

75. Seemungal TA, Donaldson GC, Paul EA, et al. Effect of exacerbation on quality of life in patients with chronic obstructive pulmonary disease. Am J Respir Crit Care Med 1998;157(5 Pt 1):1418–22.

76. Wilkinson TM, Donaldson GC, Hurst JR, et al. Early therapy improves outcomes of exacerbations of chronic obstructive pulmonary disease. Am J Respir Crit Care Med 2004;169(12):1298–303.

77. Langsetmo L, Platt RW, Ernst P, et al. Underreporting exacerbation of chronic obstructive pulmonary disease in a longitudinal cohort. Am J Respir Crit Care Med 2008;177(4):396–401.

78. Bischoff EW, Hamd DH, Sedeno M, et al. Effects of written action plan adherence on COPD exacerbation recovery. Thorax 2011;66(1):26–31.

79. Beaulieu-Genest L, Chretien D, Maltais F, et al. Self-administered prescriptions of oral steroids and antibiotics in chronic obstructive pulmonary disease: are we doing more harm than good? Chron Respir Dis 2007;4(3):143–7.

80. Walters JA, Turnock AC, Walters EH, et al. Action plans with limited patient education only for exacerbations of chronic obstructive pulmonary disease. Cochrane Database Syst Rev 2010;(5):CD005074.

81. Bourbeau J, Saad N, Joubert A, et al. Making collaborative self-management successful in COPD patients with high disease burden. Respir Med 2013;107(7):1061–5.

82. Burke RE, Coleman EA. Interventions to decrease hospital readmissions: keys for cost-effectiveness. JAMA Intern Med 2013;173(8):695–8.

83. Peytremann-Bridevaux I, Staeger P, Bridevaux PO, et al. Effectiveness of chronic obstructive pulmonary disease-management programs: systematic review and meta-analysis. Am J Med 2008; 121(5):433–43.

84. Fonarow GC, Abraham WT, Albert NM, et al. Factors identified as precipitating hospital admissions for heart failure and clinical outcomes: findings from OPTIMIZE-HF. Arch Intern Med 2008;168(8): 847–54.

85. Bosch D, Feierabend M, Becker A. COPD outpatient education programme (ATEM) and BODE index. Pneumologie 2007;61(10):629–35 [in German].

86. Chuang C, Levine SH, Rich J. Enhancing cost-effective care with a patient-centric chronic obstructive pulmonary disease program. Popul Health Manag 2011;14(3):133–6.

87. Cockburn J, Gibberd RW, Reid AL, et al. Determinants of non-compliance with short term antibiotic regimens. Br Med J (Clin Res Ed) 1987; 295(6602):814–8.

88. Pocock SJ. Ethical dilemmas and malfunctions in clinical trials research. Ann Intern Med 2012; 156(10):746–7.

89. Hurley J, Gerkin RD, Fahy B, et al. Meta-analysis of self-management education for patients with chronic obstructive pulmonary disease. Southwest J Pulm Crit Care 2012;4:194–202.

90. Puhan MA, Gimeno-Santos E, Scharplatz M, et al. Pulmonary rehabilitation following exacerbations of chronic obstructive pulmonary disease. Cochrane Database Syst Rev 2011;(10):CD005305.

91. Akinci AC, Olgun N. The effectiveness of nurse-led, home-based pulmonary rehabilitation in patients with COPD in Turkey. Rehabil Nurs 2011;36(4): 159–65.

92. Moullec G, Lavoie KL, Rabhi K, et al. Effect of an integrated care programme on re-hospitalization of patients with chronic obstructive pulmonary disease. Respirology 2012;17(4):707–14.

93. Ghanem M, Elaal EA, Mehany M, et al. Home-based pulmonary rehabilitation program: effect on exercise tolerance and quality of life in chronic obstructive pulmonary disease patients. Ann Thorac Med 2010;5(1):18–25.

94. Sridhar M, Taylor R, Dawson S, et al. A nurse led intermediate care package in patients who have been hospitalised with an acute exacerbation of chronic obstructive pulmonary disease. Thorax 2008;63(3):194–200.

95. Ninot G, Moullec G, Picot MC, et al. Cost-saving effect of supervised exercise associated to COPD self-management education program. Respir Med 2011;105(3):377–85.

96. Cosgrove D, Macmahon J, Bourbeau J, et al. Facilitating education in pulmonary rehabilitation using the living well with COPD programme for pulmonary rehabilitation: a process evaluation. BMC Pulm Med 2013;13:50.

97. Kastelik JA, Lowe D, Stone RA, et al. National audit of supported discharge programmes for management of acute exacerbations of chronic obstructive pulmonary disease 2008. Thorax 2012;67(4):371–3.

98. Steuten L, Vrijhoef B, van Merode F, et al. Evaluation of a regional disease management programme for patients with asthma or chronic obstructive pulmonary disease. Int J Qual Health Care 2006;18(6): 429–36.

99. Tinkelman D, Corsello P, McClure D, et al. One-year outcomes from a disease management program for chronic obstructive pulmonary disease. Dis Manag Health Outcome 2003;11:49–59.

100. Gadoury MA, Schwartzman K, Rouleau M, et al. Self-management reduces both short- and long-term hospitalisation in COPD. Eur Respir J 2005; 26(5):853–7.

101. Ofman JJ, Badamgarav E, Henning JM, et al. Does disease management improve clinical and economic outcomes in patients with chronic diseases? A systematic review. Am J Med 2004;117(3):182–92.

102. Dewan N, Rice K, Caldwell M, et al. Economic evaluation for a disease management program for chronic obstructive pulmonary disease. COPD 2011;8(3):153–9.

103. Gallefoss F, Bakke P. Patient satisfaction with healthcare in asthmatics and patients with COPD before and after patient education. Respir Med 2000;94(11):1057–64.

104. Tougaard L, Krone T, Sorknaes A, et al. Economic benefits of teaching patients with chronic obstructive pulmonary disease about their illness. The PASTMA Group. Lancet 1992;339(8808):1517–20.

105. Zajac B. Measuring outcomes of a chronic obstructive pulmonary disease management program. Dis Manag 2002;5(1):9–23.

106. Bourbeau J, Collet JP, Schwartzman K, et al. Economic benefits of self-management education in COPD. Chest 2006;130:1704–11.

107. Ortiz G, Fromer L. Patient-Centered Medical Home in chronic obstructive pulmonary disease. J Multidiscip Healthc 2011;4:357–65.

108. Fritzsche A, Clamor A, von Leupoldt A. Effects of medical and psychological treatment of depression in patients with COPD—a review. Respir Med 2011;105(10):1422–33.

109. Taylor SJ, Candy B, Bryar RM, et al. Effectiveness of innovations in nurse led chronic disease management for patients with chronic obstructive pulmonary disease: systematic review of evidence. BMJ 2005;331(7515):485–8.

110. Gourley G, Portner T, Gourley D, et al. Humanistic outcomes in the hypertension and COPD arms of a multicenter outcomes study. J Am Pharm Assoc (Wash) 1998;38(5):586–97.

111. Adair R, Wholey DR, Christianson J, et al. Improving chronic disease care by adding laypersons to the primary care team: a parallel randomized trial. Ann Intern Med 2013;159(3):176–84.

112. Santa J, Lipman MM. Knowledge and ignorance in the care of chronic disease. Ann Intern Med 2013; 159(3):225–6.

113. Asch DA, Muller RW, Volpp KG. Automated hovering in health care—watching over the 5000 hours. N Engl J Med 2012;367(1):1–3.

114. Linderman DJ, Koff PB, Freitag TJ, et al. Effect of integrated care on advanced chronic obstructive pulmonary disease in high-mortality rural areas. Arch Intern Med 2011;171(22):2059–61.

115. McClean S, Nurmatov U, Liu JL, et al. Telehealthcare for chronic obstructive pulmonary disease [review]. Cochrane Database Syst Rev 2011;(7). CD007718. Available at: http://onlinelibrary.wiley.com/doi/10. 1002/14651858.CD007718.pub2/pdf.

116. Au DH, Udris EM, Engelberg RA, et al. A randomized trial to improve communication about end-of-life care among patients with COPD. Chest 2012; 141(3):726–35.

117. Strand JJ, Kamdar MM, Carey EC. Top 10 things palliative care clinicians wished everyone knew about palliative care. Mayo Clin Proc 2013;88(8): 859–65.

Approaches to Outcome Assessment in Pulmonary Rehabilitation

Sally Singh, FCSP, PhD

KEYWORDS

- Pulmonary rehabilitation • Assessment • Outcomes

KEY POINTS

- A thorough, patient-centered outcome assessment is considered a necessary component of a successful pulmonary rehabilitation program.
- All tests should follow recommended procedures, including standard operating procedures for exercise testing.
- The assessments, which vary widely across centers, usually include measures of exercise performance, peripheral muscle strength, health-related quality of life, and anxiety and depression. Other aspects of outcome assessment that may be measured include functional performance, physical activity, and knowledge/self-efficacy.

INTRODUCTION

The patient-centered outcome assessment, performed before and after rehabilitation, plays an important role in delivering a successful pulmonary rehabilitation program. This assessment is conducted by a health care professional who is mindful of the complex nature of chronic obstructive pulmonary disease (COPD) and the physical and psychological comorbidities frequently associated with chronic respiratory diseases, who has experience in managing such patients, and who has experience in exercise testing. The recent American Thoracic Society/European Respiratory Society statement on pulmonary rehabilitation[1] clearly articulates the importance of the assessment.

Pulmonary rehabilitation is a comprehensive intervention based on a thorough patient assessment followed by patient-tailored therapies which include, but are not limited to, exercise training, education and behavior change, designed to improve the physical and emotional condition of people with chronic respiratory disease and to promote the long-term adherence to health-enhancing behaviors.

This article addresses several components of the assessment. There is an assumption that the individual has been screened by the referring physician and the medical director of the pulmonary rehabilitation program and deemed safe to participate in an exercise-based rehabilitation program. The construction of the assessment has not been formally cataloged, but common outcomes are exercise capacity, health-related quality of life, functional status, and anxiety and depression. There are additional outcomes that are reported with increasing frequency, such as quadriceps strength, COPD-related knowledge and self-efficacy, and physical activity.

The assessment may be completed by a single individual with expertise in the field or by an interdisciplinary team; members of the team are responsible for the components of the assessment when they have expert knowledge. There is undeniably a scientific basis to the components of the

Centre for Exercise and Rehabilitation Science, University Hospitals of Leicester NHS Trust, Groby Road, Leicester LE3 9QP, UK
E-mail address: Sally.singh@uhl-tr.nhs.uk

Clin Chest Med 35 (2014) 353–361
http://dx.doi.org/10.1016/j.ccm.2014.02.010

assessment, but personal interactions among the patients and testers that occur during the assessment may influence the assessment. Examples of this potential bias include the indirect assessment of an individual's level of motivation to participate, the discussion of barriers to rehabilitation, and the appropriate negotiation of patient-related goals to encourage engagement and active participation in rehabilitation process. Pulmonary rehabilitation has been described most widely in patients with COPD, but there is an increasing evidence base for the delivery of rehabilitation to respiratory disease other than COPD; however, the fundamental characteristics of the assessment persist.

There have been numerous studies defining the properties of the measures described later, particularly in relation to exercise tests and measures of health-related quality of life.[2,3] One important property of these outcome measures is their sensitivity to detect change after pulmonary rehabilitation. More recently, the change in outcome measure after rehabilitation is compared with published data describing the minimum clinically important difference (MCID). The MCID has been defined as the smallest difference, in either direction, that is detectable by the patient or clinician. The MCID is usually dictated by the approach taken, using a patient preference or a statistical technique.

The timing of the outcome measures largely reflects the duration of the pulmonary rehabilitation program, because few studies report interim measures.[4,5] One advantage of incorporating interim measures is that it allows for an understanding of the trajectory of the particular outcome over the course of the intervention: the dose-response curve to rehabilitation may be different for different outcome measures and different modes of delivery. Measures are often also collected after the participant has graduated from the program to understand the longevity of the response and develop strategies to enhance and maintain the benefits associated with the intervention.

PATIENT OUTCOME ASSESSMENTS FOR PULMONARY REHABILITATION
Exercise Capacity

The assessment of exercise capacity is one of the 2 most commonly reported outcome measures for pulmonary rehabilitation, alongside measures of health status.

Field walking tests are the tests of choice for most rehabilitation programs; they require little equipment and are relatively straightforward to perform for both the operator and participant. Not surprisingly, walking is a highly desired activity

by patients with COPD[6] and is therefore a clinically relevant outcome to measure in these individuals. In more sophisticated centers, cardiopulmonary exercise tests may be performed as part of the outcome assessment. The decision to incorporate this technically sophisticated test often depends on the expertise, philosophy, and available resources of the particular rehabilitation center.

In the context of pulmonary rehabilitation, the exercise test has several important functions. The referring physician should confirm that the individual referred has no significant contraindications to performing an exercise program and therefore an exercise test. The American College of Sports Medicine[7] has an exhaustive list of relative and absolute contraindications that should be considered if there are any concerns over the patient's well-being (**Box 1**).

The most established exercise test in pulmonary rehabilitation is the 6-minute walking test (6MWT). The test simply requires an individual to cover as much ground as possible over 6 minutes, being allowed to stop and rest if required.[8] The course should be 30 m long, unobstructed, and instructions and encouragement should be standardized. The test does require a practice walk to overcome any learning effect. Not performing a practice test may add a significant bias, because often, the learning effect from test 1 to test 2 is substantial. The 6MWT has been widely reported in rehabilitation studies in COPD[5–10] and other chronic respiratory diseases such as interstitial lung disease.[11] Its MCID was originally estimated to be 54 m (95% confidence interval 37–71 m),[12] but more recently, lower values have been described, using slightly different approaches from the original work.[13] Generally, the change in 6MWT distance achieved with rehabilitation is around 50 m,[14] which reflects a clinically meaningful improvement.

Box 1
Commonly cited reasons for conducting an exercise test

1. Creating an outcome measure to identify a response to therapy (ie, pulmonary rehabilitation)

2. Creating a threshold to identify suitability for further interventions (eg, surgery)

3. Identifying the reasons for exercise intolerance

4. Defining the level of disability

5. Understanding the limitation to exercise

6. Developing a prescription for an exercise training regimen

The 6MWT is included in the BODE index, which is a multidimensional grading system that includes measures of nutritional status (body mass index [BMI], calculated as weight in kilograms divided by the square of height in meters), airway obstruction (FEV_1 [forced expiratory volume in first second of expiration]), dyspnea (Modified Medical Research Council [MRC] Scale), and exercise capacity (6MWT)[15] and has been used as a marker of prognosis in COPD. The BODE index was originally created to be a better predictor of certain outcomes, such as mortality, but has also been used as a before-after outcome assessments for interventions such as pulmonary rehabilitation. It is suggested that a 1-point change in the BODE index relates to an important reduction in mortality risk. For the BODE, data from the 6MWT are divided into quartiles and each carries a different weighting. Although the BODE index is reported as an outcome for rehabilitation,[16] this has not extended to rehabilitation positively influencing survival.

Reference values for the 6MWT in healthy age-matched adults have been reported; however, they seem to vary considerably among analyses[17-19] and should be viewed with caution. It is advisable to seek values that are geographically and age appropriate. The data from the 6MWT should be reported as absolute values (meters), and percentages of normal reference values can be included. If the latter are included, the source data must be clearly identified.

An alternative to the self-paced, 6MWT is the incremental shuttle walking test (ISWT). The ISWT is an externally paced exercise test that offers an incremental protocol stressing the patient to a symptom-limited maximum performance.[20] The test is conducted around a 10-m course, identified by 2 markers placed 0.5 m from each end, presenting an elliptical course. The test has potentially 12 levels, starting at a very slow speed of walking, with 20 seconds to complete each 10-m length, increasing gradually at the end of every minute, to a speed corresponding to 8.53 km/h. The test is terminated by the patient because of intolerable symptoms or by the operator if the patient fails to reach the marker in the time allowed. The ISWT seems to be appropriate across a range of disease severities, from those with very severe disease through to those with mild disease,[21] and there are several reports of what might be an expected healthy reference value.[22-24] It is responsive to rehabilitation in COPD[25,26] and other chronic respiratory disease.[27] The MCID has been described as 47.5 m, which, in practice, is 5 shuttles (50 m).[28] Most studies of pulmonary rehabilitation that have used the ISWT have achieved this level of improvement. The ISWT has been substituted in the BODE score (the i-BODE score), and this new measure seems to retain the same properties and the old one.[29]

The endurance shuttle walking test (ESWT) can be considered a companion test to the ISWT. Like all endurance exercise tests, it cannot be performed in isolation, and a maximal test must have been performed previously.[30] The endurance test is conducted around an identical course to the ISWT, but, unlike the ISWT, the ESWT protocol uses a fixed pace. Therefore, the ESWT can be considered a constant work rate test. There are 16 predefined speeds available, with the appropriate speed selected based on performance on the ISWT. Most commonly, the ESWT is set in the range of 70% to 85% of the maximum performance. The original study describing the properties of the ESWT suggested that a practice walk was required; this would make the initial assessment require a total of 4 walks. However, if the test is to be used in the context of pulmonary rehabilitation, it seems that patients become accustomed to the externally paced protocols, and if the patient has already completed 2 ISWTs, 1 ESWT may be sufficient.[31] The ESWT has not been reported as frequently as the ISWT in rehabilitation studies, but the magnitude of change seems much greater, with improvements generally in the range of 150% to 180%. The MCID for the ESWT has also been investigated. One study[32] compared the MCID for bronchodilator treatment and pulmonary rehabilitation, and the investigators identified 2 different levels of change, which appeared to be context specific. The MCID after a short treatment with the bronchodilator was around 65 seconds, whereas after a 7-week course of rehabilitation, it was around 180 seconds.

Laboratory-based exercise tests are sometimes reported as outcome measures for rehabilitation, and, on occasion, used just at baseline to collect complex physiologic and metabolic data. Laboratory-based tests are often stationary cycle-based cardiopulmonary exercise tests, usually because the treadmill equipment requires a large amount of space and is a less stable platform to take complex physiologic measures. Nevertheless, treadmill-based exercise performance has been reported as an outcome.[33] The cycle test can be either a maximal or an endurance evaluation. An MCID has been reported for a maximal stationary cycle-based test of 4 W,[34] whereas the MCID for a cycle endurance-based test is in the region of 100 seconds.[35] The cycle endurance test is also likely to be more responsive when the training has been cycle based. This observation was apparent in a recent home-based rehabilitation study, in which patients were provided with a cycle ergometer to complete bouts of unsupervised training.[36]

Cardiopulmonary exercise tests tend to be confined to research centers. As an outcome measure, an increase in cardiorespiratory fitness (an increase in peak oxygen consumption) for a maximal test and increased endurance time might be expected. Care needs to be taken interpreting peak data from endurance tests, over and above the duration of the test. It is important to consider the physiologic and symptom reported data at isotime; otherwise, the gain made in important variables may be overlooked. For instance, a prerehabilitation to postrehabilitation reduction in minute ventilation or lactate production at identical times during cycle ergometry (ie, isotime) suggests a physiologic training effect from the intervention. This important observation may be missed by simply looking at changes in endurance time. The data from rehabilitation programs reporting laboratory-based tests are variable,[37–39] but endurance studies often show considerable improvement.

There have been, and will continue to be, variations on the commonly used exercise tests as alternative exercise outcome measures for rehabilitation, for example, the 4-m gait speed.[40] The usefulness of these tests needs further work to understand how they might be applied in rehabilitation in either the selection or assessment of patients.

The choice of exercise test for pulmonary rehabilitation is dictated by facilities, equipment, and staff skills and availability. In addition, it is important to consider the type of training regimen offered within the program. To maximize the measurable impact of the program, the test should ideally match the characteristics of the training regimen. For example, it is likely that a cycle-based training regimen shows greater benefit using a cycle-based exercise test compared with a walking-based test.[41] Overall, endurance tests, either walking or cycling, tend to be more responsive to rehabilitation than incremental exercise tests (**Box 2**).

Box 2
Commonly used exercise tests in pulmonary rehabilitation

- 6MWT
- ISWT
- ESWT
- Cycle endurance test

Strength

Declining peripheral muscle strength, particularly of the lower limbs (eg, quadriceps), is a significant manifestation of COPD and is associated with increased mortality risk.[42] Therefore, resistance training is an important component of pulmonary rehabilitation exercise training. One recommendation is to train at a level corresponding to 60% to 70% of maximum of a 1-repetition maximum test. These tests can be challenging to conduct, and an alternative approach may be to measure strength, although these measurements do require some equipment. Handheld dynamometers are readily available, or more sophisticated centers can secure measures of peripheral muscle function using isokinetic dynamometers. Given that strength training is a core component of pulmonary rehabilitation, baseline and change measures should be reported.

Health-Related Quality of Life

Although an individual's overall quality of life is obviously influenced by nonmedical as well as medical factors, the concept of health-related quality of life is confined only to health-related aspects. Health-related instruments can be generic or disease specific. For pulmonary rehabilitation, disease-specific questionnaires are generally the outcome of choice. Studies have used more generic questionnaires that examine a broader overall satisfaction with health, for example the Short-Form 36, with some success,[43] but it is increasingly common to use disease-specific questionnaires. These disease-specific questionnaires cover aspects that are of importance to those with chronic respiratory disease, such as symptoms (physical and emotional), functional limitations, and overall quality of life. Disease-specific questionnaires tend to be more sensitive to change after a course of rehabilitation compared with generic questionnaires.

The Chronic Respiratory Disease Questionnaire (CRQ)[44] and the St George's Respiratory Questionnaire (SGRQ)[3] are the most well-used disease-specific questionnaires for COPD. The CRQ has domains of dyspnea (5 questions), emotional function (7 questions), fatigue (4 questions), and mastery (4 questions); it is available as an operator-administered questionnaire,[44] taking approximately 30 minutes to complete, and as a self-reported version.[45] Each of its 20 questions is scored on a 1 to 7 scale. Both are responsive to the pulmonary rehabilitation intervention.[46,47] The SGRQ has domains measuring activities, impacts, and symptoms as well as a total score. It is also self-completed, but may require support from the health care practitioner. Both the CRQ and the SGRQ have predefined MCIDs, although the approach that determined the MCIDs was slightly different for each questionnaire. The SGRQ MCID threshold is a 4-point change in the total score, whereas for the CRQ the change is 0.5 units per question, allocated to each domain, so it is possible that after rehabilitation, a threshold has been achieved in 1 domain (eg, dyspnea) but not fatigue. Both questionnaires have been extensively and successfully applied in pulmonary rehabilitation[4,47,48]; usually, just 1 health status questionnaire is used. Both questionnaires are considered sensitive to detecting change resulting from pulmonary rehabilitation.[49]

One interesting aspect of these questionnaires to consider is the usefulness of the questionnaires to guide and influence treatment rather than using them simply to measure outcome. The dyspnea component of the CRQ allows patients to identify 5 activities that are important to them and cause difficulty. This individualization to the patient may form a useful foundation for a goal-setting regimen within the program. However, this approach has not been formally tested.

The COPD Assessment Test (CAT)[50] has recently been developed as a short (8-item), self-completed questionnaire, which is simple to score and is presented as a single number with no domains. The CAT score has been shown to be responsive to pulmonary rehabilitation in a large population with COPD.[51]

Although these questionnaires have been developed for patients with COPD (and for the SGRQ, asthma too), in the absence of other relevant validated questionnaires, their use has been extended to other chronic respiratory diseases.[11] It is likely that the questionnaires are not wholly appropriate for these individuals because there are undoubtedly other important aspects of their disease that are overlooked by these COPD-specific questionnaires.

The choice of health-related quality of life questionnaire is often based on time taken to complete, ease of scoring, and time frame to which the questionnaire makes reference (although, in reality, this is probably the least important). These questionnaires have now been translated for use into several languages.

Functional Performance

The measurement of exercise performance is arguably the outcome measure by which rehabilitation is judged; however, from the patient's perspective, functional performance may be more important. Exercise capacity usually measures what an individual can do, rather than what they do in their home environment. Of course, performance of activities of daily living and functional tasks can be influenced by a wide variety of factors. For example, the environment (stairs may not be important if you live in a ground-floor apartment) and social circumstances (carer and family attitudes and beliefs may influence participation at home) influence functional performance. Functional performance is generally assessed with questionnaires, although researchers have tested out an activities of daily living assault course.[52] Measures of functional activity have examined aspects of domestic and occupational task completion. The focus of these questionnaires is not uniform, often covering aspects such as the frequency with which the task/activity is performed, the degree of discomfort associated with that task, and the importance of that task to the individual being assessed, which may influence the desirability for that task to be resumed.

The most commonly reported questionnaires assessing functional performance are the Pulmonary Functional Status and Dyspnea Questionnaire[53] (which has been shortened to the Functional Status and Dyspnoea Questionnaire [short form]),[54] the Pulmonary Function Status Scale,[55] and the London Chest Activities of Daily Living Scale.[56] Because these questionnaires are standardized, comparisons can be made among patients and centers, but because of the standardization, the questionnaires may lose the potential to identify less common activities that are important to individual patients. This factor is of particular importance in the context of a rehabilitation program, in which the aim is to restore function.

An alternative approach to assessing functional performance is the Canadian Occupational Performance Measure. This is an operator-led measure that requires the individual to identify 5 important activities and then rate performance and satisfaction on each activity.[57] However, this test is time consuming, but it may help direct the rehabilitation process and allow for a more individual approach.[6]

Physical Activity

Compared with functional performance measures, assessment of physical activity is not so concerned with domestic task completion but rather with the measure of overall activity. This element can be assessed subjectively using questionnaires[58] or diary completion, or objectively using physical activity monitors.[59] Some suggest that the dyspnea/activity components of the health status measures do reflect domestic task completion and physical performance and so in the interest of time may be used as surrogate markers of functional performance. Physical activity is increasingly being measured as a baseline assessment for rehabilitation and again on completion of the program as an outcome measure.[10] A great deal of work is being conducted in this area, and the growth of technology will almost inevitably see an explosion of scientific data in this area. As yet, it is not at all clear which aspects of physical activity should be reported and how best to enhance this outcome through the process of rehabilitation.

Anxiety and Depression

Anxiety and depression are frequently reported symptoms in individual with COPD, so it is important that they are assessed before commencing rehabilitation. There is some research to suggest that the presence of depression may influence completion and the impact of the program, although this association is not consistent.[60,61] The most frequently reported measure of anxiety and depression used in pulmonary rehabilitation is the Hospital Anxiety and Depression Score.[62] This scale is self-completed and easy to score. A score of 8 or more indicates probable anxiety and depression symptoms, and a score in excess of 10 indicates a likely presence of anxiety and depression symptoms. In a recent report, the investigators explored a large rehabilitation database and examined the impact of rehabilitation on those with probable and likely anxiety and depression and compared the change after rehabilitation in those individuals with no proven anxiety and depression. Perhaps not surprisingly, the data showed that there was no change in anxiety and depression in those with no previously documented symptoms, but there were clinically meaningful changes in those with reported symptoms.[60]

Symptoms

Breathlessness is the most commonly reported symptom in patients with COPD. Within the context of the pulmonary rehabilitation assessment, breathlessness is typically measured at rest and on exertion during exercise testing and is also explored in health status and functional performance instruments. Dyspnea, along with fatigue, are symptoms that are captured in many of the health-related quality of life measures. Their evaluation in these questionnaires also provides information on the effect of symptoms on daily life.

At rest, breathlessness is commonly recorded using either a visual analog scale, or the Borg Breathlessness Scale.[63] The MRC dyspnea scale[64] is often used at baseline to understand the level of functional impairment associated with breathlessness. It may have been recorded on referral, because many centers define suitability for rehabilitation based on MRC score. The MRC score is also a component of the BODE[15] and i-BODE scores.[29] In addition, it is important to assess breathlessness on exertion (ie, at the end of the exercise test). For measures of exercise performance, it is also important to understand why the individual terminated the exercise or could walk no further in the time allowed. In most cases, patients stop because of shortness of breath in a walking test,[65] but before developing an exercise training regime, it is important to understand the limitation to exercise.

Knowledge and Self-Efficacy

The adoption of health-enhancing behaviors is one of the key aims of pulmonary rehabilitation; however, the subtleties of behavior change can be difficult to measure. The acquisition of knowledge is believed to be important to underpin behavior change, mediated through a change in self-efficacy for that particular behavior. Until recently, there were no specific questionnaires that formally assessed knowledge for pulmonary rehabilitation. We now have the Lung Information Needs Questionnaire (LINQ)[66] and the Bristol COPD Knowledge Questionnaire (BCKQ).[67] The LINQ is a self-administered questionnaire that has 16 items, covering topics such as medication use, exercise, and exacerbation management. The BCKQ has 65 statements, for which participants record whether they believe the statement to be true, false, or do not know. Both questionnaires have been successfully used in pulmonary rehabilitation, although they are not routinely used.

Improving self-efficacy (improving the individual's confidence to manage their disease) is also associated with knowledge improvement, but again this type of measure is not routinely used in pulmonary rehabilitation. There are a few questionnaires that measure self-efficacy. The COPD self-efficacy scale has been reported,[68] and more recently, a questionnaire has been described that addresses issues of self-efficacy pertinent to pulmonary rehabilitation, the Pulmonary Rehabilitation Adapted Index of Self-Efficacy.[69] Further work is necessary to see if these or other self-efficacy assessments add useful information to the initial evaluation or the outcome assessments.

Nutritional Status

The measurement of body composition is potentially important in COPD, because it may identify individuals who are at risk for unfavorable outcome (such as mortality) and may serve to direct the interventions during the program. Although the measurement of BMI is routine, BMI does not necessarily reflect changes in body composition, particularly a shift in fat-free mass (reflecting muscle mass) to fat mass. However, BMI is one of the 4 components of the BODE score; the composite score that is an important discriminator for mortality risk.[15] Historically, rehabilitation centers have been concerned about the potentially negative energy balance in nutritionally compromised patients. However, increasingly, the population presenting for rehabilitation has a BMI that indicates being overweight to varying degrees. The response to rehabilitation seems fairly consistent across the BMI categories, when considering conventional outcome measures.[70] To document body composition (and its changes) either bioimpedance analysis or dual-energy X-ray absorptiometry are performed. Although this type of analysis is usually a research-based endeavor, it may, at times, be helpful clinically in defining regional body composition abnormalities and in directing the pulmonary rehabilitation interventions.

Other Outcome Assessments

There are additional measures that can be taken but are not routinely used or would be part of a core dataset. These measures include upper limb strength or endurance and respiratory muscle strength or endurance. Their potential usefulness in pulmonary rehabilitation remains to be determined.

SUMMARY

It is vital that a comprehensive assessment be conducted to support the delivery of a successful pulmonary rehabilitation program. The development of a wide range of outcome measures should not detract from the main components of an assessment. It should be evident that it is not possible for a particular pulmonary rehabilitation program to incorporate all these outcome measures into its routine assessments. Rather, a limited number of assessments are made across outcome areas. Over time, there may be many developments that enhance the assessment of individuals with chronic respiratory disease before commencing a rehabilitation program. A sophisticated suit of outcomes might allow rehabilitation to be personalized.

REFERENCES

1. Spruit MA, Singh SJ, Garvey C, et al. An official American Thoracic Society/European Respiratory Society statement: key concepts and advances in pulmonary rehabilitation. Am J Respir Crit Care Med 2013;188(8):e13–64.
2. Troosters T, Vilaro J, Rabinovich R, et al. Physiological responses to the 6-min walk test in patients with chronic obstructive pulmonary disease. Eur Respir J 2002;20(3):564–9.
3. Jones PW, Quirk FH, Baveystock CM, et al. A self-complete measure of health status for chronic airflow limitation. The St. George's Respiratory Questionnaire. Am Rev Respir Dis 1992;145(6):1321–7.
4. ZuWallack R, Hashim A, McCusker C, et al. The trajectory of change over multiple outcome areas during comprehensive outpatient pulmonary rehabilitation. Chron Respir Dis 2006;3(1):11–8.
5. Pitta F, Troosters T, Probst VS, et al. Are patients with COPD more active after pulmonary rehabilitation? Chest 2008;134(2):273–80.
6. Sewell L, Singh SJ, Williams JE, et al. Can individualized rehabilitation improve functional independence in elderly patients with COPD? Chest 2005;128(3):1194–200.
7. American College of Sports Medicine. ACSM's guidelines for exercise testing and prescription. Philadelphia: Lippincott Williams & Wilkins; 2005.
8. ATS Committee on Proficiency Standards for Clinical Pulmonary Function Laboratories. ATS statement: guidelines for the six-minute walk test. Am J Respir Crit Care Med 2002;166(1):111–7.
9. Troosters T, Gosselink R, Decramer M. Short- and long-term effects of outpatient rehabilitation in patients with chronic obstructive pulmonary disease: a randomized trial. Am J Med 2000;109(3):207–12.
10. Walker PP, Burnett A, Flavahan PW, et al. Lower limb activity and its determinants in COPD. Thorax 2008;63(8):683–9.
11. Holland AE, Hill CJ, Conron M, et al. Short term improvement in exercise capacity and symptoms following exercise training in interstitial lung disease. Thorax 2008;63(6):549–54.
12. Redelmeier DA, Bayoumi AM, Goldstein RS, et al. Interpreting small differences in functional status: the Six Minute Walk test in chronic lung disease patients. Am J Respir Crit Care Med 1997;155(4):1278–82.
13. Puhan MA, Mador MJ, Held U, et al. Interpretation of treatment changes in 6-minute walk distance in patients with COPD. Eur Respir J 2008;32(3):637–43.
14. Lacasse Y, Goldstein R, Lasserson TJ, et al. Pulmonary rehabilitation for chronic obstructive pulmonary disease. Cochrane Database Syst Rev 2006;(4):CD003793.
15. Celli BR, Cote CG, Marin JM, et al. The body-mass index, airflow obstruction, dyspnea, and exercise capacity index in chronic obstructive pulmonary disease. N Engl J Med 2004;350(10):1005–12.

16. Cote CG, Celli BR. Pulmonary rehabilitation and the BODE index in COPD. Eur Respir J 2005;26(4): 630–6.

17. Enright PL, Sherrill DL. Reference equations for the six-minute walk in healthy adults. Am J Respir Crit Care Med 1998;158(5 Pt 1):1384–7.

18. Troosters T, Gosselink R, Decramer M. Six minute walking distance in healthy elderly subjects. Eur Respir J 1999;14(2):270–4.

19. Casanova C, Celli BR, Barria P, et al. The 6-min walk distance in healthy subjects: reference standards from seven countries. Eur Respir J 2011; 37(1):150–6.

20. Singh SJ, Morgan MD, Scott S, et al. Development of a shuttle walking test of disability in patients with chronic airways obstruction. Thorax 1992;47(12): 1019–24.

21. Evans RA, Singh SJ, Collier R, et al. Pulmonary rehabilitation is successful for COPD irrespective of MRC dyspnoea grade. Respir Med 2009; 103(7):1070–5.

22. Probst VS, Hernandes NA, Teixeira DC, et al. Reference values for the incremental shuttle walking test. Respir Med 2012;106(2):243–8.

23. Jurgensen SP, Antunes LC, Tanni SE, et al. The incremental shuttle walk test in older Brazilian adults. Respiration 2011;81(3):223–8.

24. Harrison SL, Greening NJ, Houchen-Wolloff L, et al. Age-specific normal values for the incremental shuttle walk test in a healthy British population. J Cardiopulm Rehabil Prev 2013;33(5):309–13.

25. Deacon SJ, Vincent EE, Greenhaff PL, et al. Randomized controlled trial of dietary creatine as an adjunct therapy to physical training in chronic obstructive pulmonary disease. Am J Respir Crit Care Med 2008;178(3):233–9.

26. Seymour JM, Moore L, Jolley CJ, et al. Outpatient pulmonary rehabilitation following acute exacerbations of COPD. Thorax 2010;65(5):423–8.

27. Johnson-Warrington V, Williams J, Bankart J, et al. Pulmonary rehabilitation and interstitial lung disease: aiding the referral decision. J Cardiopulm Rehabil Prev 2013;33(3):189–95.

28. Singh SJ, Jones PW, Evans R, et al. Minimum clinically important improvement for the incremental shuttle walking test. Thorax 2008;63(9):775–7.

29. Williams JE, Green RH, Warrington V, et al. Development of the i-BODE: validation of the incremental shuttle walking test within the BODE index. Respir Med 2012;106(3):390–6.

30. Revill SM, Morgan MD, Singh SJ, et al. The endurance shuttle walk: a new field test for the assessment of endurance capacity in chronic obstructive pulmonary disease. Thorax 1999;54(3):213–22.

31. Revill SM, Williams J, Sewell L, et al. Within-day repeatability of the endurance shuttle walk test. Physiotherapy 2009;95(2):140–3.

32. Pepin V, Laviolette L, Brouillard C, et al. Significance of changes in endurance shuttle walking performance. Thorax 2011;66(2):115–20.

33. Casaburi R, Kukafka D, Cooper CB, et al. Improvements in exercise tolerance with the combination of tiotropium and pulmonary rehabilitation in patients with COPD. Chest 2005;127(3): 809–17.

34. Kiley JP, Sri RJ, Croxton TL, et al. Challenges associated with estimating minimal clinically important differences in COPD–the NHLBI perspective. COPD 2005;2(1):43–6.

35. Casaburi R. Factors determining constant work rate exercise tolerance in COPD and their role in dictating the minimal clinically important difference in response to interventions. COPD 2005;2(1): 131–6.

36. Maltais F, Bourbeau J, Shapiro S, et al. Effects of home-based pulmonary rehabilitation in patients with chronic obstructive pulmonary disease: a randomized trial. Ann Intern Med 2008;149(12): 869–78.

37. Calvert LD, Singh SJ, Morgan MD, et al. Exercise induced skeletal muscle metabolic stress is reduced after pulmonary rehabilitation in COPD. Respir Med 2011;105(3):363–70.

38. Dolmage TE, Goldstein RS. Effects of one-legged exercise training of patients with COPD. Chest 2008;133(2):370–6.

39. Leung RW, McKeough ZJ, Peters MJ, et al. Short-form Sun-style t'ai chi as an exercise training modality in people with COPD. Eur Respir J 2013; 41(5):1051–7.

40. Kon SS, Patel MS, Canavan JL, et al. Reliability and validity of 4-metre gait speed in COPD. Eur Respir J 2013;42(2):333–40.

41. van Wetering CR, Hoogendoorn M, Mol SJ, et al. Short- and long-term efficacy of a community-based COPD management programme in less advanced COPD: a randomised controlled trial. Thorax 2010;65(1):7–13.

42. Swallow EB, Reyes D, Hopkinson NS, et al. Quadriceps strength predicts mortality in patients with moderate to severe chronic obstructive pulmonary disease. Thorax 2007;62(2):115–20.

43. Ware JE Jr, Sherbourne CD. The MOS 36-item short-form health survey (SF-36). I. Conceptual framework and item selection. Med Care 1992; 30(6):473–83.

44. Guyatt GH, Berman LB, Townsend M, et al. A measure of quality of life for clinical trials in chronic lung disease. Thorax 1987;42(10):773–8.

45. Williams JE, Singh SJ, Sewell L, et al. Development of a self-reported Chronic Respiratory Questionnaire (CRQ-SR). Thorax 2001;56(12):954–9.

46. Williams JE, Singh SJ, Sewell L, et al. Health status measurement: sensitivity of the self-reported

Chronic Respiratory Questionnaire (CRQ-SR) in pulmonary rehabilitation. Thorax 2003;58(6):515–8.

47. Griffiths TL, Burr ML, Campbell IA, et al. Results at 1 year of outpatient multidisciplinary pulmonary rehabilitation: a randomised controlled trial. Lancet 2000;355(9201):362–8.

48. Man WD, Polkey MI, Donaldson N, et al. Community pulmonary rehabilitation after hospitalisation for acute exacerbations of chronic obstructive pulmonary disease: randomised controlled study. BMJ 2004;329(7476):1209.

49. Singh SJ, Sodergren SC, Hyland ME, et al. A comparison of three disease-specific and two generic health-status measures to evaluate the outcome of pulmonary rehabilitation in COPD. Respir Med 2001;95(1):71–7.

50. Jones PW, Harding G, Berry P, et al. Development and first validation of the COPD assessment test. Eur Respir J 2009;34(3):648–54.

51. Dodd JW, Marns PL, Clark AL, et al. The COPD Assessment Test (CAT): short- and medium-term response to pulmonary rehabilitation. COPD 2012;9(4):390–4.

52. Skumlien S, Hagelund T, Bjortuft O, et al. A field test of functional status as performance of activities of daily living in COPD patients. Respir Med 2006; 100(2):316–23.

53. Lareau SC, Carrieri-Kohlman V, Janson-Bjerklie S, et al. Development and testing of the pulmonary functional status and dyspnea questionnaire (PFSDQ). Heart Lung 1994;23(3):242–50.

54. Lareau SC, Meek PM, Roos PJ. Development and testing of the modified version of the pulmonary functional status and dyspnea questionnaire (PFSDQ-M). Heart Lung 1998;27(3):159–68.

55. Weaver TE, Narsavage GL, Guilfoyle MJ. The development and psychometric evaluation of the Pulmonary Functional Status Scale: an instrument to assess functional status in pulmonary disease. J Cardiopulm Rehabil 1998;18(2):105–11.

56. Garrod R, Bestall JC, Paul EA, et al. Development and validation of a standardized measure of activity of daily living in patients with severe COPD: the London Chest Activity of Daily Living scale (LCADL). Respir Med 2000;94(6):589–96.

57. Law M, Baptiste S, McColl M, et al. The Canadian occupational performance measure: an outcome measure for occupational therapy. Can J Occup Ther 1990;57(2):82–7.

58. Garfield BE, Canavan JL, Smith CJ, et al. Stanford Seven-Day Physical Activity Recall questionnaire in COPD. Eur Respir J 2012;40(2):356–62.

59. Pitta F, Troosters T, Spruit MA, et al. Activity monitoring for assessment of physical activities in daily life in patients with chronic obstructive pulmonary disease. Arch Phys Med Rehabil 2005;86(10): 1979–85.

60. Harrison SL, Greening NJ, Williams JE, et al. Have we underestimated the efficacy of pulmonary rehabilitation in improving mood? Respir Med 2012; 106(6):838–44.

61. Garrod R, Marshall J, Barley E, et al. Predictors of success and failure in pulmonary rehabilitation. Eur Respir J 2006;27(4):788–94.

62. Zigmond AS, Snaith RP. The hospital anxiety and depression scale. Acta Psychiatr Scand 1983; 67(6):361–70.

63. Borg GA. Psychophysical bases of perceived exertion. Med Sci Sports Exerc 1982;14(5):377–81.

64. Definition and classification of chronic bronchitis for clinical and epidemiological purposes. A report to the Medical Research Council by their Committee on the Aetiology of Chronic Bronchitis. Lancet 1965;1(7389):775–9.

65. Man WD, Soliman MG, Gearing J, et al. Symptoms and quadriceps fatigability after walking and cycling in chronic obstructive pulmonary disease. Am J Respir Crit Care Med 2003;168(5):562–7.

66. Hyland ME, Jones RC, Hanney KE. The Lung Information Needs Questionnaire: development, preliminary validation and findings. Respir Med 2006; 100(10):1807–16.

67. White R, Walker P, Roberts S, et al. Bristol COPD Knowledge Questionnaire (BCKQ): testing what we teach patients about COPD. Chron Respir Dis 2006;3(3):123–31.

68. Garrod R, Marshall J, Jones F. Self efficacy measurement and goal attainment after pulmonary rehabilitation. Int J Chron Obstruct Pulmon Dis 2008;3(4):791–6.

69. Vincent E, Sewell L, Wagg K, et al. Measuring a change in self-efficacy following pulmonary rehabilitation: an evaluation of the PRAISE tool. Chest 2011;140(6):1534–9.

70. Greening NJ, Evans RA, Williams JE, et al. Does body mass index influence the outcomes of a waking-based pulmonary rehabilitation programme in COPD? Chron Respir Dis 2012;9(2):99–106.

Promoting Regular Physical Activity in Pulmonary Rehabilitation

Judith Garcia-Aymerich, MD, PhD[a],*, Fabio Pitta, PT, PhD[b]

KEYWORDS

- Physical activity • Exercise • Behavior change • Chronic obstructive pulmonary disease
- Pulmonary rehabilitation

KEY POINTS

- Physical inactivity is common in individuals with chronic respiratory diseases, and worsens their prognosis.
- Physical activity is an important outcome of pulmonary rehabilitation because it is a potentially modifiable factor that can improve prognosis.
- Current evidence from pulmonary rehabilitation studies shows inconsistent results in modifying physical activity.
- Behavioral components of pulmonary rehabilitation are a target of future research aimed at having an impact on levels of physical activity.
- The cost and logistics of pulmonary rehabilitation make difficult the adoption of strategies that could potentially improve levels of physical activity.

INTRODUCTION

As a complex behavior, physical activity is influenced by a combination of individual, sociocultural, and environmental factors (**Fig. 1**). The prevailing focus on the pathophysiologic factors limiting physical activity has led to the general knowledge that individuals with chronic respiratory diseases are physically inactive in comparison with their healthy peers. This feature has been consistently observed in patients with chronic obstructive pulmonary disease (COPD),[1,2] but not in individuals with asthma or cystic fibrosis.[3,4] A discussion of the role of pulmonary rehabilitation on physical activity needs first to review those factors that drive inactivity, and the consequences of such inactivity.

The disability resulting from COPD reflects the paradigm of a vicious cycle of disturbing symptoms such as exertional dyspnea, followed by sedentarism and immobility, followed by increased dyspnea resulting from further deconditioning. Consequently, skeletal muscle dysfunction is frequent in these patients and, in addition to respiratory and cardiac problems, further decreases exercise tolerance.[5] Physical inactivity in turn causes muscle wasting.[6] Symptoms such as dyspnea and fatigue, perceived to a greater extent by patients with COPD than by those with other diseases,[7] further limit exercise tolerance, favoring the negative trend (vicious cycle) that leads to generalized weakness, sedentary lifestyle, and, ultimately, immobility.[8] Similar mechanisms limit activity in other chronic diseases such as interstitial lung disease and bronchiectasis.[9,10]

Psychological factors likely play an important role in disability in all chronic respiratory diseases,

The authors have no conflicts of interest.
[a] Centre for Research in Environmental Epidemiology (CREAL), Doctor Aiguader 88, Barcelona 08003, Spain;
[b] Laboratory of Research in Respiratory Physiotherapy (LFIP), Departamento de Fisioterapia, Av. Robert Koch, 60, Londrina 86038-350, Brazil
* Corresponding author.
E-mail address: jgarcia@creal.cat

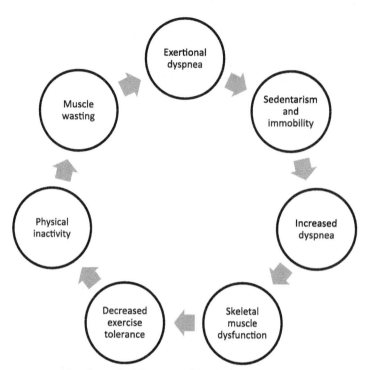

Fig. 1. Cycle of symptoms resulting from disability caused by chronic obstructive pulmonary disease.

but research on this topic is relatively scarce in respiratory disease. An example of psychological factors influencing physical activity is the finding that some asthma patients avoid participating in vigorous physical activity owing to the fear of exercise-induced bronchoconstriction.[11] It should be noted that, to date, the effects of anxiety and depression on physical-activity levels of COPD patients remain contradictory.[12,13]

The habitually low level of regular physical activity in many patients with chronic respiratory disease is of critical importance in their long-term prognosis. Again, research is more abundant for COPD than for other diseases: low levels of physical activity have been consistently demonstrated to predict higher mortality[14–17] and to increase the risk of readmission after a hospitalization for a COPD exacerbation,[14,17–20] irrespective of the setting, geographic location, cultural environment, or methods for measuring physical activity. In patients with asthma, higher levels of physical activity have been associated with reduced risk of exacerbation[21] and reduced respiratory symptoms.[22,23]

COMPONENTS OF PULMONARY REHABILITATION ADDRESSING PHYSICAL ACTIVITY

Pulmonary rehabilitation programs provide an excellent framework to enhance patients'

capabilities and promote physical activity. Rehabilitation aims to address both the pathophysiologic limitations to physical activity and the low levels of self-efficacy for regular exercise (through promoting self-management), thus addressing the 2 pillars of inactivity: physical limitation and maladaptive behavior.

Exercise Training

Exercise training is often regarded as the cornerstone of pulmonary rehabilitation. At present there is a solid body of literature clearly indicating that exercise training, by itself or as part of a pulmonary rehabilitation program, leads to improvements in a variety of negative aspects linked to chronic respiratory disease such as dyspnea, fatigue, exercise intolerance, muscle weakness, and poor health-related quality of life.[24,25] Furthermore, it is also clear that the magnitude of training effects depends on factors involved in the exercise training program, such as intensity, frequency, duration, and mode, which are described in detail in articles elsewhere in this issue. However, it must be emphasized that exercise and physical activity are not identical concepts. Physical activity comprises any bodily movement produced by skeletal muscles that results in energy expenditure, whereas exercise is a subset of physical activity that is planned, structured, repetitive, and purposeful.[26] In addition, improvements in exercise capacity (often obtained after a pulmonary rehabilitation intervention) do not necessarily result in improvements in daily physical activity in the home and community settings,[27] as discussed later in this article.

Behavioral Intervention

In addition to pathologic and physiologic factors adversely affecting exercise capacity and thereby limiting physical activity, the patient's adaptation to the illness also influences the impairment and burden of the disease.[24] For this reason, the educational component of pulmonary rehabilitation should ideally include the promotion of adaptive behavior change, especially in the area of collaborative self-management.[28] Educational interventions that address physical activity generally involve strategies such as goal setting, problem solving, decision making, taking action based on a predefined action plan, and cognitive-behavioral therapy. The latter includes techniques such as operant conditioning, changing cognitions, enhancement of self-efficacy, and addressing motivational issues.[29] It remains to be determined whether (and to what extent) these behavioral interventions are effective in improving patients' levels of physical activity.

HOW PHYSICAL ACTIVITY IS MEASURED AS AN OUTCOME OF PULMONARY REHABILITATION

Energy-expenditure assessment and the use of questionnaires and motion sensors are means used to quantify physical (in)activity. Assessment of energy expenditure aims at measuring how much energy is spent in physical activity, and not specifically at measuring the amount and intensity of the physical activity performed. Energy expended in physical activity depends on several factors such as age, gender, body mass, movement efficiency, and the energy cost of each activity.[30,31] This complexity, along with difficulties in measurement, hinders the use of energy-expenditure assessment in comparing levels of physical activity among different individuals.[30] The high cost of this measurement is also an important limitation. For these reasons, energy-expenditure assessment is not commonly used in clinical practice or even in scientific studies, leaving questionnaires and motion sensors as the most frequently used methods to measure physical activity.

Several questionnaires aim at capturing different aspects of physical activity, such as amount, type, intensity, symptom experience, and performance of activities of daily living.[32] Recent systematic reviews have described a variety of questionnaires that can be used in the context of pulmonary rehabilitation outcome assessment.[33–35] When choosing a questionnaire to be used in pulmonary rehabilitation, matching the question to be addressed with the psychometric properties of the instrument is of importance. Despite some limitations involving the instruments' validity, the frequent absence of a conceptual framework, and a potential recall bias, questionnaires are easy to use and inexpensive, which explains their common use in epidemiologic studies and large clinical trials.

Motion sensors are devices that detect body movement, and therefore can be used to objectively quantify physical activity in daily life for periods of time.[32] Most available motion sensors are small, light, and minimally intrusive. The main types of motion sensors are pedometers, which count the number of steps performed by the subject, and accelerometers, which detect body acceleration. Accelerometers are capable of estimating time spent in activity, energy expenditure, and a variety of other outcomes related to physical activity in daily life. To increase their ability to more accurately estimate daily physical activity and energy expenditure, some motion sensors combine movement data from accelerometers with physiologic data from other sensors, such as heart rate and skin temperature.[36] Recent studies on the validity of motion-sensor output have identified a few instruments that seem to be superior to others when assessing physical activity.[37,38] These devices include the DynaPort MiniMod (McRoberts, The Hague, the Netherlands), the ActiGraph GT3X (ActiGraph, Pensacola, FL), and the Sense-Wear Armband (SMT Medical, Würzburg, Germany) (all triaxial accelerometers), which were found to be valid and responsive for use in COPD in the context of pulmonary rehabilitation (**Box 1**).

EFFECTS OF PULMONARY REHABILITATION ON PHYSICAL ACTIVITY

Physical activity has only been recently included as an outcome of pulmonary rehabilitation, when

---

Box 1
Methods used to quantify physical (in)activity

1. Assessment of energy expenditure
2. Questionnaires
3. Motion sensors

the independent effects of physical activity on outcomes in chronic respiratory diseases became apparent and direct measures of activity were made available. Again, most of the available evidence comes from studies of patients with COPD. Unfortunately, the results of these studies have been inconsistent: some have demonstrated statistically significant increases in activity level after pulmonary rehabilitation,[39–41] whereas others have not.[42–45] An overall interpretation of these results is difficult because of differences in the type of patients, content of programs, duration of programs, and methods for assessing physical activity. Moreover, some of the studies had no control group[41–46] or had a control group without random allocation,[39] and many had a small sample size.[42–46]

The well-documented and consistent benefit of pulmonary rehabilitation on exercise capacity stands in stark comparison with its lack of clear-cut and consistent effects on physical activity. Several arguments, however, may explain this discrepancy. First, exercise capacity is a functional status whereas physical activity is in large part a behavior, and it should be acknowledged that this behavioral component of physical activity had been largely ignored in rehabilitation programs. This idea is supported by the fact that some recent rehabilitation programs incorporating behavioral components, such as feedback by pedometer or group activities, have shown positive effects on physical activity.[47,48] Another potential explanation for the discrepancy between impressive gains in exercise capacity and meager increases in physical activity is the relatively short duration of many pulmonary rehabilitation programs. Programs of shorter duration are usually sufficient to increase exercise performance, but are probably too brief to prompt the effective behavior changes required to increase physical activity in the home and community settings.

CHALLENGES OF PULMONARY REHABILITATION IN PROMOTING PHYSICAL ACTIVITY

The increase (or maintenance) of daily physical activity up to the recommended level of 30 minutes per day of moderate physical activity on most days of the week[49,50] should be a target of pulmonary rehabilitation programs. Ideally this goal should be set irrespective of the underlying disease or baseline levels of physical activity. However, the current organization and content of pulmonary rehabilitation programs impose some limitations and, therefore, future challenges, to achieving this target.

First, rehabilitation programs are usually of short (4–8 weeks) duration,[24] which is probably insufficient to prompt the substantial change in behavior needed for a sustained increase in physical activity. Second, little attention has focused, thus far, on the nonphysiologic determinants of physical activity. Impediments to physical activity, such as psychological factors, motivation, and social issues, are areas that may have to be addressed. Third, and related to the previous limitation, the behavioral components of pulmonary rehabilitation that may be needed to effectively increase activity need to be better defined and then implemented. Pulmonary rehabilitation is still in its infancy in this important area.

A practical and important hindrance to developing a pulmonary rehabilitation program that would better address the problem of physical inactivity in patients with chronic respiratory disease, including changes in content and duration of the intervention, is cost. Although the economic factors vary from one country to another, the cost-effectiveness of pulmonary rehabilitation remains a matter of some debate in most settings. The lack of consistency of pulmonary rehabilitation in the outcome areas of health care utilization and mortality in the stable respiratory patient has not led to its promotion by third-party payers as a routine treatment for all patients with chronic respiratory disease. The setting of traditional pulmonary rehabilitation, usually in an outpatient hospital-based setting or a highly specialized center, makes it more costly and not available for all patients at any time. One potential solution would be to promote physical activity in a structured program, based on exercise training and behavioral intervention, outside the traditional rehabilitation setting, such as in primary care offices or community centers. Obviously much more information is needed about this type of initiative with regard to development, implementation, and effectiveness.

SUMMARY

Physical activity is a strong and independent risk factor for increased health care utilization and mortality in patients with COPD and, probably, in all patients with chronic respiratory disease. As such, and because of its potential response to exercise capacity and behavioral interventions, it has become a key outcome for pulmonary rehabilitation programs. Research thus far has provided inconsistent results on the potential beneficial effects of pulmonary rehabilitation on levels of physical activity. Increased exercise performance resulting from exercise training has the potential to increase physical activity. Combining this potential with more effective behavioral interventions, resulting from additional research, may lead to a positive change in the practice of physical activity.

REFERENCES

1. Pitta F, Troosters T, Spruit MA, et al. Characteristics of physical activities in daily life in chronic obstructive pulmonary disease. Am J Respir Crit Care Med 2005;171:972–7.
2. Vorrink SN, Kort HS, Troosters T, et al. Level of daily physical activity in individuals with COPD compared with healthy controls. Respir Res 2011; 12:33.
3. Jerning C, Martinander E, Bjerg A, et al. Asthma and physical activity—a population based study results from the Swedish GA(2)LEN survey. Respir Med 2013;107(11):1651–8.
4. Savi D, Quattrucci S, Internullo M, et al. Measuring habitual physical activity in adults with cystic fibrosis. Respir Med 2013;107(12):1888–94.
5. Barnes PJ, Celli BR. Systemic manifestations and comorbidities of COPD. Eur Respir J 2009;33: 1165–85.
6. Casanova Macario C, de Torres Tajes JP, Palmero MA. COPD disease and malnutrition. Arch Bronconeumol 2009;45(Suppl 4):31–5.
7. Baghai-Ravary R, Quint JK, Goldring JJ, et al. Determinants and impact of fatigue in patients with COPD. Respir Med 2009;103:216–23.
8. ZuWallack R. How are you doing? What are you doing? Differing perspectives in the assessment of individuals with COPD. COPD 2007;3:293–7.
9. Holland AE. Exercise limitation in interstitial lung disease—mechanisms, significance and therapeutic options. Chron Respir Dis 2010;7:101–11.
10. Koulouris NG, Retsou S, Kosmas E, et al. Tidal expiratory flow limitation, dyspnoea and exercise capacity in patients with bilateral bronchiectasis. Eur Respir J 2003;21:743–8.
11. Global strategy for asthma management and prevention. Global Initiative for Asthma (GINA); 2011. Available at: http://www.ginasthma.org. Accessed October 23, 2013.
12. Garcia-Aymerich J, Felez MA, Escarrabill J, et al. Physical activity and its determinants in severe chronic obstructive pulmonary disease. Med Sci Sports Exerc 2004;36:1667–73.
13. Nguyen HQ, Fan VS, Herting J, et al. Patients with COPD with higher levels of anxiety are more physically active. Chest 2013;144:145–51.
14. Garcia-Aymerich J, Lange P, Benet M, et al. Regular physical activity reduces hospital admission and mortality in chronic obstructive pulmonary disease: a population based cohort study. Thorax 2006;61:772–8.
15. Ringbaek TJ, Lange P. Outdoor activity and performance status as predictors of survival in hypoxaemic chronic obstructive pulmonary disease (COPD). Clin Rehabil 2005;19:331–8.
16. Waschki B, Kirsten A, Holz O, et al. Physical activity is the strongest predictor of all-cause mortality in patients with COPD: a prospective cohort study. Chest 2011;140:331–42.
17. Garcia-Rio F, Rojo B, Casitas R, et al. Prognostic value of the objective measurement of daily physical activity in patients with COPD. Chest 2012; 142:338–46.
18. Garcia-Aymerich J, Farrero E, Felez MA, et al. Risk factors of readmission to hospital for a COPD exacerbation: a prospective study. Thorax 2003;58: 100–5.
19. Pitta F, Troosters T, Probst VS, et al. Physical activity and hospitalization for exacerbation of COPD. Chest 2006;129:536–44.
20. Seidel D, Cheung A, Suh ES, et al. Physical inactivity and risk of hospitalisation for chronic obstructive pulmonary disease. Int J Tuberc Lung Dis 2012;16:1015–9.
21. Garcia-Aymerich J, Varraso R, Antó JM, et al. Prospective study of physical activity and risk of asthma exacerbations in older women. Am J Respir Crit Care Med 2009;179:999–1003.
22. Ford ES, Heath GW, Mannino DM, et al. Leisuretime physical activity patterns among US adults with asthma. Chest 2003;124:432–7.
23. Kilpeläinen M, Terho EO, Helenius H, et al. Body mass index and physical activity in relation to asthma and atopic diseases in young adults. Respir Med 2006;100:1518–25.
24. Spruit MA, Singh SJ, Garvey C, et al. An official American Thoracic Society/European Respiratory Society Statement: key concepts and advances in pulmonary rehabilitation. Am J Respir Crit Care Med 2013;188:13–64.
25. Lacasse Y, Brosseau L, Milne S, et al. Pulmonary rehabilitation for chronic obstructive pulmonary disease. Cochrane Database Syst Rev 2002;(3):CD003793.
26. Caspersen CJ, Powell KE, Christenson GM. Physical activity, exercise, and physical fitness: definitions and distinctions for health-related research. Public Health Rep 1985;100:126–31.
27. Pitta F, Troosters T, Probst VS, et al. Are patients with COPD more active after pulmonary rehabilitation? Chest 2008;134:273–80.
28. Bourbeau J, Nault D, Dang-Tan T. Self-management and behaviour modification in COPD. Patient Educ Couns 2004;52:271–7.
29. Fritzsche A, Clamor A, von Leupoldt A. Effects of medical and psychological treatment of depression in patients with COPD—a review. Respir Med 2011;105:1422–33.

30. Schutz Y, Weinsier RL, Hunter GR. Assessment of free-living physical activity in humans: an overview of currently available and proposed new measures. Obes Res 2001;9:368–79.

31. Tudor-Locke CE, Myers AM. Challenges and opportunities for measuring physical activity in sedentary adults. Sports Med 2001;31:91–100.

32. Pitta F, Troosters T, Probst VS, et al. Quantifying physical activity in daily life with questionnaires and motion sensors in COPD. Eur Respir J 2006; 27:1040–55.

33. Gimeno-Santos E, Frei A, Dobbels F, et al. Validity of instruments to measure physical activity may be questionable due to a lack of conceptual frameworks: a systematic review. Health Qual Life Outcomes 2011;9:86.

34. Frei A, Williams K, Vetsch A, et al. A comprehensive systematic review of the development process of 104 patient-reported outcomes (PROs) for physical activity in chronically ill and elderly people. Health Qual Life Outcomes 2011;9:116.

35. Williams K, Frei A, Vetsch A, et al. Patient-reported physical activity questionnaires: a systematic review of content and format. Health Qual Life Outcomes 2012;10:28.

36. Patel SA, Benzo RP, Slivka WA, et al. Activity monitoring and energy expenditure in COPD patients: a validation study. COPD 2007;4:107–12.

37. Van Remoortel H, Raste Y, Louvaris Z, et al. Validity of six activity monitors in chronic obstructive pulmonary disease: a comparison with indirect calorimetry. PLoS One 2012;7:e39198.

38. Rabinovich RA, Louvaris Z, Raste Y, et al. Validity of physical activity monitors during daily life in patients with COPD. Eur Respir J 2013;42(5):1205–15.

39. Behnke M, Wewel AR, Kirsten D, et al. Exercise training raises daily activity stronger than predicted from exercise capacity in patients with COPD. Respir Med 2005;99:711–7.

40. Effing T, Zielhuis G, Kerstjens H, et al. Community based physiotherapeutic exercise in COPD self-management: a randomised controlled trial. Respir Med 2011;105:418–26.

41. Sewell L, Singh SJ, Williams JE, et al. Can individualized rehabilitation improve functional independence in elderly patients with COPD? Chest 2005;128: 1194–200.

42. Dallas MI, McCusker C, Haggerty MC, et al. Using pedometers to monitor walking activity in outcome assessment for pulmonary rehabilitation. Chron Respir Dis 2009;6:217–24.

43. Daly C, Coughlan GF, Hennessy E, et al. Effects of neuromuscular electrical stimulation on the activity levels and exercise capacity of patients with moderate to severe COPD. Physiotherapy Practice and Research 2011;32:6–11.

44. Mador MJ, Patel AN, Nadler J. Effects of pulmonary rehabilitation on activity levels in patients with chronic obstructive pulmonary disease. J Cardiopulm Rehabil Prev 2011;31:52–9.

45. Probst VS, Kovelis DT, Hernandes ND, et al. Effects of 2 exercise training programs on physical activity in daily life in patients with COPD. Respir Care 2011;56:1799–807.

46. Egan C, Deering BM, Blake C, et al. Short term and long term effects of pulmonary rehabilitation on physical activity in COPD. Respir Med 2012;106: 1671–9.

47. de Blok BM, de Greef MH, ten Hacken NH, et al. The effects of a lifestyle physical activity counseling program with feedback of a pedometer during pulmonary rehabilitation in patients with COPD: a pilot study. Patient Educ Couns 2006; 61:48–55.

48. Breyer MK, Breyer-Kohansal R, Funk GC, et al. Nordic walking improves daily physical activities in COPD: a randomised controlled trial. Respir Res 2010;11:112.

49. Nelson ME, Rejeski WJ, Blair SN, et al. Physical activity and public health in older adults: recommendation from the American College of Sports Medicine and the American Heart Association. Med Sci Sports Exerc 2007;39:1435–45.

50. Garber CE, Blissmer B, Deschenes MR, et al. American College of Sports Medicine position stand. Quantity and quality of exercise for developing and maintaining cardiorespiratory, musculoskeletal, and neuromotor fitness in apparently healthy adults: guidance for prescribing exercise. Med Sci Sports Exerc 2011;43:1334–59.

Pulmonary Rehabilitation for Respiratory Disorders Other than Chronic Obstructive Pulmonary Disease

Carolyn L. Rochester, MD[a],*, Carl Fairburn, PT, DPT[b],
Rebecca H. Crouch, PT, DPT, MS, CCS[b]

KEYWORDS

- Pulmonary rehabilitation • Pulmonary hypertension • Exercise training • Dyspnea • Quality of life
- Cystic fibrosis • Asthma • Interstitial lung disease • Lung cancer

KEY POINTS

- A strong scientific rationale exists for providing pulmonary rehabilitation (PR) to persons with many forms of respiratory disease other than chronic obstructive pulmonary disease.
- Nearly all published clinical trials have shown beneficial effects of PR for such patients.
- Evidence to date shows that PR for patients with disorders other than chronic obstructive pulmonary disease is feasible, safe, and effective.
- PR should be provided according to a disease-relevant approach to ensure patient safety and to maximize the benefits of PR.

INTRODUCTION

Pulmonary rehabilitation (PR) improves exercise tolerance, reduces symptoms and improves quality of life (QOL) for patients with chronic obstructive pulmonary disease (COPD).[1] It is now recognized increasingly that PR also improves clinical outcomes for persons with many respiratory disorders other than COPD. Although the published literature regarding PR for non-COPD disorders remains less extensive than that available for COPD, a strong scientific rationale exists for providing PR to persons with many forms of non-COPD respiratory disease, and nearly all published clinical trials have reported beneficial effects of PR for such patients. Recognition of the benefits of PR has led to consideration of PR as part of the standard of routine care in disease management guidelines for both pulmonary fibrosis and pulmonary hypertension (PH).[2,3] In the United States, payer reimbursement for PR for non-COPD disorders remains limited, and challenges remain in provision of PR to diverse patient groups. This review highlights the rationale for and documented benefits of PR for several non-COPD respiratory disorders.

RATIONALE FOR PR IN NON-COPD DISORDERS

The scientific rationale for PR for persons with COPD is that it can stabilize or reverse many systemic manifestations of the disease, including skeletal muscle dysfunction.[4,5] Participation in PR also improves exercise capacity, reduces knowledge deficits, promotes use of long-term health-enhancing behaviors, reduces depression and anxiety,[6] helps patients manage complex

[a] Section of Pulmonary, Critical Care and Sleep, Yale University School of Medicine, 333 Cedar Street, Building LCI-105, New Haven, CT 06520, USA; [b] Duke Cardiopulmonary Rehabilitation, Duke University School of Medicine, 1821 Hillandale Road, Suite 25B, Durham, NC 27705, USA
* Corresponding author.
E-mail address: carolyn.rochester@yale.edu

Clin Chest Med 35 (2014) 369–389
http://dx.doi.org/10.1016/j.ccm.2014.02.016
0272-5231/14/$ – see front matter Published by Elsevier Inc.

medical regimens and exacerbations, reduces hospitalizations,[7,8] improves patients' QOL,[1,9] and can improve physical activity levels.[1]

Many persons with respiratory disorders other than COPD also have skeletal muscle dysfunction,[10–14] with associated reduction in exercise capacity, as well as disabling symptoms such as dyspnea, cough, fatigue, anxiety, depression, and impaired QOL, in addition to abnormalities in their respiratory system per se. As is the case for COPD, these features can be improved by participation in PR. Moreover, many patients with non-COPD disorders face complex medical regimens and experience intermittent exacerbations of disease. In many disorders, including interstitial lung disease (ILD), cystic fibrosis (CF), pulmonary hypertension (PH), and lung cancer, low exercise capacity is associated with worse survival.[15–18] Improvement in exercise capacity via participation in PR has the potential to improve long-term outcomes of the disease. Consideration of PR for persons with disorders other than COPD is recommended formally in both the 2013 American Thoracic Society (ATS)/European Respiratory Society (ERS) Statement on PR[1] and in the joint American College of Chest Physicians/American Association of Cardiovascular and Pulmonary Rehabilitation evidence-based guidelines on PR.[9] Retrospective analyses of outcomes of PR have shown that participants with non-COPD respiratory disorders achieve similar improvements in exercise tolerance, symptoms, and QOL after PR to those achieved by persons with COPD.[19,20] Such findings have prompted an emerging wealth of studies showing beneficial effects of PR for individual disease groups; these are considered further below. Disorders other than COPD for which PR can be beneficial are shown in **Box 1**.

PR FOR OTHER CONDITIONS ASSOCIATED WITH AIRFLOW OBSTRUCTION
Asthma

Asthma affects all age groups and is a leading cause of chronic illness in children and adults. As a result of airflow obstruction, increased work of breathing and symptom exacerbation (including exercise-induced bronchoconstriction [EIB] for some persons), patients with asthma often experience dyspnea, show less tolerance for exercise despite optimized pharmacologic therapy, and have low physical activity levels.[21,22] Poor asthma control is associated with a greater prevalence of functional impairment, depression, sleep disturbances, and reduction in daily activities.[23] Lower fitness and physical activity levels are associated with decreased ability to perform activities of daily

---

Box 1
Non-COPD respiratory disorders for which PR may be beneficial

Other conditions associated with airflow obstruction

  Asthma

  CF

  Non-CF diffuse bronchiectasis

Respiratory disorders associated with restrictive physiology

  ILD/pulmonary fibrosis

  Acute respiratory distress syndrome survivors

  Restrictive chest wall disease (scoliosis or kyphosis)

  Selected patients with neuromuscular disease

  Obesity-related respiratory disorders

Other respiratory conditions

  PH

  Lung cancer

  Before and after lung transplantation

  Respiratory impairment related to spinal cord injury

---

living (ADLs), increased psychological distress, impaired QOL,[24–27] and increased risk of asthma exacerbations.[28] Exacerbations may lead to hospitalizations and loss of work and school days. PR has the potential to improve patients' health status and outcomes in regard to all of these issues.

Many studies have reported benefits of exercise training for patients with asthma.[22] Physical exercise has been recognized as having equal or greater importance than other interventions for the deconditioning effects of asthma. A recent systematic review of randomized controlled trials (RCTs) examined 16 studies involving 516 patients between 6 and 18 years with asthma of varying severity.[29] Aerobic capacity, as measured by maximal oxygen uptake (Vo_{2max}) improved after exercise training. Physical training can also improve QOL outcome measures. A Cochrane review published in 2012 examined 19 randomized studies (695 participants) including patients older than 8 years with diagnosed asthma.[22] These trials evaluated patients who performed physical training (ie, running, gymnastics, cycling, swimming, weights, or walking) for at least 20 minutes, 2 times per week, over a minimum period of 4 weeks. The exercise improved Vo_{2max} and maximum ventilation significantly. Physical training was well tolerated, and none of the studies reported worsening of asthma symptoms or adverse effects with training. Several studies also reported statistically and clinically significant improvements in health-related QOL.

Exercise training and PR also improve clinical outcomes for adults with asthma.[30–32] Overall, improvements in cardiovascular conditioning (as measured by Vo_{2max} and decreased maximal exercise heart rate [HR] and minute ventilation), a longer walk distance as measured by the 6-minute walk test (6MWT) or 12-minute walk tests,[22,29,31] improved symptoms,[31,32] improvement in QOL scores,[22,29,31,32] less fear of experiencing breathlessness during exercise, and less anxiety about exercising at high intensities are all gains to be expected through participation in PR.[30]

Breathing exercises such as diaphragmatic and pursed lips breathing,[33] Buteyko breathing, and pranayama breathing with yoga postures may help to reduce symptoms and improve QOL for some patients.[34] In a 2013 Cochrane review[34] incorporating a total of 13 studies of breathing exercises for asthmatic adult patients with mild to moderate disease involving 906 participants, 8 studies reported an improvement in the QOL outcomes and 7 studies showed significant differences favoring breathing exercises for asthma symptoms. However, even although most studies reported positive effects from all variations of breathing exercise, reliable conclusions could not be made concerning the use of breathing exercises for asthma in routine clinical practice.[34]

Some studies have reported that resistive or threshold inspiratory muscle training can lead to improved exercise endurance, with reduced dyspnea, dynamic hyperinflation,[35] and improved pulmonary function,[36] in persons with asthma. Further studies with more detailed protocols and outcomes measures are needed to clarify the role of general breathing exercises and inspiratory muscle training in improving clinical outcomes for asthmatic patients in PR.

The exercise training program recommended for adult patients with asthma participating in PR should ideally include both physical and breathing exercise. Cardiopulmonary exercise testing (CPET) should be considered before beginning training to assess patients for EIB. Warm-up and cool-down periods should be provided routinely to minimize the risk of EIB during training, and patients should use their inhaled bronchodilator before exercise training sessions.

In addition to patient assessment tools used traditionally in PR for patients with COPD, use of some asthma-specific tools relevant to asthma control and QOL should be considered.[27,37,38]

These tools are listed in **Box 2**. The choice of assessment tool should be age appropriate. Reduction in hospitalizations and urgent health care use, impact of PR on daily physical activity levels, and time absent from school or work may be other important outcomes to measure.

Educational topics of particular relevance to patients with asthma are shown in **Box 3**.

Cystic Fibrosis (CF)

CF is an autosomal-recessive disease characterized by impaired chloride secretion, resulting in excessively thick bronchial secretions, altered respiratory mechanics, gas exchange, and pancreatic insufficiency. Because of advances in disease management, the current median predicted survival age for patients with CF has increased steadily from age 31.3 years in 2002 to age 41.1 years as of 2012.[39]

Persons with CF have impaired exercise capacity and low physical activity levels,[40,41] which result from many factors, including pulmonary function, gas exchange and/or cardiocirculatory disturbances, EIB, and skeletal muscle weakness.[12,40] Altered expression of the CF transmembrane regulator in muscle contributes to altered exercise energy metabolism[13] and may contribute to skeletal muscle dysfunction. Moreover, the metabolic demands associated with increased effort of ventilation and pancreatic insufficiency may lead to nutritional impairment, which can contribute to skeletal muscle wasting, reduced bone density, and impaired QOL.[42] Low physical activity levels are also associated with time lost from school, work, or recreational activities,[41] and low exercise tolerance is associated with reduced survival.[15] Patients with CF also have impaired QOL.[43–45] Exacerbations of CF frequently result in hospitalizations, with associated further increase in morbidity.

Several RCTs[46–52] as well as uncontrolled trials[53,54] have reported that various forms of exercise training (including running, swimming, hiking, cycling, and strength training) can improve exercise capacity or muscle strength, regardless of disease severity, for both children and adults with CF. Aerobic training has been shown to generate significant improvements in peak aerobic capacity and QOL, whereas resistance training significantly increases fat free mass, and leg strength.[55] Inspiratory muscle training can also improve respiratory muscle strength,[56] pulmonary function, and exercise tolerance.[57,58] Respiratory muscle strength can also improve through moderate vigorous aerobic exercise.[59] Exercise rehabilitation also improves habitual physical activity[60]

Box 2
Patient assessment and outcomes measurement tools for non-COPD conditions

Asthma

    Juniper Asthma Quality of Life Questionnaire[27]

    Pediatric Asthma Quality of Life Questionnaire[37]

    Asthma Control Questionnaire[38]

CF

    6MWT[65]

    Habitual Activity Estimation Scale[60,66]

    The Cystic Fibrosis Quality of Life Questionnaire[67]

    The Cystic Fibrosis Questionnaire[68]

Non-CF diffuse bronchiectasis

    6MWT[65]

    Leicester Cough Questionnaire[76]

ILD

    CPET, 6MWT, and shuttle walk test[79]

    Borg Dyspnea Score, Medical Research Council dyspnea scale, Baseline Dyspnea Index, Transitional Dyspnea Index, dyspnea component of Chronic Respiratory Questionnaire[77,82,90,92,184]

    Short Form-36[81,86,93]

    St George's Respiratory Questionnaire[81,86]

    World Health Organization Quality of Life Assessment[81]

    IPF-specific version of St George's Respiratory Questionnaire[102]

Restrictive chest wall disease

    Scoliosis Research Society-22 Questionnaire[112]

PH

    6MWT and CPET[116]

    Borg Dyspnea Score[126]

    World Health Organization Functional Class[128]

    Short Form-36[119,123,124,126–128]

    St George's Respiratory Questionnaire[124]

    Minnesota Living with Heart Failure Questionnaire[123]

    Cambridge Pulmonary Hypertension Outcome Review[127]

    Beck Depression Inventory[119]

    Fatigue Severity Scale[135]

    Human Activity Profile[135]

Lung cancer

    Short Form-36 or Short Form-36 version 2[140,142]

    Medical Research Council dyspnea score[157]

    Cancer Dyspnea score[185]

    Functional Assessment of Cancer Therapy-Lung[162,186,187]

    Brief Fatigue Inventory[167]

    Functional Assessment of Cancer Therapy-Fatigue[146,163]

    Spielberger State Anxiety Scale[169]

    Hospital Anxiety and Depression Score[142,146]

    Center for Epidemiologic Studies Short Depression Scale[170]

    European Organization for Research and Treatment of Cancer Quality of Life Questionnaire[146,156,161,170,188]

Box 3
Educational topics for patients with respiratory disorders other than COPD

Asthma

- Recognizing and avoiding triggers
- Recognizing symptoms of exacerbations
- Monitoring peak expiratory flow rate
- Pacing
- Use of pursed lips breathing (minimize dynamic hyperinflation)
- Importance of maintaining physical activity
- Warming up before exercise
- Proper inhaler technique
- Use of action plans (age-appropriate and culture-appropriate)

CF and non-CF bronchiectasis

- Importance of maintaining physical activity
- Pacing
- Pursed lips breathing
- Proper inhaler technique
- Airway secretion clearance techniques
- Recognition and management of acute exacerbations
- Nutritional counseling
- Preparation for or recovery from lung transplantation

ILD

- Nature and expected course of disease
- Symptom management
- Pacing and energy conservation
- Benefits versus potential adverse effects of pharmacologic therapy
- Benefits and proper use of supplemental oxygen
- Body positioning to reduce work of breathing
- Nutritional counseling (avoid weight and muscle loss)
- Coping techniques for anxiety and depression
- Strategies for relaxation and recreation (eg, yoga and tai chi)
- Recognition of disease exacerbations (and when to contact health care provider)
- Preparation for and recovery from lung transplantation
- Advance directives, mechanical ventilation, and end-of-life care

Restrictive chest wall disease

- Airway secretion clearance techniques
- Thoracic mobilization and stretching exercises
- Recognizing signs of infection
- Symptoms and signs of progression of respiratory compromise
- Sleep disturbances (eg, nocturnal hypoventilation)
- Importance of and acclimatization to noninvasive positive pressure ventilation

PH

- Anatomic and physiologic basis of symptoms
- Importance and proper use of supplemental oxygen therapy
- Benefits and risks of PH-specific pharmacologic therapy
- Management of ADLs
- Pacing, energy conservation, and when to stop exercise
- Symptoms and signs of cardiorespiratory decompensation (and when to call the health care provider)
- Risks of pregnancy
- Preparation for and recovery from lung transplantation
- Advance directives/end-of-life care

Lung cancer

- Nutritional counseling
- Anxiety management
- Energy conservation and pacing
- Expected benefits versus risks of treatment (surgery, radiation, or chemotherapy)
- Familiarization with planned surgical procedure (when relevant)
- Preparation for the perioperative period
  - Secretion management
  - Controlled coughing techniques
  - Incentive spirometry
  - Chest tubes
  - Wound and pain management
  - Importance of early mobilization

Lung transplantation

Before transplant:

- Familiarization with the surgical procedure
- Preparation for the perioperative period (as indicated above for lung cancer)
- Disease-specific education topics as noted above

After transplant:

- Importance of physical activity
- Benefits and adverse effects of immunosuppressive medications
- Recognizing symptoms and signs of infection or organ rejection
- Nutritional counseling
- Postoperative physical precautions (based on individuals' needs)

and QOL[53,60] and can reduce the mechanical impedance of sputum,[61] and hence, may be important for optimization of airway clearance.

Goals of exercise training in PR are directed toward improving exercise tolerance and physical activity levels, optimizing functional capacity, increasing upper and lower body strength, optimizing bronchial hygiene, and reducing the rate of disease progression. A combination of aerobic and resistive exercise training and flexibility exercises should ideally be incorporated. Transcutaneous electrical muscle stimulation[62] or interval training[63] can be beneficial, particularly for persons who have difficulty performing conventional exercise training. Supplemental oxygen, if needed, should be titrated to maintain oxygen saturations greater than or equal to 88% to 90% during exercise. Adequate hydration must be maintained, because of the excessive salt excretion and fluid loss during activity. Careful consideration should be given to CF-related diabetes and osteoporosis when creating an exercise plan. To prevent cross-contamination and the spread of resistant organisms, strict hygiene standards, infection control measures, and isolation precautions are essential. Both standard and transmission-based precautions are recommended for all rehabilitation equipment and respiratory devices.[64]

Chest physical therapy (percussion and postural drainage) and airway clearance techniques, such as use of flutter or acapella devices or vibratory vests, are a mainstay of treatment throughout the CF patient's life span, and training regarding their use and benefits should be a core feature of PR for these patients. Precautions should be taken for patients with underlying gastroesophageal reflux, orthopnea, osteoporosis, tube feeds, and coagulopathies. Because postural deviations such as thoracic kyphosis are common among persons with CF, emphasis on postural alignment exercises and routine stretching in PR early in the course of disease may improve altered respiratory mechanics caused by thoracic kyphosis and lung hyperinflation. Outcome assessments for persons with CF may include the 6MWT,[65] CPET, modified shuttle walk test, symptom assessments, and health-related QOL questionnaires.[60,66–68] Given that CF affects both children and adults, questionnaires used must be age appropriate. Questionnaires relevant to patients with CF are shown in **Box 2**. Educational topics of particular importance to persons with CF are shown in **Box 3**.

Non-CF Diffuse Bronchiectasis

Non-CF diffuse bronchiectasis is another chronic, debilitating condition characterized by persistent cough, excessive sputum production, and recurrent chest infections.[69] Chronic airflow obstruction may be present, and intermittent acute exacerbations of symptoms and bronchoconstriction often occur. There are discernible similarities between COPD and bronchiectasis; both conditions have primary pulmonary involvement and secondary peripheral muscle, as well as nutritional and health-related QOL impairments.[70]

A prospective RCT conducted by Newall and colleagues[71] in which the outcomes of 8 weeks of high-intensity exercise training consisting of 45 minutes of stair climbing, bicycle ergometry, and walking with and without inspiratory muscle training were compared with standard medical care showed significant improvements in exercise capacity (treadmill walking endurance and the incremental shuttle walk test), but benefits in health-related QOL assessed by the St George's Respiratory Questionnaire (SGRQ) were reported

only with the combination of inspiratory muscle training and PR.[71] Retrospective studies have also shown that PR improves exercise tolerance and health status[72,73] and may improve some aspects of pulmonary function (vital capacity and residual volume)[74] for patients with non-CF bronchiectasis.

PR strategies for patients with non-CF bronchiectasis are similar to those recommended for patients with COPD and persons with CF. PR staff should implement an individualized and prescribed program of exercise training after an assessment of exercise capacity (eg, with 6MWT),[65] pulmonary hygiene, muscle function, and flexibility. Exercise program components may include endurance training (eg, ambulation, biking, water exercise, arm ergometry), strength and flexibility exercise using dumbbells, cuff weights, weight machines, and therapy bands, and functional activities to improve balance, ADLs, and energy efficiency. Activities to improve respiratory mechanics include pursed lip, diaphragmatic, and paced breathing techniques. As for patients with non-CF bronchiectasis, training regarding use of airway secretion clearance techniques is an essential component of PR.[73,75]

Outcomes measures of particular relevance for patients with non-CF bronchiectasis are shown in **Box 2**. The symptom of cough is one important outcome to assess.[76] Education sessions appropriate for patients with non-CF bronchiectasis are similar to those for persons with CF (see **Box 3**).

PR FOR CONDITIONS ASSOCIATED WITH RESTRICTIVE PHYSIOLOGY
ILD/Pulmonary Fibrosis

ILD (diffuse parenchymal lung disease) is a heterogeneous group of disorders in which the lung interstitium and/or alveolar spaces are involved with varying degrees (and differing histopathologic patterns) of inflammation or fibrosis. Typical symptoms of ILD include disabling exertional dyspnea,[77,78] nonproductive cough, and fatigue, and other symptoms may also be present when the ILD is part of a systemic disease.

Patients with ILD also have reduced exercise tolerance[79] and low physical activity levels[80] and experience depression[78] and impaired QOL.[81] Exercise limitation in ILD has a multifactorial basis,[79] including ventilatory, cardiocirculatory, and gas exchange derangements. Resting pulmonary function testing does not reliably predict exercise limitation in ILD.[79] Exercise-induced hypoxemia is often profound. In addition, skeletal muscle dysfunction can contribute to exercise impairment among patients with ILD.[10,82] In one study of 12 persons with ILD, the symptom of leg fatigue was the principal cause of cessation of exercise in 17% and led to cessation of exercise together with the symptom of dyspnea in 58% of patients.[83] Quadriceps force correlates to the symptom of leg fatigue during exercise[84] as well as to Vo_{2max} (maximal oxygen uptake),[10] 6-minute walk distance (6MWD),[85] and depression.[84] Low exercise tolerance is associated with worse QOL and lower survival.[86,87] Participation in PR has potential to improve these outcomes.

A further rationale for PR for patients with ILD lies in the fact that limited pharmacologic treatment options are available for many. Persons with end-stage pulmonary fibrosis often face consideration of and preparation for lung transplantation, yet they frequently have knowledge deficits pertaining to their disease and treatment options.[88] PR is a recommended as a component of care in the ATS/ERS guidelines on idiopathic pulmonary fibrosis (IPF)[2] and is typically required of patients before they undergo lung transplantation.

Several studies have demonstrated that patients with ILD can benefit from PR.[89] Most of the studies conducted have been fairly small cohort studies, but 2 RCTs are available.[90,91] In most of the studies, including the RCTs, PR has led to significant improvements in 6MWD.[82,91–95] Most[19,82,90,92,95–97] but not all[91,93] have also reported post-PR improvements in dyspnea, and when investigated, most have reported improvements in QOL.[19,90,91,93,96,97] Most of the PR programs in these studies have been outpatient programs of 8 to 12 weeks' duration, in which patients underwent supervised multimodality aerobic and strength training of the lower and upper extremities as well as participated in an education program. The optimal content and duration of the exercise training regimen for patients with ILD remains uncertain.

It is not yet clear whether gains in 6MWD achieved by persons with ILD are comparable with those gained by patients with COPD, because existing studies have yielded conflicting results.[19,20,98] The duration of benefit may be shorter lived than that seen after PR among patients with COPD.[90,92] Among a group of 57 persons with ILD (34 of whom had IPF), the significant gains in 6MWD that were present 9 weeks after an 8-week PR program were no longer evident at 6 months after PR.[90] Longer duration PR (24 weeks) may also lead to greater gains in 6MWD.[82] The type and severity of ILD may also influence outcomes of PR. The findings of a systematic review[99] evaluating outcomes of physical training for persons with ILD suggested that persons with a known diagnosis of IPF, persons with severe lung disease or with exertional O_2 desaturation might not achieve comparable gains in 6MWD to those without these features. A more recent study[92] confirmed these findings; among 44 patients with ILD who underwent 8 weeks of outpatient PR, those with IPF had a lesser magnitude of gains in both 6MWD and in the dyspnea component of the Chronic Respiratory Disease Questionnaire compared with other forms of ILD. Among the patients with IPF in that cohort, lesser severity of disease (as measured by forced vital capacity, degree of exercise O_2 desaturation, and right ventricular systolic pressure) was associated with greater improvements in 6MWD. The severity of baseline dyspnea assessed by the Medical Research Council dyspnea scale affects the magnitude of PR-induced gains in 6MWD, quadriceps force, and ADL scores achieved by some persons with IPF.[100] Thus, persons with IPF, particularly those with more severe lung disease, may not achieve the same magnitude of clinical benefits after PR as those with less severe disease or non-IPF ILD. Another RCT of exercise training among patients with ILD is under way.[101]

Exercise training in PR for persons with ILD generally includes aerobic (endurance) and strength training of the lower and upper extremities. Patients should be assessed for medical comorbidities such as joint involvement associated with the ILD (eg, such as can occur with autoimmune diseases), which might affect the exercise prescription. Strong emphasis on pacing and energy conservation techniques is helpful. Patients should be assessed for their supplemental O_2 requirements before and during PR, and Sao_2 (arterial oxygen saturation) should be kept greater than 88% to 90% during exercise when possible. High Fio_2 (fraction of inspired oxygen) up to 100% (or high flow) may be required to maintain adequate oxygenation during exercise.

Patient assessment and outcomes measures suitable for use among patients with ILD are shown in **Box 2**. An IPF-specific version of the SGRQ is now available for use.[102] Education topics of particular relevance to patients with ILD are shown in **Box 3**.

Restrictive Chest Wall Disease

Chest wall deformities such as scoliosis and kyphosis are common in both pediatric and adult populations. Impairments associated with these deformities include abnormal pulmonary function (restrictive physiology with limitation of lung expansion), gas exchange disturbances (principally related to hypoventilation), and cardiovascular alterations, as well as clinical symptoms of dyspnea on exertion, cough, easy fatigability, pain in the anterior chest, tachycardia, and chronic mucus expectoration.[103–105] Elderly people with hyperkyphosis experience worsened physical deconditioning[106] and are at increased risk of falls.[105] In older individuals, hyperkyphosis is also associated with earlier mortality caused by pneumonia, asthma, or COPD.[107] Thus, strategies to improve health outcomes are needed for patients with restrictive chest wall disease.

Recommended treatments of respiratory abnormalities for persons with chest wall deformities include approaches that address improvement of respiratory mechanics and improvement of the skeletal structure of the spine and rib cage. Such techniques include respiratory exercise therapy, general physical conditioning, muscle and spinal exercise-based interventions, pharmacotherapy to delay progression of kyphosis, spinal orthotics and postural taping, and surgical interventions.[104,105]

The effectiveness of exercise training in treating adolescent patients with scoliosis was examined in a systematic review.[108] Although exercise did not conclusively prevent the progression of spinal curvature, general strength, neuromotor control, and stability of the spine increased, and breathing function and postural balance improved.[108] Two more recent studies also showed that 8 to 12 weeks of aerobic exercise training, including treadmill walking, arm ergometry, and bicycling, can benefit patients with scoliosis; gains in 6MWT[109,110] and lung function[110] were noted.

Asymmetric mobilization breathing exercise therapy for scoliosis may improve spirometry measures of pulmonary function.[111] Bronchial hygiene (postural drainage and vibration), and relaxation techniques promoting decreased respiratory effort and control of dyspnea have also been effective for patients with scoliosis or pectus excavatum.[103,104] Thoracic mobilization and strengthening exercises may consist of mid to low back stretches, side-bending with arms held overhead, quadruped with unilateral arm and leg lifts, and bilateral posterior shoulder girdle exercise. The Scoliosis Research Society Questionnaire has been used to measure QOL among persons with scoliosis (see **Box 2**),[112] but it has not yet been tested in the context of PR. Educational topics of particular relevance to these patients are shown in **Box 3**.

PR FOR OTHER RESPIRATORY DISORDERS
Pulmonary Hypertension (PH)

PH, defined as an elevation in mean pulmonary artery pressure above 25 mm Hg at rest or higher than 30 mm Hg with exercise, arises from a wide variety of conditions.[113] Pulmonary arterial hypertension (PAH) is a condition that results from structural remodeling of pulmonary arteries and endothelial dysfunction in the absence of underlying left-sided cardiac disease, parenchymal lung disease or direct involvement of the pulmonary venous circulation. Currently available pharmacologic therapies have led to improved clinical outcomes for many persons with PH.[3] The principal symptoms of PH include exertional dyspnea and exercise/activity intolerance, atypical chest pain, palpitations, dizziness, and fatigue.

Exercise capacity is impaired among persons with PH[114–116] as a result of multiple factors.[114,117] In addition to pulmonary function, gas exchange, and cardiocirculatory impairments, some patients with PH, especially those with PAH, have skeletal muscle dysfunction, characterized by reduced quadriceps muscle strength, lower proportion of type I (slow twitch, endurance) muscle fibers, and altered muscle oxidative enzyme characteristics, favoring anaerobic energy metabolism compared with sedentary healthy individuals.[35] These changes correlated to exercise capacity (maximal oxygen uptake during exercise). As is true for persons with COPD, ILD, and CF, low exercise capacity in persons with PAH is associated with worse clinical outcomes.[17,116] Peak Vo_2 (oxygen consumption) of 10.4 mL/min/kg[17] or less and 6MWD less than 332 m[116] have been associated with worse survival.

In addition, patients with PAH report symptoms of fatigue,[118] anxiety, and depression,[119,120] may have cognitive impairment,[119,121] and report impaired QOL.[119,122–125] These impairments often persist despite optimized medical therapy, and many patients eventually face lung transplantation. Thus, additional strategies for patient management are needed.

Several studies have now shown that PR and exercise training administered carefully are safe, well tolerated, and can improve several of these clinical outcomes for patients with PH. A prospective RCT by Mereles and colleagues[126] first demonstrated that a 15-week program of rehabilitation (3 weeks inpatient followed by 12 weeks outpatient) led to significant gains in 6MWD, improved World Health Organization (WHO) functional class, improved peak Vo_2, and improved QOL among a cohort of 30 patients with PAH (n = 23) and PH caused by chronic thromboembolic disease (n = 7). Subsequently, other studies have also reported improvements in clinical outcomes, including increased peak work rate[127] and Vo_{2max},[128,129] improved WHO or New York Heart Association (NYHA) functional class,[128,130–132] improved exercise endurance,[127,129–131] and improved QOL.[127,128,130,131] The comparative features of these studies are shown in **Table 1**. All of these studies included fairly small numbers of patients, the mean pulmonary artery pressure in the patient populations studied did not exceed 57 mm Hg (see **Table 1**), and all patients studied were believed to be on optimized medical therapy, with no changes made in pharmacologic therapy during the course of the rehabilitation. Also, all the exercise training was supervised, and continuous HR or O_2 saturation monitoring was used during exercise training sessions in most of the studies. Supplemental oxygen was provided to avoid desaturations less than 88% to 90%,[128,129] and the intensity of exercise was limited to 60% to 80% of maximal HR identified during pretraining CPET or to 70% to 80% of HR reserve.[127] No serious adverse events occurred as a consequence of rehabilitation in most of these studies, although transient dizziness (without syncope) was reported by a few patients,[126,128,133] and an episode of syncope occurred in 1 larger cohort study by Grunig and colleagues.[130] Twelve weeks of exercise training in outpatient PR also led to improvements in skeletal muscle function, with a relative increase in the proportion of type I endurance muscle fibers and relative decrease in type IIx fibers, which correlated to reductions in isotime CO_2 output and VE (minute ventilation rate)/Vco_2 (rate of elimination of CO_2) during exercise.[133] A recent study using magnetic resonance imaging showed that exercise training was associated with increases in pulmonary blood volume and peak velocity of pulmonary blood flow.[134] A recent small RCT[135] among 24 patients with PAH also reported significant improvements in fatigue and physical activity after 10 weeks of outpatient PR. Increased patient-reported physical activity levels were also noted among an exercise training group but not a control group in a recent study by Chan and colleagues.[127]

Although no formal guidelines for exercise training and rehabilitation yet exist for patients with PH, a suggested approach based on existing evidence is shown in **Box 4**.

Patient assessment and outcomes measurement tools suitable for use with patients with PH in PR are shown in **Box 2**. Educational topics of particular importance to persons with PH are shown in **Box 3**.

Lung Cancer

There exists a strong rationale for providing PR to patients with lung cancer. First, lung cancer is present concurrently with COPD for many patients[136]; it may also complicate other forms of chronic respiratory disease and has poor overall survival.[137] Patients may have ventilatory impairment or gas exchange disturbances, and commonly have comorbidities, including anemia and cachexia, and may have knowledge deficits regarding their disease. Second, lung cancer poses a high symptom burden on patients; common symptoms include dyspnea, cough, fatigue, and pain.[138–140] Persons with lung cancer also often experience sleep disturbances, anxiety, depression, and fear[141] and report impaired QOL.[141,142]

Also, persons with lung cancer often have exercise intolerance and functional disability. In addition to structural changes in the lungs and gas exchange disturbances, skeletal muscle weakness is common. Patients are often deconditioned because of low physical activity levels.[14,143] Muscle weakness in lung patients who have lung cancer also relates to chronic systemic inflammation and cachexia[144] or may relate to paraneoplastic syndromes such as Eaton-Lambert syndrome.[145] The presence of muscle weakness has been associated with the symptom of fatigue.[146] Low exercise tolerance is associated with worse surgical outcomes after resection of malignancy,[18,147] worse responses to chemotherapy (in terms of toxicity and disease progression-free intervals)[138,148] and is associated with reduced survival.[18,147]

Low exercise tolerance (eg, $Vo_{2max} < 15$ mL/kg/min, 6MWD < 61 m [200 ft], or inability to climb a flight of stairs) is also associated with greater risk of postoperative pulmonary complications after lung resection surgery, and this parameter may be used to exclude patients from undergoing lung resection surgery.[18] PR has the potential to improve exercise capacity such that patients considered inoperable may become candidates for potentially curative surgical treatment; those with relatively low performance status may become candidates for chemotherapy. Moreover, exercise tolerance remains impaired after lung resection surgery,[149,150] and thus, interventions to improve exercise tolerance are still needed for such persons. Moreover, patients with lung cancer are often faced with making difficult choices regarding complex treatment regimens, and there is limited time for patient education in the routine clinical setting for discussions that would enable patients to make fully informed choices regarding their treatment. PR programs offer an environment

Table 1
Clinical trials of exercise training/rehabilitation for patients with PH

Reference	Number of Patients	Design	Pulmonary Artery Pressure (mm Hg)	Training Method	Continuous O$_2$, HR, or Telemetry Monitoring	Change in Outcome			
						Exercise Capacity	Dyspnea	QOL	WHO or NYHA Class
Mereles et al,[126] 2006	30	RCT	Mean 50 ± 15	Low workload, interval cycling; low-intensity strength training, respiratory muscle training, walking	Yes: O$_2$ and HR	+	NA	+	+
Mainguy et al,[133] 2010	5	Cohort	Mean 45 ± 16	Cycling, treadmill, weights, interval	Yes: O$_2$	+	NA	NA	NA
Martinez-Quintana et al,[132] 2010	8	Cohort	Systolic 101.7 ± 28	Stretching, interval cycling, low-intensity strength	Not specified	+	–	–	+
Fox et al,[129] 2011	22	Cohort	Mean 57 ± 6	Interval, continuous aerobic, step climbing, low-intensity strength	Yes: O$_2$	+	–	NA	–
Grunig et al,[128] 2011	58	Cohort	Mean 51 ± 15	Low-intensity cycling, walking, low-intensity strength, respiratory muscle training	Yes: O$_2$ and HR	+	–	+	+
Chan et al,[127] 2013	23	RCT	Mean 40 ± 13.8	Treadmill walking	Yes: O$_2$, HR	+	NA	+	NA

For each of the outcomes in the table, + indicates there was improvement, – indicates there was no improvement, and NA indicates the parameter was not measured.

in which patients' understanding of therapeutic options can be enhanced and patients can be prepared for or assisted in their recovery from treatments. Persons who are either too debilitated to tolerate selected treatments or are nonadherent to therapies can also be identified.

Several studies have documented clinical benefits of PR among persons with lung cancer. Preoperative PR before lung cancer resection surgery can lead to improved exercise endurance (6MWD or cycling endurance),[151,152] increased Vo_{2max},[151,153] and improved muscle strength,[152] and in 1 small RCT[154] was associated with shorter postoperative length of stay, fewer chest tube days, and fewer postoperative pulmonary complications compared with a breathing exercise intervention. In the study by Bobbio and colleagues,[153] some patients considered nonoperative candidates based on Vo_{2max} during baseline CPET had improvements in Vo_{2max} after PR such that

they became candidates for lung resection surgery. The duration of PR offered preoperatively in these studies ranged from 4 to 7 weeks. In one,[152] the preoperative training program was successfully implemented at home.

Postoperative PR has also led to improvements in exercise endurance,[155–160] strength,[161] peak work rate,[155,162] and reduced dyspnea.[157] Some[158,162] but not all[160] trials of postresection PR have reported improvement in QOL. Patients' postoperative pain may limit perceived improvement in QOL for some patients.[160] For patients with lung cancer undergoing chemotherapy or radiation therapy, PR can improve strength, endurance, health status, and sense of well-being.[163–166] Most of the existing studies of PR for patients with lung cancer are small, and of observational design. Larger studies are still needed to confirm their findings.

Given the complexity of patients' health care needs, a multidisciplinary PR team is desirable for patients who have lung cancer when feasible. Patients must be monitored closely for comorbidities or sequelae of treatment that might affect their safety to participate in exercise training (eg, development of anemia, thrombocytopenia, or immunocompromise after chemotherapy, involvement of long bones, spine, or brain with metastases, ataxia). The type, intensity, and duration of exercise training should be guided by the clinical circumstances. For persons who are severely debilitated, the emphasis of rehabilitation may be focused on optimizing functional independence, such that persons can continue living at home, rather than on traditional outcomes of exercise training such as improvement in 6MWD. Alternative muscle training strategies such as transcutaneous electrical muscle stimulation can be considered for persons too weak or debilitated to undergo traditional aerobic or strength exercise training or who have orthopedic issues that preclude routine training. Patient assessment and outcomes measures suitable for patients with lung cancer are shown in **Box 2**. Because fatigue, anxiety, and depression are prominent features of lung cancer, and because PR may improve these symptoms, their measurement should be considered.[167–170] Educational topics of particular relevance to patients with lung cancer are shown in **Box 3**.

PR Before and After Lung Transplantation

Before transplant

PR plays a vital role when managing lung transplant patients preoperatively. Because of the severe and progressive nature of the underlying diseases, optimization of function is essential for those awaiting transplant. Patients must be monitored closely and a disease-specific approach must be taken.

There are no formal guidelines regarding the content of pretransplant PR. Suggested content is shown in **Box 5**.

Although disease severity is typically high, pre-transplantation PR improves functional outcomes, including the 6MWT[171,172] and QOL.[172] One recent study supports that every 100-m increase in 6MWD correlates with a 2.6-day decrease in median hospital length of stay.[173] Preoperative PR may also reduce the risk of postoperative complications, and patients with characteristics that are not favorable to undergoing major surgery may also be identified.

After transplant

Regardless of the underlying diagnosis or lung disease before transplant, and despite near

---

Box 5
Suggested content and process of PR for the lung transplant patient

Before transplantation:

- Begin with initial evaluation that examines hemodynamic stability, oxygen requirements, bone health, body mass index, medical comorbidities, respiratory mechanics, and overall functional capacity

- Complete patient assessment using psychological and health-related QOL measures,[189] shortness of breath questionnaires, manual muscle testing, 30-second sit to stand test, and 6MWT[80]

- PR should consist of exercise training, including progressive aerobic exercise and upper/lower extremity strengthening under close supervision and continuous monitoring

- Exercise should begin at low intensity and be progressed gradually to the highest capacity tolerated by the individual, maintaining adequate oxygenation during activity

- Place strong emphasis on patient/caregiver education, as well as psychological and dietary support

- Frequent reassessments are necessary because of the progression of the underlying lung disease; close communication with patients' health care providers outside PR is essential

After transplantation:

- Begin ∼24 hours postoperatively, with an emphasis on early mobilization, breathing exercises, secretion clearance, and posture

- Early, inpatient postoperative rehabilitation should include breathing retraining, reassessing supplemental oxygen requirements, balancing activities, building upper and lower extremity range of motion, and managing any neuropathic pain

- Because of incisional pain and the denervated cough reflex of the donor lung, patients require direction and encouragement to cough

- Begin ambulation using a specialized walker, with careful management of chest tubes and pain

- Exercise progression should gradually incorporate upper and lower extremity resistance training. Lifting and range of motion precautions and limitations persist up to 6 weeks postoperatively dependent on the type of surgical approach. Ensure that lower extremity strength, balance, and gait are sufficient to ensure patient safety and minimize the risk of falls before hospital discharge

- Train patients and caregivers in the titration of supplemental oxygen as needed in the postoperative setting

- Necessary medical and adaptive equipment should be provided at discharge

- Outpatient PR may resume immediately after hospital discharge. Functional capacity (eg, 6MWT or CPET) and strength measurements must be performed to establish a postoperative baseline. The CPET may be used to associate exercise capacity with mortality up to 2 years after transplant[190]

- Progress the exercise training to higher intensity and duration over time (patients no longer limited by ventilatory impairment)

- Monitor underlying comorbidities such as diabetes and osteoporosis; activities that include excessive flexion and rotation should be avoided to reduce the risk of possible vertebral compression fracture. Blood glucose must be carefully monitored, because adjustments may occur frequently as a result of the influx of multiple postoperative medications and corticosteroids

normalization in lung function after transplant, activity intolerance often persists for years. Patients may reach only 50% of predicted exercise capacity 30 months postoperatively.[174] Skeletal muscle weakness and dysfunction, including reductions in type I endurance muscle fibers and altered oxidative enzymes favoring anaerobic metabolism,[175] play an important role in posttransplantation exercise impairment.[176–178] Posttransplantation skeletal muscle dysfunction likely relates, at least in part, to deconditioning associated with immobilization during hospitalization, glucocorticoid therapy, and immunosuppressive medications.[179]

Posttransplantation PR, including ambulation, resistive exercises, and cycling, can significantly improve quadriceps force, functional capacity, and QOL.[180–183] Suggested content and progress of postoperative rehabilitation are shown in **Box 5**. Education topics of particular importance for the patient recovering from lung transplantation are shown in **Box 3**.

PRACTICAL CHALLENGES OF PROVIDING PR TO PERSONS WITH RESPIRATORY DISORDERS OTHER THAN COPD

Provision of PR to persons with disorders other than COPD poses several practical challenges. First, it requires PR care providers to be familiar with the anatomic, physiologic, and clinical features of, as well as treatment options for, these diverse disorders. This in turn poses the challenge of providing educational sessions and reading materials to and assessing competencies of staff members whose clinical experience may have been limited largely to caring for patients with COPD. Second, although a multidisciplinary PR team, including a physiotherapist, exercise physiologist, nurse, respiratory therapist, occupational therapist, nutritional therapist, pharmacologist, psychologist, and the program medical director, is desirable, resources are limited at many PR programs. Close partnering between PR staff, referring health care providers, and other rehabilitation specialists in the community is, therefore, crucial. As always in PR, the interventions must be designed and implemented to meet individuals' needs and goals. Third, it can be challenging to incorporate patients with non-COPD diagnoses (often a single patient or a few patients) and varying degrees of disease severity into a group of patients with COPD undergoing PR. This issue affects staffing needs, logistics, time, and patient safety considerations, as well as the need to broaden the scope of didactic educational sessions and written educational materials. Also, it cannot be assumed that all the same patient assessment and outcomes measures tools used in PR among patients with COPD are appropriate and valid for measuring outcomes of PR among patients with disorders other than COPD. A range of disease-appropriate and age-appropriate patient assessment and outcomes measurement tools must be available for use by the PR staff, as discussed earlier and as shown in **Box 2**.

SUMMARY

PR is an important therapeutic intervention that should no longer be considered suitable only for patients with COPD. A strong rationale exists for providing PR to persons with a broad range of respiratory disorders other than COPD. Evidence shows that PR for these patients is feasible, safe, and effective. A disease-relevant approach should be undertaken based on individuals' needs. Further research is needed to better understand the optimal program content, duration, and outcomes measures, to enable patients to achieve maximal benefits of PR.

REFERENCES

1. Spruit MA, Singh SJ, Garvey C, et al. An official American Thoracic Society/European Respiratory Society statement: key concepts and advances in pulmonary rehabilitation. Am J Respir Crit Care Med 2013;188(8):e13–64.
2. Raghu G, Collard HR, Egan JJ, et al. An official ATS/ERS/JRS/ALAT statement: idiopathic pulmonary fibrosis: evidence-based guidelines for diagnosis and management. Am J Respir Crit Care Med 2011;183:788–824.
3. Galie N, Hoeper MM, Humbert M, et al. Guidelines for the diagnosis and treatment of pulmonary hypertension. Eur Heart J 2009;30:2493–537.
4. Nici L, Donner C, Wouters E, et al. American Thoracic Society/European Respiratory Society statement on pulmonary rehabilitation. Am J Respir Crit Care Med 2006;173:1390–413.
5. Skeletal muscle dysfunction in chronic obstructive pulmonary disease. A statement of the American Thoracic Society and European Respiratory Society. Am J Respir Crit Care Med 1999;159:S1–40.
6. Paz-Diaz H, Montes de Oca M, Lopez JM, et al. Pulmonary rehabilitation improves depression, anxiety, dyspnea and health status in patients with COPD. Am J Phys Med Rehabil 2007;86:30–6.
7. Puhan MA, Gimeno-Santos E, Scharplatz M, et al. Pulmonary rehabilitation following exacerbations of chronic obstructive pulmonary disease. Cochrane Database Syst Rev 2011;(10):CD005305.

8. Seymour JM, Moore L, Jolley CJ, et al. Outpatient pulmonary rehabilitation following acute exacerbations of COPD. Thorax 2010;65:423–8.

9. Ries AL, Bauldoff GS, Carlin BW, et al. Pulmonary rehabilitation: joint ACCP/AACVPR evidence-based clinical practice guidelines. Chest 2007; 131:4S–42S.

10. Nishiyama O, Taniguchi H, Kondoh Y, et al. Quadriceps weakness is related to exercise capacity in idiopathic pulmonary fibrosis. Chest 2005;127: 2028–33.

11. Mainguy V, Maltais F, Saey D, et al. Peripheral muscle dysfunction in idiopathic pulmonary arterial hypertension. Thorax 2010;65:113–7.

12. Troosters T, Langer D, Vrijsen B, et al. Skeletal muscle weakness, exercise tolerance and physical activity in adults with cystic fibrosis. Eur Respir J 2009;33(1):99–106.

13. Lamhonwah AM, Bear CE, Huan LJ, et al. Cystic fibrosis transmembrane conductance regulator in human muscle: dysfunction causes abnormal metabolic recovery in exercise. Ann Neurol 2010; 67(6):802–8.

14. Coups EJ, Park BJ, Feinstein MB, et al. Physical activity among lung cancer survivors: changes across the cancer trajectory and associations with quality of life. Cancer Epidemiol Biomarkers Prev 2009;18:664–72.

15. Nixon PA, Orenstein DM, Kelsey SF, et al. The prognostic value of exercise testing in patients with cystic fibrosis. N Engl J Med 1992;327:1785–8.

16. Kawut SM, O'Shea MK, Bartels MN, et al. Exercise testing determines survival in patients with diffuse parenchymal lung disease evaluated for lung transplantation. Respir Med 2005;99:1431–9.

17. Wensel R, Opitz CF, Anker SD, et al. Assessment of survival in patients with primary pulmonary hypertension: importance of cardiopulmonary exercise testing. Circulation 2002;106:319–24.

18. Brunelli A, Kim AW, Berger KI, et al. Physiologic evaluation of the patient being considered for lung resectional surgery: diagnosis and management of lung cancer 3rd ed., American College of Chest Physicians evidence-based clinical practice guidelines. Chest 2013;143(Suppl 5):e1665–905.

19. Ferreira G, Feuerman M, Spiegler P. Results of an 8-week, outpatient pulmonary rehabilitation program on patients with and without chronic obstructive pulmonary disease. J Cardiopulm Rehabil 2006;26:54–60.

20. Foster S, Thomas HM III. Pulmonary rehabilitation in lung disease other than chronic obstructive pulmonary disease. Am Rev Respir Dis 1990;141:601–4.

21. Ritz T, Rosenfield D, Steptoe A. Physical activity, lung function, and shortness of breath in the daily life of individuals with asthma. Chest 2010;138(4): 913–8.

22. Carson K, Chandratilleke M, Picot J, et al. Physical training for asthma (Review). Cochrane Database Syst Rev 2013;(9):CD001116.

23. Wertz DA, Pollack M, Rodgers K, et al. Impact of asthma control on sleep, attendance at work, normal activities and disease burden. Ann Allergy Asthma Immunol 2010;105(2):118–23.

24. Clark CJ, Cochrane LM. Assessment of work performance in asthma for determination of cardiorespiratory fitness and training capacity. Thorax 1988;43:745–9.

25. Adams RJ, Wilson DH, Taylor AW, et al. Psychological factors and asthma quality of life: a population based study. Thorax 2004;59:930–5.

26. Katz PP, Gregorich S, Eisner M, et al. Disability in valued life activities among individuals with COPD and other respiratory conditions. J Cardiopulm Rehabil Prev 2010;30:126–36.

27. Juniper EF, Guyatt GH, Epstein RS, et al. Evaluation of impairment of health related quality of life in asthma: development of a questionnaire for use in clinical trials. Thorax 1992;47:76–83.

28. Garcia-Aymerich J, Varraso R, Anto JM, et al. Prospective study of physical activity and risk of asthma exacerbations in older women. Am J Respir Crit Care Med 2009;179:999–1003.

29. Crosbie A. The effect of physical training in children with asthma on pulmonary function, aerobic capacity and health-related quality of life: a systematic review of randomized control trials. Pediatr Exerc Sci 2012;24(3):472–89.

30. Emtner M, Herala M, Stalenheim G. High-intensity physical training in adults with asthma: a 10-week rehabilitation program. Chest 1996;109(2):323–30.

31. Mendes FA, Goncalves RC, Nunes MP, et al. Effects of aerobic training on psychosocial morbidity and symptoms in patients with asthma. Chest 2010;138(2):331–7.

32. Turner S, Eastwood P, Cook A, et al. Improvements in symptoms and quality of life following exercise training in older adults with moderate/severe persistent asthma. Respiration 2011;81:302–10.

33. Osiadlo G, Plewa M, Zebrowska A, et al. Pulmonary physiotherapy in patients with bronchial asthma. Adv Exp Med Biol 2013;755:111–5.

34. Freitas D, Holloway E, Bruno S, et al. Breathing exercises for adults with asthma (Review). Cochrane Database Syst Rev 2013;(10):CD001277.

35. Turner LA, Mickleborough TD, McConnell AK, et al. Effect of inspiratory muscle training on exercise tolerance in asthmatic individuals. Med Sci Sports Exerc 2011;43(11):2031–8.

36. Shaw BS, Shaw I. Pulmonary function and abdominal and thoracic kinematic changes following aerobic and inspiratory resistive diaphragmatic breathing training in asthmatics. Lung 2011; 189(2):131–9.

37. Okelo SO, Wu AW, Krishnan JA, et al. Emotional quality-of-life and outcomes in adolescents with asthma. J Pediatr 2004;145(4):523–9.

38. Juniper EF, O'Byrne PM, Guyatt GH, et al. Development and validation of a questionnaire to measure asthma control. Eur Respir J 1999;14:902–7.

39. Cystic Fibrosis Foundation Patient Registry. 2012 Annual Data Report. Bethesda (MD). Available at: http://www.cff.org/UploadedFiles/research/Clinical-Research/PatientRegistryReport/2012-CFF-Patient-Registry.pdf. Accessed April 7, 2014.

40. Tejero-Garcia S, Giraldez Sanchez MA, Cejudo P, et al. Bone health, daily physical activity, and exercise tolerance in patients with cystic fibrosis. Chest 2011;140:475–81.

41. Rasekaba TM, Button BM, Wilson JW, et al. Reduced physical activity associated with work and transport in adults with cystic fibrosis. J Cyst Fibros 2013;12(3):229–33.

42. Pianosi P, Leblanc J, Almudevar A. Relationship between FEV_1 and peak oxygen uptake in children with cystic fibrosis. Pediatr Pulmonol 2005;40(4):324–9.

43. De Jong W, Kaptein AA, van der Schans CP, et al. Quality of life in patients with cystic fibrosis. Pediatr Pulmonol 1997;23:95–100.

44. Hogg M, Braithwaite M, Barley M, et al. Work disability in adults with cystic fibrosis and its relationship to quality of life. J Cyst Fibros 2007;6(3):223–7.

45. Rickert KA, Bartlett SJ, Boyle MP, et al. The association between depression, lung function and health-related quality of life among adults with cystic fibrosis. Chest 2007;132(1):231–7.

46. Schneiderman-Walker J, Pollock SL, Corey M, et al. A randomized controlled trial of a 3 year home exercise program in cystic fibrosis. J Pediatr 2000;136:304–10.

47. Selvadurai HC, Blimkie CJ, Meyers N, et al. Randomized controlled study of in-hospital exercise training programs in children with cystic fibrosis. Pediatr Pulmonol 2002;33:194–200.

48. Klijn PH, Oudshoorn A, van der Ent CK, et al. Effects of anaerobic training in children with cystic fibrosis. Chest 2004;125:1299–305.

49. Moorcroft AJ, Dodd ME, Morris J, et al. Individualised unsupervised exercise training in adults with cystic fibrosis: a 1 year randomized controlled trial. Thorax 2004;59:1074–80.

50. Hebestreit H, Kieser S, Junge S, et al. Long-term effects of a partially supervised conditioning programme in cystic fibrosis. Eur Respir J 2010;35:578–83.

51. Orenstein DM, Hovell MF, Mulvihill M, et al. Strength vs. aerobic training in children with cystic fibrosis: a randomized controlled trial. Chest 2004;126:1204.

52. Cerny FJ. Relative effects of bronchial drainage and exercise for in-hospital care of patients with cystic fibrosis. Phys Ther 1989;69:633–9.

53. Bradley J, Moran F. Physical training for cystic fibrosis. Cochrane Database Syst Rev 2008;(1):CD002768.

54. Strauss GD, Osher A, Wang C-I, et al. Variable weight training in cystic fibrosis. Chest 1987;92(2):273–6.

55. Wilkes DL, Schneiderman JE, Nguyen T, et al. Exercise and physical activity in children with cystic fibrosis. Paediatr Respir Rev 2009;10(3):105–9.

56. De Jong W, van Aalderen WM, Kraan J, et al. Inspiratory muscle training in patients with cystic fibrosis. Respir Med 2001;95(1):31–6.

57. Sawyer EH, Clanton TL. Improved pulmonary function and exercise tolerance with inspiratory muscle conditioning in children with cystic fibrosis. Chest 1993;104:1490–7.

58. Enright S, Chatham K, Ionescu AA, et al. Inspiratory muscle training improves lung function and exercise capacity in adults with cystic fibrosis. Chest 2004;126:405–11.

59. Dassios T, Katelari A, Doudounakis S, et al. Aerobic exercise and respiratory muscle strength in patients with cystic fibrosis. Respir Med 2013;107(5):684–90.

60. Paranjape SM, Barnes LA, Carson KA, et al. Exercise improves lung function and habitual activity in children with cystic fibrosis. J Cyst Fibros 2012;11(1):18–23.

61. Dwyer TJ, Alison JA, McKeough ZJ, et al. Effects of exercise on respiratory flow and sputum properties in patients with cystic fibrosis. Chest 2011;139:870–7.

62. Vivodtzev I, Decorte N, Wuyam B, et al. Benefits of neuromuscular electrical stimulation prior to endurance training in patients with cystic fibrosis and severe pulmonary dysfunction. Chest 2013;143(2):485–93.

63. Gruber W, Orenstein DM, Braumann KM, et al. Interval training in cystic fibrosis–effect on exercise capacity in severely affected adults. J Cyst Fibros 2014;13(1):86–91.

64. Saiman L, Siegel J. Infection control recommendations for patients with cystic fibrosis: microbiology, important pathogens, and infection control practices to prevent patient-to-patient transmission. Infect Control Hosp Epidemiol 2003;24:S6–52.

65. Lee AL, Button BM, Ellis S, et al. Clinical determinants of the 6 minute walk test in bronchiectasis. Respir Med 2009;103:780–5.

66. Wells GD, Wilkes DL, Schneiderman-Walker J, et al. Reliability and validity of the habitual activity estimation scale (HAES) in patients with cystic fibrosis. Pediatr Pulmonol 2008;43(4):345–53.

67. Gee L, Abbott J, Conway SP, et al. Development of a disease specific health related quality of life measure for adults and adolescents with cystic fibrosis. Thorax 2000;55:946–54.

68. Quittner AL, Buu A, Messer MA, et al. Development and validation of the cystic fibrosis questionnaire in the United States: a health-related quality-of-life measure for cystic fibrosis. Chest 2005;128:2347–54.

69. Smith MP. Non-cystic fibrosis bronchiectasis. J R Coll Physicians Edinb 2011;41:132–9 [quiz: 139].

70. Goldstein RS. Exercise training and inspiratory muscle training in patients with bronchiectasis. Thorax 2005;60(11):889–90.

71. Newall C, Stockley RA, Hill SL. Exercise training and inspiratory muscle training in patients with bronchiectasis. Thorax 2005;60(11):943–8.

72. Ong HK, Lee AL, Hill CJ, et al. Effects of pulmonary rehabilitation in bronchiectasis: a retrospective study. Chron Respir Dis 2011;8(1):21–30.

73. Mandal P, Sidhu MK, Kope L, et al. A pilot study of pulmonary rehabilitation and chest physiotherapy versus chest physiotherapy alone in bronchiectasis. Respir Med 2012;106:1647–54.

74. Van Zeller M, Mota PC, Amorim A, et al. Pulmonary rehabilitation in patients with bronchiectasis: pulmonary function, arterial blood gases and the 6-minute walk test. J Cardiopulm Rehabil 2012;32:278–83.

75. Main E, Prasad A, van der Schans C. Conventional chest physiotherapy compared to other airway clearance techniques for cystic fibrosis [review]. Cochrane Database Syst Rev 2005;(1):CD002011.

76. Murray MP, Turnbull K, MacQuarrie S, et al. Validation of the Leicester cough questionnaire in non-cystic fibrosis bronchiectasis. Eur Respir J 2009;34:125–31.

77. Collard HR, Pantilat SZ. Dyspnea in interstitial lung disease. Curr Opin Support Palliat Care 2008;2:100–4.

78. Ryerson CJ, Berkeley J, Carrieri-Kohlman VL. Depression and functional status are strongly associated with dyspnea in interstitial lung disease. Chest 2011;139:609–16.

79. Holland AE. Aspects of interstitial lung disease: exercise limitation in interstitial lung disease-mechanisms, significance and therapeutic options. Chron Respir Dis 2010;7:101–11.

80. Langer D, Cebria I, Iranzo MA, et al. Determinants of physical activity in daily life in candidates for lung transplantation. Respir Med 2012;106:747–54.

81. Swigris JJ, Kuschner WG, Jacobs SS, et al. Health-related quality of life in patients with idiopathic pulmonary fibrosis: a systematic review. Thorax 2005;60:588–94.

82. Salhi B, Troosters T, Mahaegel M, et al. Effects of pulmonary rehabilitation in patients with restrictive lung diseases. Chest 2010;137(2):273–9.

83. O'Donnell DE, Chau LK, Webb KA. Qualitative aspects of exertional dyspnea in patients with interstitial lung disease. J Appl Physiol 1998;84(6):2000–9.

84. Spruit M, Thomeer MJ, Gosselink R, et al. Skeletal muscle weakness in patients with sarcoidosis and its relationship with exercise intolerance and reduced health status. Thorax 2005;60:32–8.

85. Watanabe F, Taniguchi H, Sakamoto K, et al. Quadriceps weakness contributes to exercise capacity in nonspecific interstitial pneumonia. Respir Med 2013;107(4):622–8.

86. Chang JA, Curtis JR, Patrick DL, et al. Assessment of health-related quality of life in patients with interstitial lung disease. Chest 1999;116:1175–82.

87. Caminati A, Bianchi A, Cassandro R. Walking distance on 6-MWT is a prognostic factor in idiopathic pulmonary fibrosis. Respir Med 2008;103:117–23.

88. Collard HR, Tino G, Noble PW, et al. Patient experiences with pulmonary fibrosis. Respir Med 2007;101:1350–4.

89. Ryerson CJ, Garvey C, Collard HR. Pulmonary rehabilitation for interstitial lung disease. Chest 2010;138(1):240–1.

90. Holland AE, Hill CJ, Conron M, et al. Short-term improvement in exercise capacity and symptoms following exercise training in interstitial lung disease. Thorax 2008;63:549–54.

91. Nishiyama O, Kondoh Y, Kimura T, et al. Effects of pulmonary rehabilitation in patients with idiopathic pulmonary fibrosis. Respirology 2008;13:394–9.

92. Holland AE, Hill CJ, Glaspole I, et al. Predictors of benefit following pulmonary rehabilitation for interstitial lung disease. Respir Med 2012;106:429–35.

93. Huppmann P, Sczepanski B, Boensch M, et al. Effects of in-patient pulmonary rehabilitation in patients with interstitial lung disease. Eur Respir J 2012. http://dx.doi.org/10.1183/09031936.00081512.

94. Swigris JJ, Fairclough DL, Morrison M, et al. Benefits of pulmonary rehabilitation in idiopathic pulmonary fibrosis. Respir Care 2011;56(6):783–9.

95. Ferreira A, Garvey C, Connors GL, et al. Pulmonary rehabilitation in interstitial lung disease: benefits and predictors of response. Chest 2009;135:442–7.

96. Jastrzebski D, Gumola A, Gawlik R, et al. Dyspnea and quality of life in patients with pulmonary fibrosis after six weeks of respiratory rehabilitation. J Physiol Pharmacol 2006;57(Suppl 4):139–48.

97. Naji NA, Connor MC, Donnelly SC, et al. Effectiveness of pulmonary rehabilitation in restrictive lung disease. J Cardiopulm Rehabil 2006;26:237–43.

98. Kozu R, Senjyu H, Jenkins SC, et al. Differences in response to pulmonary rehabilitation in idiopathic pulmonary fibrosis and chronic obstructive pulmonary disease. Respiration 2011;81:196–205.

99. Holland A, Hill C. Physical training for interstitial lung disease. Cochrane Database Syst Rev 2008;(1):CD006322.

100. Kozu R, Jenkins S, Senjyu H. Effect of disability level on response to pulmonary rehabilitation in patients with idiopathic pulmonary fibrosis. Respirology 2011;16:1196–202.

101. Dowman L, McDonald CF, Hill C, et al. The benefits of exercise training in interstitial lung disease: protocol for a multicentre randomized controlled trial. BMC Pulm Med 2013;13:8.

102. Yorke J, Jones PW, Swigris JJ. Development and validity testing of an IPF-specific version of the St George's respiratory questionnaire. Thorax 2010; 65:921–6.

103. Solache-Carrando A, Sanchez-Bringas M. Evaluation of a respiratory rehabilitation program in children with scoliosis. Cir Cir 2012;80(1):11–7.

104. Canavan P, Cahalin L. Integrated physical therapy intervention for a person with pectus excavatum and bilateral shoulder pain: a single-case study. Arch Phys Med Rehabil 2008;89:2195–203.

105. Kado D. The rehabilitation of hyperkyphotic posture in the elderly. Eur J Phys Rehabil Med 2009;45:583–93.

106. Kado D, Huang M, Barrett-Connor E. Hyperkyphotic posture and poor physical functional ability in older community-dwelling men and women: the Rancho Bernardo study. J Gerontol A Biol Sci Med Sci 2005;60:633–7.

107. Kado D, Huang M, Karlamangla A, et al. Hyperkyphotic posture predicts mortality in older community-dwelling men and women: a prospective study. J Am Geriatr Soc 2004;52:1662–7.

108. Negrini S, Antonini G, Carabalona R, et al. Physical exercise as a treatment for adolescent idiopathic scoliosis. A systematic review. Pediatr Rehabil 2003;6(3–4):227–35.

109. Moamary M. Impact of a pulmonary rehabilitation programme on respiratory parameters and health care utilization in patients with chronic lung diseases other than COPD. East Mediterr Health J 2012;18(2):120–6.

110. dos Santos Alves V, Stirbulov R, Avanzi O. Impact of physical rehabilitation program on the respiratory function of adolescents with idiopathic scoliosis. Chest 2006;130:500–5.

111. Fabian K. Evaluation of the effectiveness of asymmetric breathing exercises according to Dobosiewicz on chosen functional parameters of the respiratory system in girls with scoliosis. Fizjoterapia (Physiotherapy) 2010;18(4):21–6.

112. Berliner JL, Verma K, Lonner BS, et al. Discriminative validity of the Scoliosis Research Society 22 Questionnaire among five curve-severity subgroups of adolescents with idiopathic scoliosis. Spine J 2013;13(2):27–33.

113. Simmonneau G, Robbins I, Beghetti M, et al. Updated clinical classification of pulmonary hypertension. J Am Coll Cardiol 2009;54(Suppl 1):S43–54.

114. Desai SA, Channick RN. Exercise in patients with pulmonary arterial hypertension. J Cardiopulm Rehabil Prev 2008;28:12–6.

115. Sun XG, Hansen JE, Oudiz RJ, et al. Exercise pathophysiology in patients with primary pulmonary hypertension. Circulation 2001;104:429–35.

116. Miyamoto S, Nagaya N, Satoh T, et al. Clinical correlates and prognostic significance of six-minute walk test in patients with primary pulmonary hypertension: comparison with cardiopulmonary exercise testing. Am J Respir Crit Care Med 2000; 161:487–92.

117. Palange P, Ward SA, Carlsen KH, et al. Recommendations on the use of exercise testing in clinical practice. Eur Respir J 2007;29:185–209.

118. Matura LA, McDonough A, Carroll DL. Cluster analysis of symptoms in pulmonary arterial hypertension: a pilot study. Eur J Cardiovasc Nurs 2012; 11:51–61.

119. White J, Hopkins RO, Glissmeyer EW, et al. Cognitive, emotional and quality of life outcomes in patients with pulmonary arterial hypertension. Respir Res 2006;7:55–64.

120. Lowe B, Grafe K, Ufer C, et al. Anxiety and depression in patients with pulmonary hypertension. Psychosom Med 2004;66:831–6.

121. Hopkins RO, Morton J, Glissmeyer EW. Cognitive dysfunction in patients with pulmonary arterial hypertension. Am J Respir Crit Care Med 2003;167: A273.

122. Shafazand S, Goldstein MK, Doyle RL, et al. Health-related quality of life in patients with pulmonary arterial hypertension. Chest 2004;126:1452–9.

123. Chua R, Keogh AM, Byth K, et al. Comparison and validation of three measures of quality of life in patients with pulmonary hypertension. Intern Med J 2006;36:705–10.

124. Taichman DB, Shin J, Hud L, et al. Health-related quality of life in patients with pulmonary arterial hypertension. Respir Res 2005;6:92–101.

125. Cenedese E, Speich R, Dorschner L, et al. Measurement of quality of life in pulmonary hypertension and its significance. Eur Respir J 2006;28: 808–15.

126. Mereles D, Ehlken N, Kreuscher S, et al. Exercise and respiratory training improve exercise capacity and quality of life in patients with severe chronic pulmonary hypertension. Circulation 2006;114: 1482–9.

127. Chan L, Chin LM, Kennedy M, et al. Benefits of intensive treadmill exercise training on cardiorespiratory function and quality of life in patients with pulmonary hypertension. Chest 2013;143(2): 333–43.

128. Grunig E, Ehlken N, Ghofrani A, et al. Effect of exercise and respiratory training on clinical progression and survival in patients with severe chronic

pulmonary hypertension. Respiration 2011;81:394–401.

129. Fox BD, Kassirer M, Weiss I, et al. Ambulatory rehabilitation improves exercise capacity in patients with pulmonary hypertension. J Card Fail 2011;17:196–200.

130. Grunig E, Lichtblau M, Ehlken N, et al. Safety and efficacy of exercise training in various forms of pulmonary hypertension. Eur Respir J 2012;40(1):84–92.

131. de Man FS, Handoko ML, Groepenhoff H, et al. Effects of exercise training in patients with idiopathic pulmonary arterial hypertension. Eur Respir J 2009;34(3):669–75.

132. Martinez-Quintana E, Miranda-Calderin G, Ugarte-Lopetegui A, et al. Rehabilitation program in adult congenital heart disease patients with pulmonary hypertension. Congenit Heart Dis 2010;5:44–50.

133. Mainguy V, Maltais F, Saey D, et al. Effects of a rehabilitation program on skeletal muscle function in idiopathic pulmonary arterial hypertension. J Cardiopulm Rehabil Prev 2010;30:319–23.

134. Ley S, Fink C, Risse F, et al. Magnetic resonance imaging to assess the effect of exercise training on pulmonary perfusion and blood flow in patients with pulmonary hypertension. Eur Radiol 2013;23(2):324–31.

135. Weinstein AA, Chin LM, Keyser RE, et al. Effect of aerobic exercise training on fatigue and physical activity in patients with pulmonary arterial hypertension. Respir Med 2013;107(5):778–84.

136. Maione P, Perrone F, Gallo C, et al. Pretreatment quality of life and functional status assessment significantly predict survival of elderly patients with advanced non-small-cell lung cancer receiving chemotherapy: a prognostic analysis of the multicenter Italian lung cancer in the elderly study. J Clin Oncol 2005;23:6865–72.

137. Available at: http://www.cancer.gov/cancertopics/types/lung. Accessed April 7, 2014.

138. Spiro SG, Douse J, Read C, et al. Complications of lung cancer treatment. Semin Respir Crit Care Med 2008;29(3):302–17.

139. Temel J, Pirl WF, Lych TJ. Comprehensive symptom management in patients with advanced-stage non-small-cell lung cancer. Clin Lung Cancer 2006;7(4):241–9.

140. Ostroff JS, Krebs P, Coups EJ, et al. Health-related quality of life among early-stage, non-small cell, lung cancer survivors. Lung Cancer 2011;71:103–8.

141. Smith EL, Hann DM, Ahles TA, et al. Dyspnea, anxiety, body consciousness, and quality of life in patients with lung cancer. J Pain Symptom Manage 2001;21:323–9.

142. Myrdal G, Valtysdottir S, Lambe M, et al. Quality of life following lung cancer surgery. Thorax 2003;58:194–7.

143. Novoa N, Varela G, Jimenez MF, et al. Influence of major pulmonary resection on postoperative daily ambulatory activity of the patients. Interact Cardiovasc Thorac Surg 2009;9:934–8.

144. MacDonald N. Cancer cachexia and targeting chronic inflammation: a unified approach to cancer treatment and palliative/supportive care. J Support Oncol 2007;5:157–62 [discussion: 164–6, 183].

145. Mareska M, Gutmann L. Lambert-Eaton myasthenic syndrome. Semin Neurol 2004;24(2):149–53.

146. Brown DJ, McMillan DC, Milroy R. The correlation between fatigue, physical function, the systemic inflammatory response, and psychological distress in patients with advanced lung cancer. Cancer 2005;103:377–82.

147. Datta D, Lahiri B. Preoperative evaluation of patients undergoing lung resection surgery. Chest 2003;123(6):2096–103.

148. Ruckdeschel C, Finkelstein DM, Mason BA, et al. Chemotherapy for metastatic non-small-cell bronchogenic carcinoma: EST 2575, generation V–a randomized comparison of four cisplatin-containing regimens. J Clin Oncol 1985;3:72–9.

149. Nagamatsue Y, Maeshiro K, Kimura NY, et al. Long-term recovery of exercise capacity and pulmonary function after lobectomy. J Thorac Cardiovasc Surg 2007;134:1273–8.

150. Win T, Groves AM, Ritchie AJ, et al. The effect of lung resection on pulmonary function and exercise capacity in lung cancer patients. Respir Care 2007;52(6):720–6.

151. Jones LW, Peddle CJ, Eves ND, et al. Effects of presurgical exercise training on cardiorespiratory fitness among patients undergoing thoracic surgery for malignant lung lesions. Cancer 2007;110:590–8.

152. Coats V, Maltais F, Simard F, et al. Feasibility and effect of a home-based exercise training program before lung resection surgery. Can Respir J 2013;20(2):e10–6.

153. Bobbio A, Chetta A, Ampollini L, et al. Preoperative pulmonary rehabilitation in patients undergoing lung resection for non-small cell lung cancer. Eur J Cardiothorac Surg 2008;33:95–8.

154. Morano MT, Araujo AS, Nascimento FB, et al. Preoperative pulmonary rehabilitation versus chest physical therapy in patients undergoing lung cancer resection: a pilot randomized controlled trial. Arch Phys Med Rehabil 2013;94:53–8.

155. Spruit MA, Janssen PP, Willemsen SC, et al. Exercise capacity before and after an 8-week multidisciplinary inpatient pulmonary rehabilitation program in lung cancer patients: a pilot study. Lung Cancer 2006;52:257–60.

156. Riesenberg H, Lubbe AS. In-patient rehabilitation of lung cancer patients–a prospective study. Support Care Cancer 2010;18:877–82.

157. Glattki GP, Manika K, Sichletidis L, et al. Pulmonary rehabilitation in non-small cell lung cancer patients after completion of treatment. Am J Clin Oncol 2012;35:120–5.

158. Granger CL, McDonald CF, Berney S, et al. Exercise intervention to improve exercise capacity and health related quality of life for patients with non-small cell lung cancer: a systematic review. Lung Cancer 2011;72:139–53.

159. Cesario A, Ferri L, Galetta D, et al. Post-operative respiratory rehabilitation after lung resection for non-small cell lung cancer. Lung Cancer 2007;57: 175–80.

160. Stigt JA, Uil SM, van Riesen SJ, et al. A randomized controlled trial of post-thoracotomy pulmonary rehabilitation in patients with resectable lung cancer. J Thorac Oncol 2013;8(2):214–21.

161. Arbane G, Tropman D, Jackson D, et al. Evaluation of an early exercise intervention after thoracotomy for non-small cell lung cancer (NSCLC), effects on quality of life, muscle strength and exercise tolerance: randomised controlled trial. Lung Cancer 2011;71:229–34.

162. Jones LW, Eves ND, Peterson BL, et al. Safety and feasibility of aerobic training on cardiopulmonary function and quality of life in postsurgical nonsmall cell lung cancer patients: a pilot study. Cancer 2008;113:3430–9.

163. Dimeo F, Schwartz S, Wesel N, et al. Effects of an endurance and resistance exercise program on persistent cancer-related fatigue after treatment. Ann Oncol 2008;19:1495–9.

164. Benzo R, Wigle D, Novotny P, et al. Preoperative pulmonary rehabilitation before lung cancer resection: results from two randomized studies. Lung Cancer 2011;74:441–5.

165. Temel JS, Greer JA, Goldberg S, et al. A structured exercise program for patients with advanced non-small cell lung cancer. J Thorac Oncol 2009;4: 595–601.

166. Quist M, Rorth M, Langer S, et al. Safety and feasibility of a combined exercise intervention for inoperable lung cancer patients undergoing chemotherapy: a pilot study. Lung Cancer 2012; 75:203–8.

167. Mendoza TR, Wang X, Cleeland CS, et al. The rapid assessment of fatigue severity in cancer patients: use of the brief fatigue inventory. Cancer 1999;85:1186–96.

168. Webster K, Cella D, Yost K. The functional assessment of chronic illness therapy (FACIT) measurement system: properties, applications and interpretation. Health Qual Life Outcomes 2003;1:79.

169. Marteau TM, Bekker H. The development of a six-item short-form of the State Scale of the Spielberger State-Trait Anxiety Inventory (STATI). Br J Clin Psychol 1992;31:301–6.

170. Aukst Margetić B, Kukulj S, Santić Z. Predicting depression with temperament and character in lung cancer patients. Eur J Cancer Care (Engl) 2013;22(6):807–14.

171. Jastrzebski D, Ochman M, Ziora D, et al. Pulmonary rehabilitation in patients referred for lung transplantation. In: Pokorski M, editor. Respiratory regulation-clinical advances, advances in experimental medicine and biology. Dordrecht (The Netherlands): Springer Science and Business Media; 2013. p. 19–25.

172. Florian J, Rubin A, Mattiello R, et al. Impact of pulmonary rehabilitation on quality of life and functional capacity in patients on waiting lists for lung transplantation. J Bras Pneumol 2013;39(3):349–56.

173. Li M, Mathur S, Chowdhury NA, et al. Pulmonary rehabilitation in lung transplant candidates. J Heart Lung Transplant 2013;32(6):626–32.

174. Bartels MN, Armstrong HF, Gerardo RE, et al. Evaluation of pulmonary function and exercise performance by cardiopulmonary exercise testing before and after lung transplantation. Chest 2011; 140(6):1604–11.

175. Wang XN, Williams TJ, McKenna MJ, et al. Skeletal muscle oxidative capacity, fiber type, and metabolites after lung transplantation. Am J Respir Crit Care Med 1999;160:57–63.

176. Mathur S, Reid WD, Levy RD. Exercise limitation in recipients of lung transplants. Phys Ther 2004;84: 1178–87.

177. Pantoja JG, Andrade FH, Stoki DS, et al. Respiratory and limb muscle function in lung allograft recipients. Am J Respir Crit Care Med 1999;160: 1205–11.

178. Reinsma GD, ten Hacken NH, Grevink RG, et al. Limiting factors of exercise performance 1 year after lung transplantation. J Heart Lung Transplant 2006;25(11):1310–6.

179. Sanchez H, Zoll J, Bigard X, et al. Effect of cyclosporine A and its vehicle on cardiac and skeletal muscle mitochondria: relationship to efficiency of the respiratory chain. Br J Pharmacol 2001;133: 781–8.

180. Langer D, Burtin C, Schepers L, et al. Exercise training after lung transplantation improves participation in daily activity: a randomized controlled trial. Am J Transplant 2012;12(6):1584–92.

181. Maury G, Langer D, Verleden G, et al. Skeletal muscle force and functional exercise tolerance before and after lung transplantation: a cohort study. Am J Transplant 2008;8:1275–81.

182. Wickerson L, Mathur S, Brooks D. Exercise training after lung transplantation: a systematic review. J Heart Lung Transplant 2010;29:497–503.

183. Munro PE, Holland AE, Bailey M, et al. Pulmonary rehabilitation following lung transplantation. Transplant Proc 2009;41:292–5.

184. Ryerson CJ, Donesky D, Pantilat SZ, et al. Dyspnea in idiopathic pulmonary fibrosis: a systematic review. J Pain Symptom Manage 2012;43: 771–82.

185. Tanaka K, Akechi T, Okuyama T, et al. Development and validation of the Cancer Dyspnea Scale: a multidimensional, brief, self-rating scale. Br J Cancer 2000;82(4):800–5.

186. Butt Z, Webster K, Eisenstein AR. Quality of life in lung cancer: the validity and cross-cultural applicability of the functional assessment of cancer therapy-lung scale. Hematol Oncol Clin North Am 2005;19:389–420.

187. Peddle-McIntyre C, Bell G, Fenton D, et al. Feasibility and preliminary efficacy of progressive resistance exercise training in lung cancer survivors. Lung Cancer 2012;75:126–32.

188. Available at: http://groups.eortc.be/qol/eortc-qlq-c30. Accessed April 7, 2014.

189. Parekh PI, Blumenthal JA, Babyak MA, et al. Psychiatric disorder and quality of life in patients awaiting lung transplantation. Chest 2003;124:1682–8.

190. Armstrong HF, Garber CE, Bartels MN. Exercise testing parameters associated with post lung transplant mortality. Respir Physiol Neurobiol 2012; 181(2):118–22.

Pulmonary Rehabilitation at the Time of the COPD Exacerbation

Roger Goldstein, MB ChB, FRCP[a,b,c,d,]*,
Dina Brooks, PhD, PT[a,b,d]

KEYWORDS

- Pulmonary rehabilitation • COPD • Exercise • Physical therapy • Acute exacerbation

KEY POINTS

- Pulmonary rehabilitation (PR) is associated with improvements in exercise capacity, health-related quality of life, psychological symptoms, and resource utilization.
- Acute exacerbations threaten these PR improvements.
- An awareness of the clinical sequelae of acute exacerbation of chronic obstructive pulmonary disease enables approaches, such as early post-exacerbation rehabilitation to mitigate its negative effects.

INTRODUCTION

In chronic obstructive pulmonary disease (COPD), severe exacerbations, especially when multiple, are an independent adverse prognostic variable[1] with an adjusted risk of death being 4 times higher than for those free of exacerbation. Therefore, a reduction in the number and the impact of exacerbations has become a priority in the management of COPD. There is growing evidence that pulmonary rehabilitation (PR) is an effective and safe intervention to improve health-related quality of life, peripheral muscle function, and exercise capacity as well as to reduce hospital admission and possibly mortality in patients with COPD post-exacerbation.[2] Despite this growing evidence, authoritative reviews of exacerbations in COPD make scant mention of nonpharmacologic approaches[3,4] such as rehabilitation. This article discusses the definition of an acute exacerbation (AE), the rationale, and evidence for post-exacerbation

PR and how the program might be modified to take into consideration the more frail state of such patients.

DEFINITION, CAUSE, AND PATHOPHYSIOLOGY OF ACUTE EXACERBATION
Definition

An AE was originally defined[5] based on symptoms and characterized by a change in purulence, viscosity, or volume of sputum production and/or an increase in dyspnea, which may be associated with nasal discharge, sore throat, fever, and increased cough or wheeze. Other experts have modified this definition or provided alternative definitions, for example, adding a duration for the symptoms of at least 2 consecutive days.[6] An international working group defined AE more broadly as "a sustained worsening of a patient's condition from stable state, and beyond the usual

a Graduate Department of Rehabilitation Science, Faculty of Medicine, University of Toronto, Toronto, Ontario, Canada; b Department of Physical Therapy, University of Toronto, Toronto, Ontario, Canada; c Department of Medicine, Faculty of Medicine, University of Toronto, Toronto, Ontario, Canada; d Department of Respiratory Medicine, West Park Healthcare Centre, 82 Buttonwood Avenue, Toronto, Ontario, M6M 2J5, Canada
* Corresponding author. West Park Healthcare Centre, 82 Buttonwood Avenue, Toronto, Ontario, M6M 2J5, Canada.
E-mail address: rgoldstein@westpark.org

Clin Chest Med 35 (2014) 391–398
http://dx.doi.org/10.1016/j.ccm.2014.02.005
0272-5231/14/$ – see front matter © 2014 Elsevier Inc. All rights reserved.

day-to-day variation, that is acute in onset and necessitates a change in regular medication in a patient with underlying COPD."[7] In the GOLD guidelines for treatment,[8] a definition of AE severity was developed based on the need for a therapeutic intervention (event-based definition). AEs were termed mild if they were managed at home by increased bronchodilator therapy without additional health care contact. Moderate exacerbations were also managed at home through unscheduled health care contact and/or the initiation of treatment with oral glucocorticosteroids, whereas severe exacerbations were managed in the emergency room and/or in hospital.[8]

The availability of multiple definitions, whether symptom or event-based, is problematic and has hampered the assessment of efficacy of treatment.[9] In fact, a systematic review found that less than 20% of trials used a symptom-based definition of AE, such as those mentioned earlier.[5,6] In half the trials, definition of AE was limited to those requiring new treatment with pharmacotherapy and/or hospitalization. The article concluded that clinical trials used varied definitions and analysis of AE, leading to biased estimates of treatment effects for new treatments for AEs.[10]

Cause and Incidence

The triggers of AEs are infections of the tracheobronchial tree, environmental exposures, or unidentified.[6,8,11–13] Infections account for up to 80% of acute exacerbation of COPD (AECOPD) and can be bacterial or viral.[12,14–17] The relative risk of hospital admissions for AECOPD increases with higher levels of air pollutants.[18,19] Although infections are the prime precipitating factors, a primary physiologic mechanism that contributes to the impact of an AE is dynamic hyperinflation. Dynamic hyperinflation refers to an acute increase in the retained air at the end of expiration that occurs during exercise in patients with airway obstruction such as COPD.[20] During AE, with increased airway obstruction, dynamic hyperinflation occurs as the respiratory rate increases and the expiratory flow rate decreases and can lead to increased mechanical disadvantage of the respiratory musculature, marked dyspnea, anxiety, and negative cardiovascular consequences.[20]

The frequency of AECOPD for severe COPD is 1 to 4 per year.[6,11,21] Hospitalization occurs in up to 16% of those with AE.[6,22] In those with severe AEs, mortality has been reported between 3% and 10%[23,24] and much higher (at 15%–24%) in those admitted to the intensive care unit.[25,26] In a 6-month longitudinal study of 1016 patients hospitalized for COPD, death during the AE was

11% and 2-year mortality was 49%. Hospital readmission rates were as high as 50% in the first 6 months after discharge.[24] In a study of 377 post-exacerbation COPD patients, the worst quality of life scores were associated with the highest readmission to hospital.[27] In a retrospective study of 551 post-exacerbation hospital discharges of whom 59% were readmitted within 12 months, dependency in self-care[28] was identified as an independent contributor to readmission.

ACUTE EXACERBATIONS—THE ENEMY OF REHABILITATION

In addition to the short- and long-term threat to mortality as a result of AECOPD, especially among those requiring hospitalization, the result of a single episode may threaten many of the gains achieved by PR. The positive impact of PR on exercise tolerance and health-related quality of life is well established, and as a result, PR is considered standard practice for COPD and recommended by professional societies around the world.[29] Much of this positive impact is the result of decreased dyspnea and improved peripheral muscle function.[30] In addition, functional activities of daily living and other secondary impairments such as anxiety and depression are improved by PR.[31] Health resource utilization in terms of unscheduled emergency room visits and reduced hospitalization is also reduced.[32,33]

Impact on Lung Function

To establish the impact of exacerbations on lung function, one study followed 109 patients with COPD over 4 years. The investigators noted that those with frequent exacerbations had a faster decline in FEV_1 (-40 mL/y) compared with those who experience fewer exacerbations (-32 mL/y),[34] even when adjusted for smoking status. Moreover, among 20 of 46 frequent exacerbators, the rate of hospitalization was 1.5 per annum in contrast to admissions on one occasion for only 7 of 63 infrequent exacerbators.

Impact on Muscle Strength

In addition to the consequences of bed rest, the multifactorial changes in metabolic and inflammatory states, as well as nutritional, oxidative, pharmacologic (eg, steroids), and gas exchange (eg, hypoxia) alterations associated with an AECOPD, all will affect peripheral muscle function. In 2003, investigators studied the impact of hospitalization for an AECOPD on muscle force[35] and reported that on admission the quadriceps peak torque (QPT) among hospitalized patients was 66% ($\pm 22\%$) of the values measured in healthy age-matched elderly subjects, declining by 5% between days 3 and 8 and partially recovering 3 months later (**Fig. 1**). There was an inverse correlation between QPT and levels of the inflammatory marker interleukin 8, which were increased in AECOPD patients compared with stable COPD and healthy elderly. These observations have led to interest in starting rehabilitation during the exacerbation, using resistance training to counterbalance the deterioration in quadriceps function during an AECOPD.[36] In fact, resistance training is feasible and effective. In 40 hospitalized patients with a COPD exacerbation, resistance training enhanced quadriceps force on discharge (+9% ± 16%) compared to untrained subjects (−1 ± 13%). The improvement was maintained at 1 month post-discharge (**Fig. 2**).

Impact on Health-related Quality of Life

In contrast to the gains made in PR, investigators[37] noted that among a group of COPD patients followed for 12 years, those labeled as frequent exacerbators (≥3 per annum) experienced a lower health-related quality of life as reflected by the total and component (symptoms, activities, and impact) scores on the disease-specific St George's Respiratory Questionnaire. Predictors of frequent exacerbations included daily cough, wheeze, and sputum production, as well as frequent exacerbations in the previous year. Subsequently, these same investigators described a prodromal preexacerbation period during which time subjective measurements of dyspnea

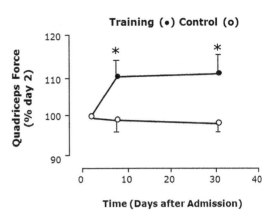

Training (•) Control (o)

Fig. 2. Resistance training and quadriceps muscle function during AECOPD. * = *p<0.05.* (*Data from* Troosters T, Probst VS, Crul T, et al. Resistance training prevents deterioration in quadriceps muscle function during acute exacerbations of chronic obstructive pulmonary disease. Am J Respir Crit Care Med 2010;181(10):1072.)

increased. Subsequent to the AE, recovery of peak expiratory flow to baseline levels was complete after a week in only 75% of exacerbations, and in 7% of exacerbations, recovery to baseline had still not occurred at 3 months.[6] Although the investigators did not track activities during the period of observation, it is very likely that the increase in dyspnea and other symptoms would have reduced physical activities both during the prodromal period and subsequent to the exacerbation itself.

Impact on Physical Activity

A study looking at[38] the impact of exacerbations on the behavior of patients with COPD used diary card measures of time spent outside the home as a marker of physical activity. Of 147 patients followed for approximately 4 years, time indoors increased gradually. At baseline, patients spent all day at home for 2.1 days per week (34% of their days). After exacerbation they spent 2.5 days at home (44% of their days), decreasing gradually over the next few weeks. This study highlighted the negative impact of exacerbations on time spent outside the home, exactly the opposite of one of the goals of PR. In 2006, a group of investigators[39] studied whether the lower time spent in physical activity associated with bed rest during an AECOPD could contribute to the reductions in muscle force. Activity monitors were applied at the beginning and end of hospitalization for an AECOPD and again after 1 month. Compared to stable COPD patients who spent approximately one-third of their time during the day in weight bearing activities,[40] the time spent in physical

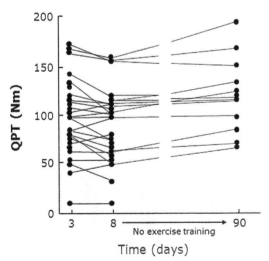

Fig. 1. QPT during hospitalization for AECOPD. (*Adapted from* Spruit MA, Gosselink R, Troosters T, et al. Muscle force during an acute exacerbation in hospitalized patients with COPD and its relationship with CXCL8 and IGF-I. Thorax 2003;58(9):752; with permission.)

activities such as walking and standing was low both on the second and seventh day of hospitalization (**Fig. 3**). Moreover, these activities were still reduced 1 month after discharge. These investigators further observed that the time spent in weight bearing activities after a week correlated positively with measurements of quadriceps force and that the reduction in quadriceps force correlated with a smaller improvement in walking time at 1 month. Although at the beginning of the exacerbation there were no differences in clinical characteristics, those hospitalized in the previous year walked for less time after 1 month compared with those who had not been hospitalized.

Impact on Hospital Readmission

Exacerbations that subsequently reduce physical activity not only reverse the gains made by PR but may also promote hospital readmission from further exacerbations. Of 340 patients recruited at the time of admission to hospital and followed for just over a year,[41] 63% of patients were readmitted at least once and 29% died. The investigators reported that more than 3 admissions for an AECOPD increased the risk of readmission (hazard ratio [HR] 1.66, 95% confidence interval [CI] 1.16–2.39). The investigators also showed for the first time that involvement in higher levels of usual physical activity was protective (HR 0.54, 95%CI 0.34–0.86). Physical activity was derived from a questionnaire, the results of which were converted to kcal/d. This strong association has important therapeutic implications, because the third of patients who reported activities equivalent to walking for more than 60 min/d had a reduction of almost 50% in risk of admission to hospital. Recent studies[42–44] are encouraging as to the impact of PR on domestic function and physical activity, especially when administered in a way that will promote longer-term adherence. A systematic review of the impact of exercise on physical activity noted the need for larger randomized controlled trial in which activity is measured in absolute units such as steps or activity counts.[45]

PSYCHOLOGICAL IMPACT OF ACUTE EXACERBATION

AECOPDs have been associated with an increase in anxiety and depression.[46] In a series of home-based interviews and focus groups among 25 post-AECOPD patients, anxiety and depression was noted in 64% and 40%, respectively. Patients also expressed fear of another episode and uncertainty regarding the availability of social and medical care. In a Nordic study of the prevalence of psychological symptoms among 416 patients hospitalized with an AECOPD,[47] a high prevalence of anxiety and depression was noted (**Fig. 4**).

A recent interpretive meta-synthesis compiled the results of 8 qualitative studies exploring the perspectives of patients with COPD after an exacerbation.[48] AECOPD resulted in a "heightened patient arousal, vigilance and powerlessness". Breathlessness with an AE resulted in fear and anxiety and patients often perceived that their symptoms were dismissed by the medical team. Patients also felt that they lacked the knowledge on discharge from hospital to handle their medical condition. Concerns were also expressed about the impact of the AE on their caregiver's health and the strain of the illness on their relationship with the caregiver.[46,48] Of note, when asked to describe their experiences of an AE, in addition to the usual symptoms of dyspnea and cough, more than 80% of patients experienced fatigue and more than 40% experienced a change in mood.[49] These findings indicate that there is a need to address the psychological needs of the patients, design intervention to acknowledge their

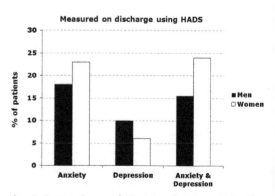

Fig. 4. Depression and anxiety after hospitalization for AECOPD. (*Adapted from* Gudmundsson G, Gislason T, Janson C, et al. Depression, anxiety and health status after hospitalisation for COPD: a multicentre study in the Nordic countries. Respir Med 2006; 100(1):87; with permission.)

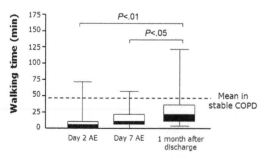

Fig. 3. Hospitalization and physical activity post-AECOPD. (*Adapted from* Pitta F, Troosters T, Probst VS, et al. Physical activity and hospitalization for exacerbation of COPD. Chest 2006;129(3):536; with permission.)

fears, and manage the high levels of anxiety and depression after AE. Such screening and intervention can occur during post-exacerbation rehabilitation.

REHABILITATION AFTER ACUTE EXACERBATION: THE EVIDENCE, PRACTICE, AND COMPONENTS

The gains of PR, especially dyspnea reduction, increased exercise capacity, and physical activities of daily living are diminished by AECOPD. Therefore, there is growing interest in the initiation of PR during or soon after an AECOPD to reverse the loss of peripheral muscle function, improve dyspnea and health-related quality of life, decrease depression, and increase physical activity. PR post-exacerbation includes physical exercise in patients recently managed for an AE.[2]

Airway Clearance Techniques for Acute Exacerbation

The evidence for airway clearance techniques as a component of rehabilitation is unclear because of conflicting findings and poor methodological rigor.[50] Airway clearance techniques may include "postural drainage or gravity assisted positioning, breathing exercises, chest wall percussion and/or vibration, forced expiratory technique, coughing maneuvers and the use of devices such as positive expiratory pressure (PEP) masks."[51] Two systematic reviews examined the safety and effectiveness of airway clearance techniques in the management of AECOPD.[51,52] Both systematic reviews included studies with patients who were breathing spontaneously; although only one[51] reviewed randomized controlled trials or randomized cross over, the other[52] included cohort studies as well. Airway clearance techniques were found not to result in improvement in lung function or

changes in measures of gas exchange or hospital length of stay.[51] In fact, chest wall percussion in gravity-assisted positions for approximately 5 minutes resulted in a reduction of forced expiratory volume in 1 second.[51] All other airway clearance techniques were reported to be safe.[51,52] In patients with copious secretions, mechanical vibration and PEP mask were beneficial in encouraging sputum expectoration.[51,52] There was insufficient evidence regarding effectiveness of breathing exercises.[52]

Consistent with the evidence, surveys of practice patterns on the management of patients with COPD hospitalized for AE have shown that treatment focuses on mobilization and much less on airway clearance techniques.[50,53] However, despite the lack of evidence to support their effectiveness techniques like purse lip breathing, active cycle breathing techniques and diaphragmatic breathing were used by most therapists.[50,53] These findings may indicate that patients hospitalized with an AECOPD require assistance to improve ventilation but not to clear secretions.

Pulmonary Rehabilitation

In a single-center randomized controlled trial evaluating early post-hospitalization community-based PR, investigators[54] reported on significant between-group improvements in the endurance shuttle walk (60 m 95% CI 27–93 m), the St. George's Respiratory Questionnaire (−12.7, −5 to −20), and all 4 components of the chronic respiratory questionnaire, noting that early PR is both feasible and effective (**Fig. 5**). Subsequently, a similar study by the same group[55] noted a reduction in hospital readmissions subsequent to PR with 33% of the control group and only 7% of the rehabilitation group being admitted during the subsequent 3 months. A Cochrane review[2] assessed the effects of PR after AE in individuals with COPD on future hospital admissions, exercise

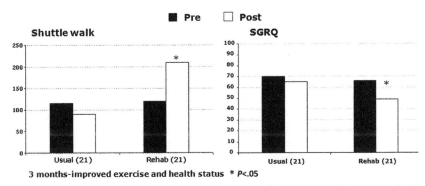

Fig. 5. Early rehabilitation post-AECOPD. (*Data from* Man WD, Polkey MI, Donaldson N, et al. Community pulmonary rehabilitation after hospitalisation for acute exacerbations of chronic obstructive pulmonary disease: randomised controlled study. BMJ 2004;329(7476):1209.)

capacity, health-related quality of life, and mortality. PR was defined as any inpatient and/or outpatient PR program, started either immediately after initiation of AE treatment or up to 3 weeks after AE. PR resulted in a reduction in the odds of hospital readmission. There was also a favorable effect on health-related quality of life that exceeded the minimal clinically important difference. PR also resulted in improvement in 6-minute walk test and shuttle walk test, despite substantial differences between trials. There were no adverse effects in any of the studies. Although the pooled relative risk of death was decreased in the rehabilitation groups, this result requires confirmation because 2 of the 3 trials did not show an effect, and one study was reported only in abstract form. Although the limitation of this systematic review is the small total number of patients and methodological shortcomings of the study, the effect of PR after AE appears to be substantial.

Despite the evidence in support of PR, less than 25% of patients are referred to PR on discharge from hospital.[50] This absence of referral may be the result of lack of availability of PR or lack of awareness of its effectiveness.[50] In a recent clinical audit in the UK,[56] of 448 post-exacerbation discharges, 286 were eligible for post-hospitalization PR, but only 31% were referred and of the 60 who began the course only 43 finished. Studies are required to investigate patient, staff, and organizational barriers to post-hospitalization PR. It is not clear what the optimal time or setting for initiation of PR is. In almost half the studies in the Cochrane systematic review, PR was initiated within 3 to 8 days of hospital admission and the setting included inpatient, outpatient, and home.

PROGRAM MODIFICATION POST-EXACERBATION

The extent to which the rehabilitation program will require modification post-AE depends on the severity of the exacerbation. For mild exacerbations little or no modifications are required. For moderate and severe exacerbations, dyspnea and fatigue will be markedly increased and exercise endurance will be decreased. It is advisable to encourage all patients to continue with their breathing exercises as they require only a modest effort and they improve flexibility, ventilation, and secretion clearance as well as promoting relaxation. For upper extremity strength training, the increased respiratory demands of the AE and the use of upper limbs as accessory muscles of respiration may require program modification with fewer sets, fewer repetitions, or longer rests in between. Similar adaptations may be required for lower-extremity resistance training. Self-paced leisure walking as a mechanism of increased physical activity should be encouraged and determined by patient tolerance, with eventual progression to more specific aerobic prescription using cycle or treadmill. The use of supplemental oxygen may be indicated for some patients, although oxygen has to be prescribed with care in those who are carbon dioxide retainers.

The multidisciplinary treatment team should be aware of the increase in anxiety, which stems from but may also increase dyspnea during and after an AE. For individuals with COPD who have received education on self-management, breathing control and energy conservation may be able to manage symptoms better that those without such education. For some, the combination of severe dyspnea and anxiety may result in panic that requires hospitalization. For patients with COPD who have previous experience of PR during stable periods, resuming activities post-exacerbation is important. However, getting back on track may be a slow process. Deconditioning occurs relatively quickly, and attempts by the patient to resume aerobic training at the same work rate as before will be met with frustration. Aerobic exercise may need to be resumed at a lower level of intensity. This information should be provided on completion of a PR program during stable periods so that subsequent patient expectations are realistic.

SUMMARY

PR is associated with improvements in exercise capacity, health-related quality of life, psychological symptoms, and resource utilization. AEs threaten each of these improvements. An awareness of the clinical sequelae of AECOPD enables approaches such as early post-exacerbation rehabilitation to mitigate the negative effects of the exacerbation. Such approaches should occur alongside pharmacologic management to maximize success and reduce the likelihood of repeat hospitalization.

REFERENCES

1. Soler-Cataluna JJ, Martinez-Garcia MA, Roman Sanchez P, et al. Severe acute exacerbations and mortality in patients with chronic obstructive pulmonary disease. Thorax 2005;60(11):925–31.
2. Puhan MA, Gimeno-Santos E, Scharplatz M, et al. Pulmonary rehabilitation following exacerbations of chronic obstructive pulmonary disease. Cochrane Database Syst Rev 2011;(10):CD005305.

3. Celli BR, Barnes PJ. Exacerbations of chronic obstructive pulmonary disease. Eur Respir J 2007;29(6):1224–38.

4. Bach PB, Brown C, Gelfand SE, et al, American College of Physicians-American Society of Internal Medicine, American College of Chest Physicians. Management of acute exacerbations of chronic obstructive pulmonary disease: a summary and appraisal of published evidence. Ann Intern Med 2001;134(7):600–20.

5. Anthonisen NR, Manfreda J, Warren CP, et al. Antibiotic therapy in exacerbations of chronic obstructive pulmonary disease. Ann Intern Med 1987; 106(2):196–204.

6. Seemungal TA, Donaldson GC, Bhowmik A, et al. Time course and recovery of exacerbations in patients with chronic obstructive pulmonary disease. Am J Respir Crit Care Med 2000;161(5):1608–13.

7. Rodriguez-Roisin R. Toward a consensus definition for COPD exacerbations. Chest 2000;117(5 Suppl 2):398S–401S.

8. Global Strategy for the Diagnosis, Management and Prevention of COPD, Global Initiative for Chronic Obstructive Lung Disease (GOLD). 2013. Available at: http://www.goldcopd.org/. Accessed March 4, 2013.

9. Pauwels R, Calverley P, Buist AS, et al. COPD exacerbations: the importance of a standard definition. Respir Med 2004;98(2):99–107.

10. Aaron SD, Fergusson D, Marks GB, et al. Counting, analysing and reporting exacerbations of COPD in randomised controlled trials. Thorax 2008;63(2): 122–8.

11. Wedzicha JA. Airway infection accelerates decline of lung function in chronic obstructive pulmonary disease. Am J Respir Crit Care Med 2001; 164(10 Pt 1):1757–8.

12. Wedzicha JA. Exacerbations: etiology and pathophysiologic mechanisms. Chest 2002;121(5 Suppl): 136S–41S.

13. Hogg JC. Role of latent viral infections in chronic obstructive pulmonary disease and asthma. Am J Respir Crit Care Med 2001;164(10 Pt 2):S71–5.

14. Sethi S. Infectious etiology of acute exacerbations of chronic bronchitis. Chest 2000;117(5 Suppl 2): 380S–5S.

15. Sethi S, Murphy TF. Bacterial infection in chronic obstructive pulmonary disease in 2000: a state-of-the-art review. Clin Microbiol Rev 2001;14(2): 336–63.

16. Sethi S, Evans N, Grant BJ, et al. New strains of bacteria and exacerbations of chronic obstructive pulmonary disease. N Engl J Med 2002;347(7): 465–71.

17. Seemungal T, Harper-Owen R, Bhowmik A, et al. Respiratory viruses, symptoms, and inflammatory markers in acute exacerbations and stable chronic obstructive pulmonary disease. Am J Respir Crit Care Med 2001;164(9):1618–23.

18. Anderson HR, Spix C, Medina S, et al. Air pollution and daily admissions for chronic obstructive pulmonary disease in 6 European cities: results from the APHEA project. Eur Respir J 1997;10(5): 1064–71.

19. Donaldson GC, Seemungal T, Jeffries DJ, et al. Effect of temperature on lung function and symptoms in chronic obstructive pulmonary disease. Eur Respir J 1999;13(4):844–9.

20. O'Donnell DE, Parker CM. COPD exacerbations. 3: pathophysiology. Thorax 2006;61(4):354–61.

21. Burge S, Wedzicha JA. COPD exacerbations: definitions and classifications. Eur Respir J Suppl 2003;41:46S–53S.

22. Miravitlles M, Espinosa C, Fernandez-Laso E, et al. Relationship between bacterial flora in sputum and functional impairment in patients with acute exacerbations of COPD. Study Group of Bacterial Infection in COPD. Chest 1999; 116(1):40–6.

23. Mushlin AI, Black ER, Connolly CA, et al. The necessary length of hospital stay for chronic pulmonary disease. JAMA 1991;266(1):80–3.

24. Connors AF Jr, Dawson NV, Thomas C, et al. Outcomes following acute exacerbation of severe chronic obstructive lung disease. The SUPPORT investigators (Study to Understand Prognoses and Preferences for Outcomes and Risks of Treatments). Am J Respir Crit Care Med 1996;154(4 Pt 1):959–67.

25. Afessa B, Morales IJ, Scanlon PD, et al. Prognostic factors, clinical course, and hospital outcome of patients with chronic obstructive pulmonary disease admitted to an intensive care unit for acute respiratory failure. Crit Care Med 2002;30(7): 1610–5.

26. Seneff MG, Wagner DP, Wagner RP, et al. Hospital and 1-year survival of patients admitted to intensive care units with acute exacerbation of chronic obstructive pulmonary disease. JAMA 1995; 274(23):1852–7.

27. Osman IM, Godden DJ, Friend JA, et al. Quality of life and hospital re-admission in patients with chronic obstructive pulmonary disease. Thorax 1997;52(1):67–71.

28. Lau AC, Yam LY, Poon E. Hospital re-admission in patients with acute exacerbation of chronic obstructive pulmonary disease. Respir Med 2001; 95(11):876–84.

29. Spruit MA, Singh SJ, Garvey C, et al. An official american thoracic society/european respiratory society statement: key concepts and advances in pulmonary rehabilitation. Am J Respir Crit Care Med 2013;188(8):e13–64.

30. Troosters T, Gosselink R, Decramer M. Short- and long-term effects of outpatient rehabilitation in

patients with chronic obstructive pulmonary disease: a randomized trial. Am J Med 2000;109(3): 207–12.

31. Emery CF, Leatherman NE, Burker EJ, et al. Psychological outcomes of a pulmonary rehabilitation program. Chest 1991;100(3):613–7.

32. Bourbeau J, Collet JP, Schwartzman K, et al. Economic benefits of self-management education in COPD. Chest 2006;130(6):1704–11.

33. Bourbeau J, Julien M, Maltais F, et al. Reduction of hospital utilization in patients with chronic obstructive pulmonary disease: a disease-specific self-management intervention. Arch Intern Med 2003; 163(5):585–91.

34. Donaldson GC, Seemungal TA, Bhowmik A, et al. Relationship between exacerbation frequency and lung function decline in chronic obstructive pulmonary disease. Thorax 2002;57(10):847–52.

35. Spruit MA, Gosselink R, Troosters T, et al. Muscle force during an acute exacerbation in hospitalised patients with COPD and its relationship with CXCL8 and IGF-I. Thorax 2003;58(9):752–6.

36. Troosters T, Probst VS, Crul T, et al. Resistance training prevents deterioration in quadriceps muscle function during acute exacerbations of chronic obstructive pulmonary disease. Am J Respir Crit Care Med 2010;181(10):1072–7.

37. Seemungal TA, Donaldson GC, Paul EA, et al. Effect of exacerbation on quality of life in patients with chronic obstructive pulmonary disease. Am J Respir Crit Care Med 1998;157(5 Pt 1):1418–22.

38. Donaldson GC, Wilkinson TM, Hurst JR, et al. Exacerbations and time spent outdoors in chronic obstructive pulmonary disease. Am J Respir Crit Care Med 2005;171(5):446–52.

39. Pitta F, Troosters T, Probst VS, et al. Physical activity and hospitalization for exacerbation of COPD. Chest 2006;129(3):536–44.

40. Pitta F, Troosters T, Spruit MA, et al. Characteristics of physical activities in daily life in chronic obstructive pulmonary disease. Am J Respir Crit Care Med 2005;171(9):972–7.

41. Garcia-Aymerich J, Farrero E, Felez MA, et al. Risk factors of readmission to hospital for a COPD exacerbation: a prospective study. Thorax 2003;58(2): 100–5.

42. Sewell L, Singh SJ, Williams JE, et al. Can individualized rehabilitation improve functional independence in elderly patients with COPD? Chest 2005;128(3):1194–200.

43. de Blok BM, de Greef MH, ten Hacken NH, et al. The effects of a lifestyle physical activity counseling program with feedback of a pedometer during pulmonary rehabilitation in patients with COPD: a pilot study. Patient Educ Couns 2006; 61(1):48–55.

44. Pitta F, Troosters T, Probst VS, et al. Are patients with COPD more active after pulmonary rehabilitation? Chest 2008;134(2):273–80.

45. Cindy Ng LW, Mackney J, Jenkins S, et al. Does exercise training change physical activity in people with COPD? A systematic review and meta-analysis. Chron Respir Dis 2012;9(1):17–26.

46. Gruffydd-Jones K, Langley-Johnson C, Dyer C, et al. What are the needs of patients following discharge from hospital after an acute exacerbation of chronic obstructive pulmonary disease (COPD)? Prim Care Respir J 2007;16(6):363–8.

47. Gudmundsson G, Gislason T, Janson C, et al. Depression, anxiety and health status after hospitalisation for COPD: a multicentre study in the Nordic countries. Respir Med 2006;100(1):87–93.

48. Harrison SL, Horton EJ, Smith R, et al. Physical activity monitoring: addressing the difficulties of accurately detecting slow walking speeds. Heart Lung 2013;42(5):361–4.e1.

49. Costi S, Brooks D, Goldstein RS. Perspectives that influence action plans for chronic obstructive pulmonary disease. Can Respir J 2006;13(7):362–8.

50. Harth L, Stuart J, Montgomery C, et al. Physical therapy practice patterns in acute exacerbations of chronic obstructive pulmonary disease. Can Respir J 2009;16(3):86–92.

51. Hill K, Patman S, Brooks D. Effect of airway clearance techniques in patients experiencing an acute exacerbation of chronic obstructive pulmonary disease: a systematic review. Chron Respir Dis 2010; 7(1):9–17.

52. Tang CY, Taylor NF, Blackstock FC. Chest physiotherapy for patients admitted to hospital with an acute exacerbation of chronic obstructive pulmonary disease (COPD): a systematic review. Physiotherapy 2010;96(1):1–13.

53. Yohannes AM. Health status and quality of life after acute exacerbations of chronic obstructive pulmonary disease. Qual Life Res 2007;16(2):357–8.

54. Man WD, Polkey MI, Donaldson N, et al. Community pulmonary rehabilitation after hospitalisation for acute exacerbations of chronic obstructive pulmonary disease: randomised controlled study. BMJ 2004;329(7476):1209.

55. Seymour JM, Moore L, Jolley CJ, et al. Outpatient pulmonary rehabilitation following acute exacerbations of COPD. Thorax 2010;65(5):423–8.

56. Jones SE, Green SA, Clark AL, et al. Pulmonary rehabilitation following hospitalisation for acute exacerbation of COPD: referrals, uptake and adherence. Thorax 2014;69(2):181–2.

Anxiety, Depression, and Cognitive Impairment in Patients with Chronic Respiratory Disease

Vincent S. Fan, MD, MPH[a],*, Paula M. Meek, RN, PhD[b]

KEYWORDS

- Anxiety • Depression • Cognitive impairment • Chronic respiratory disease

KEY POINTS

- Depression, anxiety and cognitive impairment are common among persons with COPD, and psychological symptoms are associated with worse outcomes.
- Psychological symptoms may affect adherence to pulmonary rehabilitation programs, and screening for these symptoms should be considered.
- Pulmonary rehabilitation may improve depression and anxiety symptoms although the effect on cognitive function is not as clear.

INTRODUCTION

Feelings, beliefs, and expectations are important influences on the outcomes from pulmonary rehabilitation. Depression, anxiety, and cognitive impairment are common among patients with chronic obstructive pulmonary disease (COPD) and may both affect the delivery of pulmonary rehabilitation and be modified by pulmonary rehabilitation. Evaluation for these conditions should therefore be considered during the baseline assessment for pulmonary rehabilitation.[1,2]

There has been increasing awareness that depression is a common feature of many chronic illnesses, including respiratory conditions.[3] In lung disease, the psychological comorbidity of anxiety also seems to play an important role, given the relationship between anxiety and dyspnea. In recent years, the links between chronic illness, decreases in cognitive function, and these emotional states have begun to be made. The interrelationships among the physiologic aspects of

pulmonary rehabilitation and these psychological and cognitive concerns are complex. In addition, it is not clear how and to what degree pulmonary rehabilitation modifies, ameliorates, or eliminates these emotional states or decreases in cognitive function.

A goal of pulmonary rehabilitation is to change patient health behaviors. This change can be facilitated by increasing physical activity in a supervised setting, ideally maintaining this increased physical activity after the formal pulmonary rehabilitation sessions are complete. Changing health behaviors in chronic illness is challenging, and there is increasing evidence that addressing comorbid psychological symptoms such as depression is an important component of health behavior change.[4]

In this article, the prevalence of depression, anxiety, and cognitive impairment in persons with COPD, and the extent to which these conditions limit or modify the effectiveness of pulmonary rehabilitation, are reviewed; in addition, whether

VA Statement: The views expressed in this article are those of the authors and do not necessarily reflect the position or policy of the Department of Veterans Affairs or the United States Government. *This material is the result of work supported by resources from the VA Puget Sound Health Care System, Seattle, Washington.*
a Veterans Affairs Puget Sound Health Care System, Department of Medicine, University of Washington, Seattle, WA, USA; b College of Nursing, University of Colorado, CO, USA
* Corresponding author.
E-mail address: Vincent.fan@va.gov

pulmonary rehabilitation may ameliorate these psychological and cognitive impairments is discussed.

Depression

Depression is an adjustment disorder that exists on a continuum from feelings of being blue or sad to major depressive illness. Simple mood disturbance such as mild anxiety or depression is typically associated with an identifiable life stressor, which is commonplace in chronic disease. An individual with a simple mood disturbance who begins pulmonary rehabilitation should be able to adequately participate in the program and, with encouragement, have positive outcomes. However, someone with a major depressive disorder needs to be treated aggressively within and beyond the rehabilitation program. Unless this major depression is recognized and addressed, patients probably do not realize their potential gains in pulmonary rehabilitation outcomes.

The defined criteria for the diagnosis of a major depressive disorder are that at least 5 of the symptoms in **Box 1** must be present nearly every day during a 2-week period.

To meet the diagnostic criteria for depression, these symptoms need to have caused clinically significant distress or impairment in social,

---

Box 1
Symptoms used to diagnose a major depressive disorder

- Depressed mood most of the day or markedly diminished interest or pleasure in all, or almost all, activities most of the day (must be one of the symptoms)
- Significant weight loss when not dieting or weight gain (eg, 5%) or decrease or increase in appetite
- Insomnia or hypersomnia
- Psychomotor agitation or retardation
- Fatigue or loss of energy
- Feelings of worthlessness or excessive or inappropriate guilt (not merely self-reproach or guilt about being sick)
- Diminished ability to think or concentrate
- Recurrent thoughts of death (not just fear of dying), recurrent suicidal ideation without a specific plan, or a suicide attempt or a specific plan

Data from Diagnostic and statistical manual of mental disorders, fourth edition text revision. Washington, DC: American Psychiatric Association; 2000.

---

occupational, or other important areas of functioning. If one of these symptoms existed previously, then it must have changed from the previous occurrence to be considered in the assessment. The symptoms must not be caused by the direct physiologic effects of a substance or a general medical condition or be associated with bereavement unless it has persisted for 2 months.

Some of the symptoms of depression such as poor appetite, sleep disturbance and fatigue are also associated with COPD and, therefore, may present a challenge to providers who are evaluating patients. Also, few studies of the impact of depressive symptoms on COPD outcomes have used strict *Diagnostic and Statistical Manual of Mental Disorders* (DSM) criteria for depression but instead have relied on symptom scales such as the Hospital Anxiety and Depression Scale (HADS)[5] or the Beck Depression Inventory (BDI) scale.[6]

PREVALENCE OF DEPRESSION

Depression and anxiety are the most common psychosocial concerns seen in chronic pulmonary patients enrolled in pulmonary rehabilitation.[7] Estimates of the prevalence of depression range from 10% to close to 80% (depending on the instrument and method used to screen), although the prevalence is most commonly reported as between 25% and 50%.[8–10] The higher percentages likely reflect the presence of symptom burden rather than clinically defined disease. Also, the prevalence of depression may be higher in patients with more severe COPD.[11,12] Some estimates suggest that patients with COPD are 2.5 times more likely to have anxiety and depression than healthy individuals.[11] Cross-sectional studies suggest that women, those with a body mass index less than 21 kg/m^2, and those who experience more significant dyspnea or disability are more likely to have symptoms of depression.[3,13] Patients with COPD without depression also are more than twice as likely to subsequently develop depression compared with those without COPD.[14]

Depressive symptoms in COPD are associated with worse clinical outcomes, including worse health-related quality of life,[9,15] decreased functional performance measured with the 6-minute walk test,[16] increased risk of COPD exacerbations,[17] and a higher risk of death.[18–20] Although it is not known whether treatment of depression may decrease the risk of these adverse outcomes, because there are effective treatments, it seems reasonable to address as an important potentially modifiable comorbid condition in COPD.

Psychological disorders such as depression are also common among patients with other lung diseases undergoing rehabilitation, including interstitial lung disease[21,22] and pulmonary hypertension.[23–25] It is therefore important to understand that depression is common in individuals with chronic lung disease, and most likely, it is an issue for all those enrolled in pulmonary rehabilitation.

Depression Treatment

In general, outside the setting of pulmonary rehabilitation, patients with depression are typically treated with either antidepressant medications or psychotherapy. Although a complete review of antidepressant therapy is beyond the scope of this article, there are few randomized trials specifically assessing the efficacy of antidepressants in COPD. An early study[26] found that nortriptyline improved depressed mood and anxiety. A small randomized trial[27] of a serotonin selective reuptake inhibitor, paroxetine, in 28 patients with COPD found no improvement during the 6-week trial, but improvement in depression and quality of life in a 3-month follow-up open-labeled period. In terms of psychotherapy, cognitive behavioral therapy has been studied in COPD, and the results have been mixed, with 1 randomized trial[28] showing no benefit compared with education alone, and another[29] showing significant improvements in anxiety and depression, which were maintained at 8 months. Although there are limited data of treating depression in COPD specifically,[30] the data on treating depression in older adults with other chronic illness[31] suggest that a comprehensive intervention with antidepressants and psychotherapy is likely to be effective in this population.

DOES DEPRESSION AFFECT PARTICIPATION AND THE LIKELIHOOD OF BENEFITTING FROM PULMONARY REHABILITATION?

Depression may affect patients' ability to engage in self-care behaviors,[32] and in diabetes and heart disease depression, it is associated with worse adherence to medications used to treat the disease.[33,34] In COPD, it is not known whether depression affects adherence to medications, but there is increasing evidence that depression affects whether patients initiate or complete a pulmonary rehabilitation program. For example, an analysis of participants in a large randomized controlled trial of lung volume reduction surgery (National Emphysema Treatment Trial)[35] showed that baseline mild depression and anxiety were both associated with decreased likelihood to complete the 10 required pulmonary rehabilitation sessions: 27% did not complete all of the sessions, and those with mild depressive symptoms (BDI≥5) were less likely to complete the pulmonary rehabilitation program. Depression measured with the HADS was also found to be associated with noncompletion of both a 7-week[36] and an 8-week pulmonary rehabilitation program[37] and with decreased likelihood to be adherent to home pulmonary rehabilitation at 1 year.[38] Although not all studies have found that depression decreases adherence to pulmonary rehabilitation,[39] these results indicate that depressed patients may be less likely to initiate and complete a pulmonary rehabilitation program.

There is also evidence that patients with depression may require more intensive self-management interventions than nondepressed patients. A randomized trial of dyspnea self-management combined with either 4 weeks or 24 weeks of supervised exercise found that those with significant depressive symptoms (Center for Epidemiologic Studies Depression [CES-D] Scale >15) experienced a significant reduction in dyspnea with 24 weeks of exercise, whereas those without depression improved with only 4 weeks.[40]

The finding that depression may adversely affect COPD self-management behaviors by potentially decreasing the participation and completion of pulmonary rehabilitation is consistent with evidence from a recent large randomized controlled trial of patients with depression who also had either diabetes or heart disease.[4] In this trial, concurrent treatment of both depression and chronic medical illness improved both depressive symptoms and the management of the chronic illness. Treatment of depression may therefore have the potential to improve clinical outcomes and also to improve self-management and increase participation in pulmonary rehabilitation programs.

Improvement in Depressive Symptoms as a Result of Pulmonary Rehabilitation

By improving dyspnea, increasing exercise tolerance, and reducing disability, pulmonary rehabilitation may itself contribute to improvement in psychological symptoms such as depression. Pulmonary rehabilitation programs often incorporate education and self-management components to improve patients' ability to manage their dyspnea and stress, which may also contribute to improved psychological symptoms. Several instruments have been used to measure psychological outcomes after a pulmonary rehabilitation program. Desirable instruments are tools that do not rely on physical symptoms (such as fatigue or tiredness), so that the mood and emotional issues can be separated from physical changes that typically result from the disease and the exercise components of pulmonary rehabilitation.

Some of the possible tools include the CES-D,[41] the BDI,[42] the Geriatric Depression Scale (GDS),[43] and the HADS.[5] The CES-D, a 20-item tool using a 0 (rarely) to 3 (most of the time) scoring, also has limited physical items and follows the DSM-III (DSM third edition) criteria.[41] A score less than 16 is considered normal, 16 to 24 shows borderline increase of depressed symptoms and should be considered for referral, and 24 and higher must be immediately referred for evaluation. The BDI has 21 items and has a score with a range from 0 to 63 with a score of 10 or higher corresponding to mild to moderate depressive symptoms. The BDI has been used extensively in the cardiovascular literature, as well as in pulmonary studies.[20] However, a disadvantage of both the BDI and the CES-D instruments is that they were not designed specifically for patients with chronic disease.

The HADS and the GDS are examples of depression symptom scales designed for chronically ill older adults. The GDS is a 15-item tool that is answered with yes or no, so it is quick to administer.[43] A score on the GDS of 5 or greater should trigger further evaluation, whereas a score of 10 or greater requires immediate referral. The HADS has 14 questions (7 depression related and 7 anxiety related), and the depression scale ranges from 0 to 21, with 8 or higher corresponding to mild symptoms, and 11 or higher corresponding to moderate to severe depression.

Several randomized controlled trials of pulmonary rehabilitation have assessed depressive symptoms before and after completion of the intervention program. An early 3-arm trial compared exercise combined with stress management education, stress management education alone, and usual care.[44] This study found that only the group who received the combined exercise and stress management program had a reduction in depression and anxiety. Another small study[45] randomized 24 patients to either an 8-week pulmonary rehabilitation program or control, and found that the intervention group had significant improvement in depressive symptoms measured with the BDI, and improvement in anxiety measured with the Spielberger State-Trait Anxiety Index (STAI). A larger trial of 200 patients with COPD[46] compared pulmonary rehabilitation (including stress management) with usual care and found improvement in both depression and anxiety measured with the HADS at 6 weeks; it also found that depression continued to be improved compared with the intervention group

at 1 year. A meta-analysis in 2007 and updated in 2009 that included 5 clinical trials[47,48] also found that comprehensive pulmonary rehabilitation improved depressive and anxiety symptoms among older patients with COPD. Clinical trial data therefore suggest that a comprehensive pulmonary rehabilitation program that includes stress management can improve psychological outcomes in COPD.

A small randomized trial of 30 patients[49] specifically addressed the question of whether 24 sessions of pulmonary rehabilitation combined with 12 sessions of psychotherapy would improve psychological outcomes compared with pulmonary rehabilitation alone and found that the addition of psychotherapy sessions resulted in a greater reduction in depression and anxiety measured with the BDI and Beck Anxiety Inventory. This finding therefore supports the approach of treating psychological symptoms at the same time as the exercise program and incorporating staff with expertise in psychotherapy to the pulmonary rehabilitation team to improve depressive and anxiety symptoms. This approach requires corroboration from further studies.

Several nonrandomized observational studies have been performed using a pre-post study design to address whether patients' depressive symptoms improve with pulmonary rehabilitation. Two observational studies[36,50] found no improvement in HADS depression or HADS anxiety scores after pulmonary rehabilitation. In contrast, several studies have found improvement in depression or anxiety,[37,51,52] and improvement was seen regardless of severity of COPD.[53] These observational data seem to support the general finding that psychological symptoms may improve after pulmonary rehabilitation.

An important consideration when assessing whether pulmonary rehabilitation improves psychological outcomes is the proportion of participants with depression or anxiety on entry into the program. A study of 334 patients with COPD who completed a pulmonary rehabilitation program found an improvement in mean HADS anxiety and depression scores after completion of the rehabilitation program, although these were less than the traditional minimum clinically important difference (MCID) of 1.5.[39] However, when the results were stratified by whether the baseline HADS scores were abnormal (≥8), it was found that those with abnormal baseline HADS anxiety or HADS depression scores had a significant improvement in their postpulmonary rehabilitation HADS scores. These findings are supported by another large study of 257 patients who completed a pulmonary rehabilitation program, in which the mean HADS anxiety and depression scores improved significantly, although the anxiety scores did not meet the MCID threshold.[37] However, when the investigators focused on abnormal anxiety or depression scores (HADS $\geq$10 for both scales) at baseline, they found that the proportion of anxious patients decreased from 25% to 9% (P<.001), and the proportion of patients with depressive symptoms decreased from 17% to 6% (<0.001) after the intervention.

These 2 studies make the compelling case that the effect of pulmonary rehabilitation on psychological outcomes is likely underestimated, because patients without baseline depression or anxiety who are unlikely to experience an improvement in these areas are included in the analysis. To more rigorously assess whether pulmonary rehabilitation improves depression or anxiety, randomized controlled trials should avoid looking at mean improvement in psychological symptom for all patients regardless of whether they have significant depression or anxiety at baseline. Instead, studies should consider analyzing data by looking at whether the proportion of patients with significant depressive or anxiety symptoms decreases with pulmonary rehabilitation or should restrict the analysis to those who had significant depressive or anxiety symptoms at baseline.

Should Screening for Depression be Performed Before Entry into a Pulmonary Rehabilitation Program?

Given the potential effect of depressive symptoms on completion of pulmonary rehabilitation programs as well as the potential beneficial effect of pulmonary rehabilitation on depressive symptoms, the American Thoracic Society (ATS)/European Respiratory Society statement on the key concepts of pulmonary rehabilitation states that "screening questionnaires for anxiety, depression, and/or cognitive impairment may be undertaken."[2] Little is known in the United States or Europe about whether pulmonary rehabilitation programs consistently screen for and treat depression. A survey of 22 programs in Australia[54] found that most were not using depression-specific or anxiety-specific instruments to screen for psychological comorbidity, and 36% did not offer specific psychological support. Of those programs that did provide support, 41% offered informal support (patients were referred to mental health), and only 5 (23%) provided formal psychological support. A greater awareness in pulmonary rehabilitation programs of the potential benefits of screening for depression is needed to ensure that patients are referred to licensed health professionals for accurate diagnosis and for consideration of antidepressant medications or psychotherapy.

In the United States, the US Preventative Services Taskforce review on screening for depression lists several potential depression screen instruments, which include the BDI, the GDS, and the Primary Care Evaluation of Mental Disorders (PRIME-MD).[55] The PRIME-MD brief screen includes 2 questions that are able to adequately screen those who need further evaluation.[56,57] These 2 questions are:

In the past month, have you felt bothered a lot by:

1. Little interest or pleasure in doing things?

2. Feeling down, depressed or hopeless?

These questions have proved to be sensitive and reasonably predictive of depression that requires further evaluation. An affirmative answer to either or both of these questions should trigger a further evaluation by a mental health professional. Although it is not known whether screening for depression among patients referred to pulmonary rehabilitation changes outcomes, screening with the PRIME-MD or another depression symptom measure used in chronically ill adults such as the GDS or HADS should be considered.

Anxiety

Like depression, anxiety can be considered on a continuum from generalized anxiety to panic disorder. Anxiety can frequently be present along with depression, and some recent reports have suggested that they may be interrelated. Generalized anxiety can be defined as an apprehensive anticipation of danger or a stressful situation. It may be associated with excessive feelings of somatic stress, such as fatigue, restlessness, irritability, rapid speech, sleep disturbances, tachycardia, dyspnea, and sweating. Generalized anxiety would be present if these symptoms and the apprehension are present more days than not over a 6-month period. Because respiratory patients commonly have fatigue, dyspnea, tachycardia, and sleep disturbance, their interpretation in the context of anxiety assessment can be problematic.

An additional difficulty is that there is also a condition called an adjustment disorder with generalized anxiety, which is adjustment to major life events (eg, recent severe exacerbation of a disease requiring hospitalization). The problematic piece is that there may not have been 6 months between the event and when the individual is enrolled in a pulmonary rehabilitation program. In this case, it is important to ascertain whether there were troubling symptoms present for a substantial period before hospitalization.

Panic attacks are further along the continuum, defined as intense episodes of acute anxiety, with dyspnea and cognitive fears. The dyspnea associated with a panic attack must be separated from an acute, severe episode of dyspnea resulting from underlying physical illness, but this may be difficult. A panic disorder is recurrent unexpected episodes (panic attacks) that are coupled with persistent concern about other attacks and worry about implications of such attacks. Panic attacks and panic disorder are serious issues that require further evaluation and treatment outside pulmonary rehabilitation. They can clearly interfere with maximizing benefits from rehabilitation. However, with appropriate support, the rehabilitation environment can be therapeutic to these patients.

Prevalence of Anxiety in COPD

In general, there has been less literature on the role of anxiety in COPD and therefore fewer studies to estimate the prevalence of this condition. The estimated prevalence varies widely, from 6% and 74%, and similar to studies of depression, most studies have used symptom measures and not a clinical diagnosis of anxiety,[58] and the prevalence varies with the severity of COPD and the instrument used to measure anxiety symptoms. Although the results are not consistent, anxiety may increase with worsening disease severity, as measured with a multidimensional index of COPD severity.[59]

What is the Relationship Between Anxiety and Pulmonary Rehabilitation?

Several of the studies that have already been mentioned in this article also assessed the impact of anxiety on adherence to pulmonary rehabilitation. In NETT (National Emphysema Treatment Trial), anxiety was measured with the STAI, which has a range of 20 to 80.[35] Patients with an STAI trait score of more than 36 were less likely to complete pulmonary rehabilitation after adjusting for disease severity. However, in a different study,[38] anxiety measured with the HADS anxiety scale was not associated with adherence to pulmonary rehabilitation in study of long-term follow-up. Anxiety affects patients' ability to exercise, and there is evidence that those with increased anxiety have decreased results on the 6-minute walk test after adjusting for disease severity.[59,60] Although there are fewer studies in this area, the literature

suggests that anxiety may lead to worse adherence to pulmonary rehabilitation and limit functional performance measured with the 6-minute walk test.

As described earlier for depression, participants in pulmonary rehabilitation may have an improvement in anxiety symptoms at the end of the intervention period. Many of the studies that have shown improvements in depressive symptoms after pulmonary rehabilitation have also reported a beneficial impact on anxiety symptoms.[44,45,49] Pulmonary rehabilitation therefore seems to improve both depressive and anxiety symptoms for patients with COPD.

Screening for Panic Disorder and Generalized Anxiety

As with depression, it is important to be aware of diagnostic criteria for anxiety, although the diagnosis is generally made by a licensed professional. The ATS statement on key concepts and advances in pulmonary rehabilitation states that "management of anxiety/panic in pulmonary rehabilitation has the potential to reduce such events and improve patient outcomes." To determine whether patients referred to pulmonary rehabilitation have significant anxiety symptoms, adequately screening for anxiety is important. The same study that used the PRIME-MD to screen for depression also successfully used the following 3 questions to adequately screen those who need further evaluation for significant anxiety.[56,57] The first 2 questions are similar to the depression screening questions, but the third question attempts to capture more severe episodes such as panic attacks.

In the past month, have you felt bothered *a lot* by:

1. "Nerves" or feeling anxious or edge?
2. Worrying about a lot of different things?

In the last month:

3. Have you had an anxiety attack (suddenly feeling fear or panic)?

An affirmative answer to any one of these questions should prompt the pulmonary rehabilitation staff to refer the patient for further evaluation by a mental health professional. These questions are also sensitive, with reasonable predictive properties for the detection of generalized anxiety that requires further evaluation. The controlled exercise sessions associated with pulmonary rehabilitation are a perfect venue to help determine if panic attacks are a feature associated with dyspnea episodes and should also be considered part of an assessment of anxiety.

Measures Used to Assess Anxiety as an Outcome in Pulmonary Rehabilitation

Although the 3 PRIME-MD questions are adequate screening questions for rehabilitation programs, there are established anxiety measures that can be used both to screen for anxiety and to assess anxiety outcomes after pulmonary rehabilitation. A recent tool developed for use in primary care holds promise for screening and outcome measurement, the General Anxiety Disorder-7 (GAD-7).[61] The GAD-7 is a 7-item tool that is answered on a 0 to 3 (nearly every day) scale, with an eighth question on how distressing the symptoms are. A score on the GAD-7 of 5 or greater indicates mild anxiety and a score of 10 or greater indicates the need for referral. The Penn State Worry Questionnaire is also a public domain questionnaire that could be used to screen and measure outcomes.[62] The tool originally had 16 items scored on a 1 (not at all typical of me) to 4 (very typical of me) scale, but recent analysis has reduced it to 8 items.[63] The 8-item tool has performed well, but does not have a clear cutoff score, although a mean score of 30 is considered normal for the 16-item version. Other measures that have been used in COPD include the HADS-anxiety scale with 7 questions and a score between 0 and 21 with a cutoff of 8 or more for mild symptoms and 10 or more for moderate to severe symptoms.[5] The STAI has also been used, which has a range of 20 to 80.[64] Symptom measures may also be used successfully as a screening and an outcome variable.

Cognitive function

Cognitive function can be defined as the mental process of knowing, including awareness, perception, reasoning, and judgment. Cognitive function improves as we develop from childhood, then declines as we age. Normal aging has been associated with declines in cognitive function involving memory, language, thinking, and judgment but does not interfere with overall functioning. Mild cognitive impairment is an intermediate stage between the expected cognitive decline of normal aging and dementia. Mild cognitive impairment goes beyond slips of the memory or not being able to find the right word, and many individuals may be aware that their memory or mental function has slipped or it may be noticed by family and friends. In general, normal aging changes and even mild cognitive impairment may not be severe

enough to interfere with a person's day-to-day life or their ability to self-manage their illness or affect their usual activities.

However, chronic illness such as COPD can accelerate the normal aging process and lead to important deficits. Clearly, cognitive impairments have implications for pulmonary rehabilitation in terms of education and self-management strategies. Some have suggested that cognitive impairment should be considered a primary component of hypoxemic COPD and not a mere comorbidity of this disease. Hypoxemia can influence cognitive decline but is neither sufficient nor required for an individual with COPD to show decline.

Prevalence of cognitive decline in COPD

Deficits in cognitive function are prevalent in COPD and can be complicated by chronic hypoxemia.[65–68] Cognitive deficiencies worsen along with disease progression,[69] with some reporting abnormalities (such as scores <24 in the Mini-Mental State Examination [MMSE]) in 64% of those with severe COPD.[70] The percentage of patients with abnormalities in the MMSE included verbal recall (26%), construction (39%), attention (31%), language (13%), and orientation (current date or location, 24%). In addition, impairment in test performance that requires a drawing task, such as producing an analog clock with a set time, or other complex goal-directed tasks indicates problems associated with judgment and complexity[71] and has been proposed to be prognostic in hypoxemic patients with COPD.[72]

A recent investigation in nonhypoxemic individuals with COPD that combined multiple modes to assess cognitive function including magnetic resonance imaging and standard neuropsychological tests found reduced white matter integrity, disturbance in the function of gray matter, and lower neuropsychiatric test scores compared with age-related controls.[73] In this investigation, there were deficits in processing speed and executive function as well as episodic and working memory, which corresponds to the deficits seen on the MMSE. Recent findings from the Rotterdam Study[74] have found on high-resolution magnetic resonance imaging greater frequency of cerebral microbleeds in individuals with COPD. This finding supports the proposition that the cognitive function changes seen are at least in part caused by cerebral microbleeds, a novel marker for cerebral small-vessel disease. Although all the cognitive function changes found are important, working memory is particularly relevant to individuals who participate in pulmonary rehabilitation programs; this topic is reviewed in the next section.

Working memory

Working memory in the past was referred to as short-term memory; however, its functions are more complex than first proposed.[75–78] Originally, it was believed that short-term memory collected all sensory information to be stored in a single collection. We know now that there are different systems for different types of information, such as visual and verbal.[79] Working memory consists of a central executive that controls and coordinates the operation of 2 subsystems that process and store information: one for spoken and written material and one for visual or spatial information.[80] Also, the central executive is involved in other cognitive tasks like problem solving and mental arithmetic. Working memory becomes critical in any intervention designed to increase knowledge and change behavior as it applies to real-life tasks. Specifically, working memory is essential to reading and understanding educational materials and navigation of daily activities requiring visual and spatial processing and problem solving central to self-care.

There is some evidence that working memory is linked to the ability to focus attention on a task or information and disregard distractions.[81,82] However, some of the literature that tested working memory training has been drawn into question, and improvements may simply be caused by increasing ability to focus. One study did show improvements in working memory by high-intensity exercise. In this study of both sedentary and active young women,[83] the participants were exercised to the point of exhaustion and working memory was measured during, immediately after, and on recovery. Working memory in these participants decreased during and immediately after the exercise but increased after recovery.

Although specific working memory training has not been performed in individuals with COPD, general cognitive training aimed at stimulating attention, learning, and logical-deductive thinking has been attempted without success.[84] Consequently, it is not clear that extensive cognitive training as opposed to classic strategies that improve the quality of educational materials and improve working memory strategies such as focusing attention is any better. In general, working memory is improved via increased attention to task or information, limitation of distraction, and, potentially, exercise.

Pulmonary rehabilitation as an intervention to improve depression, anxiety, and cognitive impairment

Pulmonary rehabilitation has a real advantage when it comes to treating many psychosocial concerns, because exercise is one of the best interventions for anxiety, depression, and stress relief. Even a short course of pulmonary rehabilitation has shown improvements in depression, verbal memory, and visuospatial functioning.[85]

Besides participating in the exercise portion of the rehabilitation program, there are specific medications and psychotherapy interventions that may improve depression and lower anxiety. The specific medications are not reviewed here, but most of these medications do not take immediate effect and can take as long as several weeks before the individual feels the impact. Unless otherwise indicated by the individual's health care provider, participation in a program should not be restricted. However, anxiety, depression, and cognitive impairments can all affect the individual's ability to focus and learn from any formal educational classes. Care must be given to individualizing the program when the individual has these psychosocial concerns.

It seems that exercise training produces little if any improvement in cognitive function in hypoxic COPD. Therefore, it may be necessary to adapt and tailor the program so that individuals with cognitive impairment can obtain the essential knowledge needed to self-manage their disease. If the individual's cognitive impairments are such that retention of information and judgment are impaired, then a significant other or caregiver needs to be an integral part of the rehabilitative process. Further, the age-old strategy of repetition, repetition, repetition can go a long, long, long way toward helping reinforce information retention.

REFERENCES

1. Nici L, Donner C, Wouters E, et al. American Thoracic Society/European Respiratory Society statement on pulmonary rehabilitation. Am J Respir Crit Care Med 2006;173(12):1390–413.
2. Spruit MA, Singh SJ, Garvey C, et al. An official American Thoracic Society/European Respiratory Society statement: key concepts and advances in pulmonary rehabilitation. Am J Respir Crit Care Med 2013;188(8):e13–64.
3. Schane RE, Walter LC, Dinno A, et al. Prevalence and risk factors for depressive symptoms in persons with chronic obstructive pulmonary disease. J Gen Intern Med 2008;23(11):1757–62.
4. Katon WJ, Lin EH, Von Korff M, et al. Collaborative care for patients with depression and chronic illnesses. N Engl J Med 2010;363(27):2611–20.
5. Zigmond AS, Snaith RP. The hospital anxiety and depression scale. Acta Psychiatr Scand 1983; 67(6):361–70.

6. Beck AT, Ward CH, Mendelson M, et al. An inventory for measuring depression. Arch Gen Psychiatry 1961;4:561–71.

7. Maurer J, Rebbapragada V, Borson S, et al. Anxiety and depression in COPD: current understanding, unanswered questions, and research needs. Chest 2008;134(Suppl 4):43S–56S.

8. Ng TP, Niti M, Tan WC, et al. Depressive symptoms and chronic obstructive pulmonary disease: effect on mortality, hospital readmission, symptom burden, functional status, and quality of life. Arch Intern Med 2007;167(1):60–7.

9. Norwood R. Prevalence and impact of depression in chronic obstructive pulmonary disease patients. Curr Opin Pulm Med 2006;12(2):113–7.

10. van Ede L, Yzermans CJ, Brouwer HJ. Prevalence of depression in patients with chronic obstructive pulmonary disease: a systematic review. Thorax 1999;54(8):688–92.

11. van Manen JG, Bindels PJ, Dekker FW, et al. Risk of depression in patients with chronic obstructive pulmonary disease and its determinants. Thorax 2002;57(5):412–6.

12. Watz H, Waschki B, Boehme C, et al. Extrapulmonary effects of chronic obstructive pulmonary disease on physical activity: a cross-sectional study. Am J Respir Crit Care Med 2008;177(7):743–51.

13. Chavannes NH, Huibers MJ, Schermer TR, et al. Associations of depressive symptoms with gender, body mass index and dyspnea in primary care COPD patients. Fam Pract 2005;22(6):604–7.

14. Polsky D, Doshi JA, Marcus S, et al. Long-term risk for depressive symptoms after a medical diagnosis. Arch Intern Med 2005;165(11):1260–6.

15. Yohannes AM, Roomi J, Waters K, et al. Quality of life in elderly patients with COPD: measurement and predictive factors. Respir Med 1998;92(10): 1231–6.

16. Al-shair K, Dockry R, Mallia-Milanes B, et al. Depression and its relationship with poor exercise capacity, BODE index and muscle wasting in COPD. Respir Med 2009;103(10):1572–9.

17. Xu W, Collet JP, Shapiro S, et al. Independent effect of depression and anxiety on chronic obstructive pulmonary disease exacerbations and hospitalizations. Am J Respir Crit Care Med 2008;178(9): 913–20.

18. Almagro P, Calbo E, Ochoa de Echaguen A, et al. Mortality after hospitalization for COPD. Chest 2002;121(5):1441–8.

19. de Voogd JN, Wempe JB, Koeter GH, et al. Depressive symptoms as predictors of mortality in patients with COPD. Chest 2009;135(3):619–25.

20. Fan VS, Ramsey SD, Giardino ND, et al. Sex, depression, and risk of hospitalization and mortality in chronic obstructive pulmonary disease. Arch Intern Med 2007;167(21):2345–53.

21. Akhtar AA, Ali MA, Smith RP. Depression in patients with idiopathic pulmonary fibrosis. Chron Respir Dis 2013;10(3):127–33.

22. Ryerson CJ, Arean PA, Berkeley J, et al. Depression is a common and chronic comorbidity in patients with interstitial lung disease. Respirology 2012;17(3):525–32.

23. Harzheim D, Klose H, Pinado FP, et al. Anxiety and depression disorders in patients with pulmonary arterial hypertension and chronic thromboembolic pulmonary hypertension. Respir Res 2013;14(1): 104.

24. McCollister DH, Beutz M, McLaughlin V, et al. Depressive symptoms in pulmonary arterial hypertension: prevalence and association with functional status. Psychosomatics 2010;51(4):339–339.e8.

25. Batal O, Khatib OF, Bair N, et al. Sleep quality, depression, and quality of life in patients with pulmonary hypertension. Lung 2011;189(2):141–9.

26. Borson S, McDonald GJ, Gayle T, et al. Improvement in mood, physical symptoms, and function with nortriptyline for depression in patients with chronic obstructive pulmonary disease. Psychosomatics 1992;33(2):190–201.

27. Eiser N, Harte R, Spiros K, et al. Effect of treating depression on quality-of-life and exercise tolerance in severe COPD. COPD 2005;2(2):233–41.

28. Kunik ME, Veazey C, Cully JA, et al. COPD education and cognitive behavioral therapy group treatment for clinically significant symptoms of depression and anxiety in COPD patients: a randomized controlled trial. Psychol Med 2008;38(3): 385–96.

29. Hynninen MJ, Bjerke N, Pallesen S, et al. A randomized controlled trial of cognitive behavioral therapy for anxiety and depression in COPD. Respir Med 2010;104(7):986–94.

30. Alexopoulos GS, Kiosses DN, Sirey JA, et al. Personalised intervention for people with depression and severe COPD. Br J Psychiatry 2013;202(3): 235–6.

31. Unutzer J, Katon W, Callahan CM, et al. Collaborative care management of late-life depression in the primary care setting: a randomized controlled trial. JAMA 2002;288(22):2836–45.

32. Katon WJ. Clinical and health services relationships between major depression, depressive symptoms, and general medical illness. Biol Psychiatry 2003;54(3):216–26.

33. Ciechanowski PS, Katon WJ, Russo JE. Depression and diabetes: impact of depressive symptoms on adherence, function, and costs. Arch Intern Med 2000;160(21):3278–85.

34. Carney RM, Freedland KE, Eisen SA, et al. Major depression and medication adherence in elderly patients with coronary artery disease. Health Psychol 1995;14(1):88–90.

35. Fan VS, Giardino ND, Blough DK, et al. Costs of pulmonary rehabilitation and predictors of adherence in the National Emphysema Treatment Trial. COPD 2008;5(2):105–16.

36. Lewko A, Bidgood PL, Jewell A, et al. Evaluation of multidimensional COPD-related subjective fatigue following a pulmonary rehabilitation programme. Respir Med 2014;108(1):95–102.

37. Bhandari NJ, Jain T, Marolda C, et al. Comprehensive pulmonary rehabilitation results in clinically meaningful improvements in anxiety and depression in patients with chronic obstructive pulmonary disease. J Cardiopulm Rehabil Prev 2013;33(2):123–7.

38. Heerema-Poelman A, Stuive I, Wempe JB. Adherence to a maintenance exercise program 1 year after pulmonary rehabilitation: what are the predictors of dropout? J Cardiopulm Rehabil Prev 2013;33(6):419–26.

39. Harrison SL, Greening NJ, Williams JE, et al. Have we underestimated the efficacy of pulmonary rehabilitation in improving mood? Respir Med 2012;106(6):838–44.

40. Nguyen HQ, Carrieri-Kohlman V. Dyspnea self-management in patients with chronic obstructive pulmonary disease: moderating effects of depressed mood. Psychosomatics 2005;46(5):402–10.

41. Radloff L. The CES-D Scale: a self-report depression scale for research in the general population. Appl Psychol Meas 1977;1:385–401.

42. Beck AT, Steer RA, Garbin M. Psychometric properties of the Beck depression inventory: twenty-five years of evaluation. Clin Psychol Rev 1988;8:77–100.

43. Yesavage JA, Brink TL, Rose TL, et al. Development and validation of a geriatric depression screening scale: a preliminary report. J Psychiatr Res 1982;17(1):37–49.

44. Emery CF, Schein RL, Hauck ER, et al. Psychological and cognitive outcomes of a randomized trial of exercise among patients with chronic obstructive pulmonary disease. Health Psychol 1998;17(3):232–40.

45. Paz-Diaz H, Montes de Oca M, Lopez JM, et al. Pulmonary rehabilitation improves depression, anxiety, dyspnea and health status in patients with COPD. Am J Phys Med Rehabil 2007;86(1):30–6.

46. Griffiths TL, Burr ML, Campbell IA, et al. Results at 1 year of outpatient multidisciplinary pulmonary rehabilitation: a randomised controlled trial. Lancet 2000;355(9201):362–8.

47. Coventry PA, Hind D. Comprehensive pulmonary rehabilitation for anxiety and depression in adults with chronic obstructive pulmonary disease: systematic review and meta-analysis. J Psychosom Res 2007;63(5):551–65.

48. Coventry PA. Does pulmonary rehabilitation reduce anxiety and depression in chronic obstructive pulmonary disease? Curr Opin Pulm Med 2009;15(2):143–9.

49. de Godoy DV, de Godoy RF. A randomized controlled trial of the effect of psychotherapy on anxiety and depression in chronic obstructive pulmonary disease. Arch Phys Med Rehabil 2003;84(8):1154–7.

50. Bentsen SB, Wentzel-Larsen T, Henriksen AH, et al. Anxiety and depression following pulmonary rehabilitation. Scand J Caring Sci 2013;27(3):541–50.

51. Pirraglia PA, Casserly B, Velasco R, et al. Association of change in depression and anxiety symptoms with functional outcomes in pulmonary rehabilitation patients. J Psychosom Res 2011;71(1):45–9.

52. von Leupoldt A, Taube K, Lehmann K, et al. The impact of anxiety and depression on outcomes of pulmonary rehabilitation in patients with COPD. Chest 2011;140(3):730–6.

53. Tselebis A, Bratis D, Pachi A, et al. A pulmonary rehabilitation program reduces levels of anxiety and depression in COPD patients. Multidiscip Respir Med 2013;8(1):41.

54. Doyle C, Dunt D, Ames D, et al. Managing mood disorders in patients attending pulmonary rehabilitation clinics. Int J Chron Obstruct Pulmon Dis 2013;8:15–20.

55. O'Connor EA, Whitlock EP, Gaynes B, et al. Screening for Depression in Adults and Older Adults in Primary Care: An Updated Systematic Review [Internet]. Rockville (MD): Agency for Healthcare Research and Quality (US); 2009 Dec. Report No.: 10-05143-EF-1. U.S. Preventive Services Task Force Evidence Syntheses, formerly Systematic Evidence Reviews. PMID: 20722174 [PubMed].

56. Kunik ME, Azzam PN, Souchek J, et al. A practical screening tool for anxiety and depression in patients with chronic breathing disorders. Psychosomatics 2007;48(1):16–21.

57. Spitzer RL, Williams JB, Kroenke K, et al. Utility of a new procedure for diagnosing mental disorders in primary care. The PRIME-MD 1000 study. JAMA 1994;272(22):1749–56.

58. Yohannes AM, Willgoss TG, Baldwin RC, et al. Depression and anxiety in chronic heart failure and chronic obstructive pulmonary disease: prevalence, relevance, clinical implications and management principles. Int J Geriatr Psychiatry 2010;25(12):1209–21.

59. Eisner MD, Blanc PD, Yelin EH, et al. Influence of anxiety on health outcomes in COPD. Thorax 2010;65(3):229–34.

60. Giardino ND, Curtis JL, Andrei AC, et al. Anxiety is associated with diminished exercise performance

and quality of life in severe emphysema: a cross-sectional study. Respir Res 2010;11:29.

61. Spitzer RL, Kroenke K, Williams JB, et al. A brief measure for assessing generalized anxiety disorder: the GAD-7. Arch Intern Med 2006;166(10):1092–7.

62. Meyer TJ, Miller ML, Metzger RL, et al. Development and validation of the Penn State Worry Questionnaire. Behav Res Ther 1990;28(6):487–95.

63. Hopko DR, Stanley MA, Reas DL, et al. Assessing worry in older adults: confirmatory factor analysis of the Penn State Worry Questionnaire and psychometric properties of an abbreviated model. Psychol Assess 2003;15(2):173–83.

64. Spielberger CE, Goruch RL. Manual for the state-trait anxiety inventory. Palo Alto (CA): Consulting Psychologists Press; 1970.

65. Incalzi RA, Gemma A, Marra C, et al. Verbal memory impairment in COPD: its mechanisms and clinical relevance. Chest 1997;112(6):1506–13.

66. Incalzi RA, Gemma A, Marra C, et al. Chronic obstructive pulmonary disease. An original model of cognitive decline. Am Rev Respir Dis 1993;148(2):418–24.

67. Kozora E, Filley CM, Julian LJ, et al. Cognitive functioning in patients with chronic obstructive pulmonary disease and mild hypoxemia compared with patients with mild Alzheimer disease and normal controls. Neuropsychiatry Neuropsychol Behav Neurol 1999;12(3):178–83.

68. Chang SS, Chen S, McAvay GJ, et al. Effect of coexisting chronic obstructive pulmonary disease and cognitive impairment on health outcomes in older adults. J Am Geriatr Soc 2012;60(10):1839–46.

69. Li J, Huang Y, Fei GH. The evaluation of cognitive impairment and relevant factors in patients with chronic obstructive pulmonary disease. Respiration 2013;85(2):98–105.

70. Ozge C, Ozge A, Unal O. Cognitive and functional deterioration in patients with severe COPD. Behav Neurol 2006;17(2):121–30.

71. Royall DR. Double jeopardy. Chest 2006;130(6):1636–8.

72. Antonelli-Incalzi R, Corsonello A, Pedone C, et al. Drawing impairment predicts mortality in severe COPD. Chest 2006;130(6):1687–94.

73. Dodd JW, Chung AW, van den Broek MD, et al. Brain structure and function in chronic obstructive pulmonary disease: a multimodal cranial magnetic resonance imaging study. Am J Respir Crit Care Med 2012;186(3):240–5.

74. Lahousse L, Vernooij MW, Darweesh SK, et al. Chronic obstructive pulmonary disease and cerebral microbleeds. The Rotterdam Study. Am J Respir Crit Care Med 2013;188(7):783–8.

75. Baddeley AD. Working memory. Oxford (United Kingdom), New York: Clarendon Press, Oxford University Press; 1986.

76. Hitch GJ, Baddeley AD. Verbal reasoning and working memory. Q J Exp Psychol 1976;28:603–21.

77. Dales RE, Cakmak S, Leech J, et al. The association between personal care products and lung function. Ann Epidemiol 2013;23(2):49–53.

78. Vogiatzis I, Zakynthinos S. The physiological basis of rehabilitation in chronic heart and lung disease. J Appl Physiol (1985) 2013;115(1):16–21.

79. Baddeley AD, Hitch GJ, Allen RJ. Working memory and binding in sentence recall. J Mem Lang 2009;61(3):438–56.

80. Polkey MI, Spruit MA, Wouters E, et al. Reply: minimal or maximal clinically important difference: using death to define MCID. Am J Respir Crit Care Med 2013;187(12):1392.

81. Zanto TP, Gazzaley A. Neural suppression of irrelevant information underlies optimal working memory performance. J Neurosci 2009;29(10):3059–66.

82. Berry AS, Zanto TP, Rutman AM, et al. Practice-related improvement in working memory is modulated by changes in processing external interference. J Neurophysiol 2009;102(3):1779–89.

83. Bue-Estes CL, Willer B, Burton H, et al. Short-term exercise to exhaustion and its effects on cognitive function in young women. Percept Mot Skills 2008;107(3):933–45.

84. Incalzi RA, Corsonello A, Trojano L, et al. Cognitive training is ineffective in hypoxemic COPD: a six-month randomized controlled trial. Rejuvenation Res 2008;11(1):239–50.

85. Kozora E, Tran ZV, Make B. Neurobehavioral improvement after brief rehabilitation in patients with chronic obstructive pulmonary disease. J Cardiopulm Rehabil 2002;22(6):426–30.

Palliative Care and Pulmonary Rehabilitation

Daisy J.A. Janssen, MD, PhD[a,b,*], James R. McCormick, MD, FCCP[c]

KEYWORDS

- Palliative care • Advance care planning • Education • Hospice • End of life
- Pulmonary rehabilitation

KEY POINTS

- Patients with advanced chronic obstructive pulmonary disease (COPD) commonly have unmet needs, such as dealing with a high daily symptom burden, emotional distress, needs of family caregivers, and requirements for advance care planning. Each of these can be addressed in the context of a palliative care program.
- Palliative care and pulmonary rehabilitation are both important components of integrated care for patients with chronic respiratory diseases and share some similarities.
- Pulmonary rehabilitation provides the opportunity to introduce palliative care by implementing education about advance care planning as an integral part of its program.

INTRODUCTION

A century ago, most deaths occurred suddenly, caused by infectious diseases, accidents, and childbirth.[1] Demographic transitions, like aging of the population and a shift in causes of death to chronic diseases, have had major consequences for the experience of dying and palliative care needs.[2,3] The experience of dying has increasingly become a feature of old age.[2] Many people acquire progressive chronic diseases toward the end of life.[1,2] Chronic obstructive pulmonary disease (COPD) is a highly prevalent chronic disease and is the third leading cause of death worldwide.[4]

Management of COPD includes reduction of risk factors, like smoking cessation; appropriate immunizations; attention to nutrition; pharmacologic treatment, such as inhaled bronchodilators and glucocorticosteroids; and nonpharmacologic treatment, such as pulmonary rehabilitation, long-term oxygen therapy, and surgery.[5]

Pulmonary rehabilitation is indicated for patients who are symptomatic or who complain of having decreased daily life activities.[6] The American Thoracic Society/European Respiratory Society Statement *Key Concepts and Advances in Pulmonary Rehabilitation*[7] defines pulmonary rehabilitation as "a comprehensive intervention based on a thorough patient assessment followed by patient-tailored therapies which include, but are not limited to, exercise training, education and behavior change, designed to improve the physical and psychological condition of people with chronic respiratory disease and to promote the long-term adherence to health-enhancing behaviors." Pulmonary rehabilitation has been shown to reduce dyspnea, increase exercise capacity, and improve quality of life in patients with COPD and other chronic respiratory diseases.[7]

Quality of life in patients with COPD is even more greatly affected by their disease than quality of life

[a] Program Development Centre, CIRO+, Centre of Expertise for Chronic Organ Failure, Hornerheide 1, Horn 6085 NM, The Netherlands; [b] Centre of Expertise for Palliative Care, Maastricht University Medical Centre+ (MUMC+), P. Debyelaan 25, 6229 HX, Maastricht, The Netherlands; [c] Department of Internal Medicine, Division of Pulmonary, Critical Care and Sleep Medicine, University of Kentucky Medical School, Kentucky Clinic, L543, 740 S. Limestone, Lexington, KY 40536, USA
* Corresponding author. Program Development Centre, CIRO+, Centre of Expertise for Chronic Organ Failure, Hornerheide 1, Horn 6085 NM, The Netherlands.
E-mail address: daisyjanssen@ciro-horn.nl

Clin Chest Med 35 (2014) 411–421
http://dx.doi.org/10.1016/j.ccm.2014.02.006
0272-5231/14/$ – see front matter © 2014 Elsevier Inc. All rights reserved.

of patients with cancer.[8] Therefore, palliative care has been recognized as an important approach for patients with advanced COPD.[8–10] Palliative care is defined by the World Health Organization (WHO) as "an approach that improves the quality of life of patients and their families facing the problem associated with life-threatening illness, through the prevention and relief of suffering by means of early identification and impeccable assessment and treatment of pain and other problems, physical, psychosocial and spiritual" (**Box 1**).[11]

Palliative care and pulmonary rehabilitation are both important components of integrated care for patients with chronic respiratory diseases and share some similarities. Palliative care, like pulmonary rehabilitation, aims to decrease symptom burden and improve quality of life and uses an interdisciplinary approach to achieve this. Despite the similarities, several differences distinguish these approaches.[12] For example, palliative care focuses on decreasing symptoms, whereas pulmonary rehabilitation intends to modify the disease and promote the long-term adherence to health-enhancing behaviors. In addition, palliative care includes several aspects that do not receive attention during pulmonary rehabilitation, such as bereavement counseling and spiritual care. Exercise training is the cornerstone of pulmonary rehabilitation but receives little attention in palliative care.[12]

The needs of patients with advanced respiratory disease are complex and should be addressed by integrating curative-restorative and palliative care.[13] In this article, an overview of the complex needs and barriers involved in the provision of palliative care is provided, and how advance care planning education as a component of palliative care can be introduced during pulmonary rehabilitation is described.

Box 1
WHO definition of palliative care

Palliative care is an approach that improves the quality of life of patients and their families facing the problem associated with life-threatening illness, through the prevention and relief of suffering by means of early identification and impeccable assessment and treatment of pain and other problems, physical, psychosocial and spiritual

Palliative care:

- Provides relief from pain and other distressing symptoms
- Affirms life and regards dying as a normal process
- Intends neither to hasten nor postpone death
- Integrates the psychological and spiritual aspects of patient care
- Offers a support system to help patients live as actively as possible until death
- Offers a support system to help the family cope during the patient's illness and in their own bereavement
- Uses a team approach to address the needs of patients and their families, including bereavement counseling, if indicated
- Will enhance quality of life and may also positively influence the course of illness
- Is applicable early in the course of illness, in conjunction with other therapies that are intended to prolong life, such as chemotherapy or radiation therapy, and includes those investigations needed to better understand and manage distressing clinical complications

From World Health Organization. WHO definition of palliative care. Available at: http://www.who.int/cancer/palliative/definition/en. Accessed December 01, 2013.

DISEASE TRAJECTORY AND THE PALLIATIVE CARE MODEL IN ADVANCED COPD

The course of advanced COPD is typically marked by a gradual decline in health status, punctuated by acute exacerbations. Every exacerbation can be life threatening and is associated with an increased risk of dying.[1] About 10% of patients with COPD admitted to the hospital because of an acute exacerbation die during their stay in the hospital.[14] Moreover, almost half of these patients die within 4 years of discharge.[15] Progressive respiratory failure is the primary cause of death in patients with COPD hospitalized for an exacerbation.[16] In addition, patients with COPD often suffer from comorbidities, which may further compromise survival.[17] Cardiovascular events are an important cause of death for patients with COPD.[18]

Even the best models of 6-month survival in patients with nonmalignant diseases have a limited ability to predict death for individual patients.[19,20] As a result, introducing palliative care should not depend on the physician's estimation of a limited life expectancy. The traditional dichotomous model of curative and palliative care, in which curative care ends and palliative care starts at a certain moment, is not appropriate for patients with chronic life-limiting diseases like COPD. The Official American Thoracic Society Clinical Policy Statement *Palliative Care for Patients with Respiratory Diseases and Critical Illnesses* describes an individualized integrated model of palliative care, in which palliative care starts when a patient suffering from a progressive respiratory disease becomes symptomatic.[13] Palliative care needs to be offered concurrently with curative-restorative care, and the intensity of palliative care is titrated to the needs of the patient and the patient's family.[13]

PALLIATIVE CARE NEEDS IN ADVANCED COPD

Patients with advanced COPD have palliative care needs comparable with the palliative care needs of patients with advanced cancer.[8] These palliative care needs occur in the following domains: symptoms, daily care, family caregiving, comorbidities and advance care planning (**Fig. 1**).

Symptoms

The high symptom burden and impaired quality of life of patients with advanced COPD was described more than a decade ago. Quality of life in these patients is even more greatly affected by their disease than quality of life of patients with cancer.[8] Moreover, patients with COPD reported more severe symptoms of anxiety and depression than patients with lung cancer.[8] It has been shown that, according to bereaved relatives, common symptoms reported in the last year of life by patients with chronic lung disease include dyspnea, pain, low mood, anorexia, insomnia, and cough.

The proportion of patients experiencing dyspnea is higher among those with chronic lung disease than among those with lung cancer (94% vs 78%, respectively).[9] In-depth interviews with bereaved relatives of patients with COPD showed that dyspnea had major consequences in terms of physical functioning, lifestyle restrictions, and anxiety.[21] A questionnaire survey including bereaved relatives suggested that symptom control is poor in the last year of life of patients with COPD. Moreover, patients may receive inadequate services from primary and secondary health care providers.[22] Patients with advanced COPD suffer from dyspnea (94%), fatigue (71%–89%), mouth problems (60%), coughing (56%–58%), low mood (52%), and anxiety (51%).[23,24] Nevertheless, only a few of them received symptom-related treatment and those receiving treatment described only moderate satisfaction. In addition, involvement of allied health care professionals was low, and palliative medication was scarcely prescribed.[24]

Care Needs

Patients with advanced COPD often experience impairment in performing normal daily tasks.[25,26] A study of patients with COPD admitted to the hospital showed that patients may not only need assistance with instrumental activities of daily living, like grocery shopping, house working, doing laundry and traveling, but also with basic activities

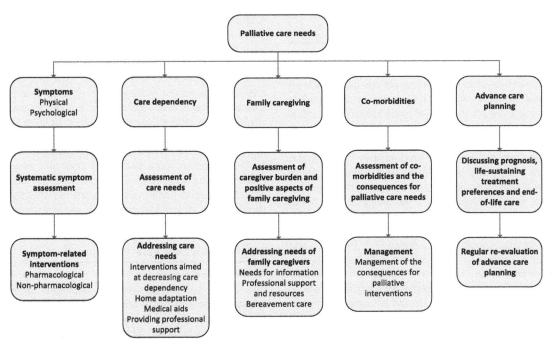

Fig. 1. Palliative care needs of patients with advanced chronic organ failure: symptoms, care dependency, family caregiving, comorbidities, and advance care planning.

of daily living, like bathing and dressing.[26] About half of outpatients with advanced COPD need help with personal care.[27] Care dependency is an important correlate of impaired health status and even predicts 2-year survival among patients with advanced disease.[27,28] Furthermore, care dependency may lead to feelings of frustration and social isolation and is often difficult to deal with for both the patient and their loved ones.[25,29] Therefore, palliative management programs should assess impairments in basic and instrumental activities of daily living and should try to minimize care dependency and provide support as needed. Studies have shown that there are difficulties with accessing appropriate health and social care services for patients with advanced COPD.[8,30,31] Provision of aids and appliances could be improved, for instance, by obtaining support earlier in the course of the disease.[31] Interdisciplinary care, including occupational interventions, may have an important role in improvement of daily functioning.[32,33] For example, patients with COPD use a higher proportion of their peak aerobic capacity and peak ventilation to perform normal daily tasks than healthy elderly persons.[34] The use of energy conservation techniques has been shown to reduce energy cost and the perception of dyspnea during activities of daily living in patients with moderate to very severe COPD.[35] These interventions may increase the ability to perform daily tasks and should be considered for patients with advanced COPD.

Family Caregiving

Family caregivers have a crucial role in providing care for patients with advanced COPD.[22,27,36] A qualitative study of bereaved relatives showed that patients with COPD became increasingly dependent on their loved ones toward the end of life.[21] Caring for a loved one with advanced disease may have significant consequences for the family caregiver(s). Qualitative studies have shown that a decline in patients' health status can lead to a range of physical, social, and emotional consequences for their caregivers.[25,37] Adapting to functional limitations may be difficult for both patients and caregivers.[25] Nevertheless, family caregiving can also be a positive experience.[36,38] Partners and family caregivers of patients with psychological symptoms and of patients suffering from comorbidities are at increased risk for a higher caregiver burden and, therefore, should be assessed themselves for both burden and benefits of caregiving.[36] Family caregivers of patients with life-limiting illnesses have reported that they desire information about the expected course of the disease, physical

and psychological care, and information about medical aids and other resources such as hospice care and how to deal with an emergency.[39]

For many loved ones of patients with COPD, death is unexpected.[22] Previous investigators have shown that loved ones of patients with COPD were less likely to be present at the death of the patient than loved ones of patients with lung cancer, despite most wanting to be present.[9] Therefore, loved ones of deceased patients with COPD may be at risk for the development of complicated grief. A qualitative study among bereaved caregivers of patients with COPD reported that some loved ones experienced feelings of guilt, for example, because of not being with the patient at the time of death. In addition, loved ones expressed the need for information about bereavement support services.[37] Nevertheless, only a few of the loved ones of deceased patients with COPD requested bereavement care.[40]

Comorbidities

Comorbidities are prevalent in patients with COPD[41] and may influence palliative care needs. It is reasonable to assume that comorbid conditions are associated with additional symptom burden or care needs. Moreover, comorbidities may negatively influence health status in patients with COPD.[42,43] Comorbidities may also influence the experience of family caregiving.[36] Therefore, careful analysis of comorbidities, including polypharmacy, is important in offering palliative care. Comorbidities and polypharmacy need to be taken into account in symptom-related interventions. For example, chronic kidney disease is highly prevalent and underdiagnosed in elderly patients with COPD.[44] Because of the complex pharmacokinetics of opioids in patients with chronic kidney disease,[45] the presence of chronic kidney disease should be considered when prescribing opioids for the treatment of dyspnea in these patients. Management of palliative care needs in patients with multiple medical conditions and complex polypharmacy is challenging. Therefore, coordination of care between health professionals such as the medical specialist, nurse specialist, general practitioner, and palliative care physician is essential.

Need for Advance Care Planning

Advance care planning is defined as "planning for and about preference-sensitive decisions often arising at the end-of-life and implemented usually by means of effective patient-provider communication and education. This may involve discussions regarding goals of care, resuscitation and life support, palliative care options, surrogate decision making as well as living wills and medical directives."[46] In recent years, several studies have shown the benefits of advance care planning for patients, as well as for their loved ones. Advance care planning improves concordance between patient's wishes for end-of-life care and the end-of-life care received.[47] Moreover, advance care planning improves quality of end-of-life care and reduces symptoms of anxiety and depression among bereaved loved ones.[48] Therefore, advance care planning is an important component of palliative care for patients with COPD and their closest relatives.[10,49] The unpredictable disease trajectory demands early discussions concerning preferences for end-of-life care and life-sustaining treatments. It has been shown that patients with COPD desire communication about end-of-life care and education about topics such as diagnosis and disease process, treatment, prognosis, and the dying process.[50] Although patients with advanced COPD have clear opinions about their willingness to undergo life-sustaining treatments, these preferences and their preferences for end-of-life care are rarely discussed with their physician.[51] Moreover, patients rate their physician's skills to communicate about end-of-life care as poor and report that topics such as prognosis, the dying process, and spiritual issues are not discussed at all.[52,53]

BARRIERS TOWARD PROVISION OF PALLIATIVE CARE

Despite a patient's need for these services, access to palliative care remains limited for patients with nonmalignant diseases.[8,54] The first step in improving access to palliative care for patients with advanced respiratory disease is to gain insight into barriers to receiving palliative care. The following section discusses barriers to optimal symptom management and advance care planning (**Box 2**).

Barriers to Optimal Symptom Management

Daily symptom burden of patients with COPD often remains unrecognized. Patients with advanced COPD may not actively express a wish for help for their symptoms, because they adapt to their situation, attribute their symptoms to getting older, or believe that there are no treatments to improve their situation.[55] Therefore, a systematic assessment of symptom distress should be part of regular clinical care. Recognition and acknowledgment of symptoms might be the first step to alleviate symptoms of patients with advanced COPD and improve function and quality of life. The lack of consensus about standardization of symptom

---

Box 2
Patient-related and clinician-related barriers to implementing effective palliative care

Barriers toward optimal symptom management

Patient
- Lack of help-seeking behavior for daily symptoms

Clinician
- Lack of standardized and regular symptom assessment
- Insufficient knowledge concerning pharmacologic symptom management

Barriers toward advance care planning

Patient
- Failure to understand the course and prognosis of COPD
- Feeling not ready to talk about end-of-life care
- Assumption that clinician will initiate advance care planning when needed
- Being unaware of preferences for life-sustaining treatments and end of life

Clinician
- Disease trajectory of COPD and the difficulty in predicting prognosis of survival
- Limited skills in communication about end-of-life care
- Fear to diminish hope
- Lack of time during regular clinic visits
- Lack of continuity in care

---

assessment in palliative care may limit the widespread use of instruments to assess symptom burden.

Many instruments for symptom assessment in palliative care were previously developed for patients with cancer.[56] Although previous research has shown that, in general, symptom distress of patients with advanced COPD is comparable with symptom distress of patients with cancer, prevalence and severity of individual symptoms may be different.[9,57] Furthermore, disease-specific tools for patients with nonmalignant disease, for example, multidimensional instruments for symptom assessment in COPD, are often not validated in patients with advanced disease.[58] In turn, these instruments may not be sensitive enough to detect small but significant changes that may occur in the symptoms of patients with advanced disease.[58] These instruments may also not detect symptoms caused by comorbid conditions. Therefore, further research is necessary to develop an instrument for multidimensional symptom assessment in patients with advanced COPD. The instrument should be easy to use on a regular basis in clinical practice and should provide a clear insight into the presence and severity of symptoms, with the aim of identifying the need for symptom-related interventions.

Another factor contributing to undertreatment of symptoms may be that many questions remain concerning optimal symptom management. For example, most patients with advanced COPD suffer from severe dyspnea, and yet, only a few patients are prescribed opioids,[24,59] although prescription of opioids is recommended for management of severe dyspnea.[13] Although previous studies support the use of opioids to treat dyspnea in patients with advanced disease,[60–62] knowledge about which patients suffering from dyspnea are likely to respond to opioids is scarce.[63,64] Furthermore, no randomized clinical trials are available comparing the effect of different opioids or administration routes on the sensation of dyspnea in advanced COPD. Adequately powered randomized clinical trials are needed to identify patients who are likely to benefit from the prescription of opioids and to provide recommendations about when to prescribe opioids, which opioids to prescribe, administration routes, and dosage regimes. Physicians often report insufficient knowledge, as well as lack of education and guidelines as barriers to the prescription of opioids.[65] Concerns about the safety of opioid prescription and the fear of respiratory depression are important barriers to prescribing opioids in these patients.[66] Current studies provide no evidence for significant respiratory depression caused by opioids.[62,67,68]

Barriers Toward Advance Care Planning

The disease trajectory of COPD and the difficulty in predicting prognosis are an important barrier to advance care planning.[46] Although clinicians acknowledge that the appropriate timing for these discussions is when patients are well enough to participate in decision making, these discussions are often initiated when patients are too ill to participate.[69] Patients with COPD are frequently not informed that they have a life-limiting illness.[69] Only 31% of the individuals with advanced COPD estimated their life expectancy to be less than 1 year in the month before their death.[70] This failure to understand the likelihood of death is reported as a barrier to initiating discussions about end-of-life care.[69] Patients also report not being

ready to talk about end-of-life care and preferring to concentrate on staying alive.[53,71] This observation reflects that most patients with COPD experience their disease as a way of life, without anticipating the end of their life.[30] Therefore, most patients do not initiate advance care planning discussions and do wait for their clinician to initiate these discussions.[72] Clinicians clearly need skills to be able to discuss a difficult topic like care at the end of life.[71] Reflecting this need, the official American Thoracic Society Clinical Policy Statement *Palliative Care for Patients with Respiratory Diseases and Critical Illnesses* has recommended advance care planning as a core competency for chest physicians.[13] Nevertheless, only 23% of the patients with severe COPD reported "my doctor is very good at talking about end-of-life care."[71]

Studies have identified barriers and facilitators to patient-clinician communication about end-of-life care in COPD.[53,71] The most frequently reported clinician-related barrier was lack of time during regular appointments to discuss end-of-life care.[71] Clearly, these discussions require both preparation and careful organization for the right time and place.[49] However, these conversations may save time during future care.[73] Other health care professionals can also support physicians in initiating advance care planning. For example, a randomized controlled trial has shown the benefits of an advance care planning intervention by nonphysician facilitators.[48] In addition, a qualitative study has highlighted the important role of nurses in communication about end-of-life care.[74]

Another barrier to end-of-life discussions reported by physicians is fear of taking away patients' hope.[71] A study among dialysis patients has shown that hope has a central role in the process of advance care planning. Hope is highly individual and helps to determine future goals of care and a patient's willingness to engage in discussions concerning end-of-life care.[75] Patients report that information about prognosis is vital in maintaining the ability to hope.[75] For patients who are uncomfortable with talking about prognosis, a more indirect approach to discussing prognosis may be warranted, such as discussing prognosis in terms of outcomes for groups instead of individuals.[76]

An additional barrier to end-of-life planning reported by patients is not knowing which care they prefer if they become very ill.[53] However, most clinically stable outpatients with advanced COPD have explicit opinions about the use of life-sustaining treatments. Patients are able to discuss their treatment preferences based on treatment burden, treatment outcome, and the likelihood of a negative outcome.[51] On the other hand, patients with COPD, in general, lack knowledge about the likelihood of a negative outcome of life-sustaining treatment interventions, such as resuscitation.[77] Therefore, education about life-sustaining treatment preferences is clearly needed.

Patients report not knowing which doctor will be responsible for them if they become severely ill as a barrier to effective end-of-life planning.[53,71] Continuity of care is an important aspect in palliative care. Therefore, physicians should try to provide continuity of expertise as well as continuity in the patient-physician relationship.[78]

ADVANCE CARE PLANNING EDUCATION DURING PULMONARY REHABILITATION

Pulmonary rehabilitation programs is a suitable venue for educating patients with COPD about advanced directives and promoting patient initiative to enter into a dialogue with their loved ones and health care provider(s) regarding these issues. The American Thoracic Society/European Respiratory Society Statement *Key Concepts and Advances in Pulmonary Rehabilitation*[7] describes several educational topics concerning advance care planning, such as prognosis, life-sustaining treatments, advanced directives, and discussing advance care planning with health care professionals and family caregivers (**Box 3**).

Studies in the United States have shown the need for advance care planning education in

patients entering pulmonary rehabilitation. Only 25% to 42% of the patients enrolled in pulmonary rehabilitation programs had written advanced directives.[72,79] Nonetheless, 61% of the patients expected that they might need intubation or mechanical ventilation in the future, and almost all patients had opinions about whether they wanted to accept this intervention or not.[72] However, only one-fifth of the patients had discussed advanced directives with their treating physician. Moreover, only 15% of the patients discussed life support with their physician, and 14% believed that their physician understood their current wishes for life-sustaining treatments.[72] Almost all patients found discussions with their physician about advanced directives acceptable and wanted to learn more about advanced directives, intubation, and mechanical ventilation.[72]

A cross-sectional survey of 346 pulmonary and cardiopulmonary rehabilitation programs showed that, in 82% of the 218 responding programs, prognosis and natural history of lung disease were discussed during the rehabilitation program. However, only 33% of the programs asked whether patients had completed a living will or durable power of attorney for health care (DPAHC), and only 17% of the programs kept a copy of advanced directives in their patient files. Educational sessions in which issues concerning living wills or DPAHC were addressed were present in one-third of the programs. However, only 8% of the programs offered advanced directives education in structured sessions that exposed all patients to these issues. In addition, 42% of the programs distributed some form of written materials on living wills and DPAHC. Of the programs, 58% did not know how many of their patients had completed a living will.[80]

In a nonrandomized study on the effect of an educational workshop on advance care planning, as part of an outpatient pulmonary rehabilitation program,[81] the proportion of patients who completed a living will increased significantly in both the intervention and the control groups during the study (52%–72% in the educational group and 30%–44% in the control group). However, the proportion of patients with DPAHC increased significantly (from 34% to 86%) only in the educational group. Patient-physician discussions about advanced directives were increased significantly in both groups, but the effect was stronger in the educational group (22%–58% in the educational group and 19%–37% in the control group, odds ratio 2.9 [1.1–8.3]), with these patients having an increased sense that their physician understood their preferences for life-sustaining treatments (from 14% to 44%).[81]

Box 3
Educational topics concerning advance care planning

- Diagnosis and disease process
- Prognosis
- Patient autonomy in medical decision making
- Life-sustaining treatments
- Advance directives
- Surrogate decision making
- Durable powers of attorney for health care
- Discussing advance care planning with health care professionals and family caregivers
- Process of dying
- Prevention of suffering

Adapted from Spruit MA, Singh SJ, Garvey C, et al. An Official American Thoracic Society/European Respiratory Society statement: key concepts and advances in pulmonary rehabilitation - an executive summary. Am J Respir Crit Care Med 2013;188(8):1011–27.

Education in advance care planning as part of a pulmonary rehabilitation program may be an effective strategy to increase the proportion of patients with advanced directives.[81] These patient-physician discussions may improve the physicians' understanding of the patients' preferences for life-sustaining treatments. Offering palliative care education during pulmonary rehabilitation might not only address the information needs of patients but can also be an effective strategy to promote patient-physician discussion about palliative or end-of-life care.[72]

SUMMARY

Patients with advanced COPD have unmet palliative care needs, such as high daily symptom burden, daily care needs, needs of family caregivers, and needs for advance care planning. Numerous barriers exist toward the timely introduction of palliative care in this patient population. The complex needs of patients with advanced COPD require the integration of curative-restorative care and palliative care. Palliative care and pulmonary rehabilitation are both important components of integrated care for patients with chronic respiratory diseases. Pulmonary rehabilitation provides the opportunity to introduce palliative care by implementing education about advance care planning. Education about advance care planning addresses the information needs of patients and can be an effective strategy to promote patient-physician discussion about these issues.

REFERENCES

1. Murray SA, Kendall M, Boyd K, et al. Illness trajectories and palliative care. BMJ 2005;330(7498): 1007–11.
2. Seale C. Changing patterns of death and dying. Soc Sci Med 2000;51(6):917–30.
3. Murray CJ, Lopez AD. Alternative projections of mortality and disability by cause 1990-2020: Global Burden of Disease Study. Lancet 1997; 349(9064):1498–504.
4. Lozano R, Naghavi M, Foreman K, et al. Global and regional mortality from 235 causes of death for 20 age groups in 1990 and 2010: a systematic analysis for the Global Burden of Disease Study 2010. Lancet 2012;380(9859):2095–128.
5. Vestbo J, Hurd SS, Agusti AG, et al. Global strategy for the diagnosis, management, and prevention of chronic obstructive pulmonary disease: GOLD executive summary. Am J Respir Crit Care Med 2013;187(4):347–65.
6. Spruit MA, Vanderhoven-Augustin I, Janssen PP, et al. Integration of pulmonary rehabilitation in COPD. Lancet 2008;371(9606):12–3.
7. Spruit MA, Singh SJ, Garvey C, et al. An official American Thoracic Society/European Respiratory society statement: key concepts and advances in pulmonary rehabilitation–an Executive Summary. Am J Respir Crit Care Med 2013;188(8):1011–27.
8. Gore JM, Brophy CJ, Greenstone MA. How well do we care for patients with end stage chronic obstructive pulmonary disease (COPD)? A comparison of palliative care and quality of life in COPD and lung cancer. Thorax 2000;55(12):1000–6.
9. Edmonds P, Karlsen S, Khan S, et al. A comparison of the palliative care needs of patients dying from chronic respiratory diseases and lung cancer. Palliat Med 2001;15(4):287–95.
10. Curtis JR. Palliative and end-of-life care for patients with severe COPD. Eur Respir J 2008;32(3): 796–803.
11. World Health Organization. WHO definition of palliative care. Available at: http://www.who.int/cancer/palliative/definition/en. Accessed December 01, 2013.
12. Reticker AL, Nici L, ZuWallack R. Pulmonary rehabilitation and palliative care in COPD: two sides of the same coin? Chron Respir Dis 2012;9(2): 107–16.
13. Lanken PN, Terry PB, Delisser HM, et al. An official American Thoracic Society clinical policy statement: palliative care for patients with respiratory diseases and critical illnesses. Am J Respir Crit Care Med 2008;177(8):912–27.
14. Steer J, Gibson J, Bourke SC. The DECAF Score: predicting hospital mortality in exacerbations of chronic obstructive pulmonary disease. Thorax 2012;67(11):970–6.
15. Piquet J, Chavaillon JM, David P, et al. High-risk patients following hospitalisation for an acute exacerbation of COPD. Eur Respir J 2013;42(4):946–55.
16. Groenewegen KH, Schols AM, Wouters EF. Mortality and mortality-related factors after hospitalization for acute exacerbation of COPD. Chest 2003; 124(2):459–67.
17. Wouters EF, Celis MP, Breyer MK, et al. Co-morbid manifestations in COPD. Resp Med COPD Update 2007;3:135–51.
18. Sin DD, Anthonisen NR, Soriano JB, et al. Mortality in COPD: role of comorbidities. Eur Respir J 2006; 28(6):1245–57.
19. Fox E, Landrum-McNiff K, Zhong Z, et al. Evaluation of prognostic criteria for determining hospice eligibility in patients with advanced lung, heart, or liver disease. SUPPORT Investigators. Study to Understand Prognoses and Preferences for Outcomes and Risks of Treatments. JAMA 1999; 282(17):1638–45.

20. Coventry PA, Grande GE, Richards DA, et al. Prediction of appropriate timing of palliative care for older adults with non-malignant life-threatening disease: a systematic review. Age Ageing 2005;34(3):218–27.

21. Elkington H, White P, Addington-Hall J, et al. The last year of life of COPD: a qualitative study of symptoms and services. Respir Med 2004;98(5):439–45.

22. Elkington H, White P, Addington-Hall J, et al. The healthcare needs of chronic obstructive pulmonary disease patients in the last year of life. Palliat Med 2005;19(6):485–91.

23. Blinderman CD, Homel P, Andrew Billings J, et al. Symptom distress and quality of life in patients with advanced chronic obstructive pulmonary disease. J Pain Symptom Manage 2009;38(1):115–23.

24. Janssen DJ, Spruit MA, Uszko-Lencer NH, et al. Symptoms, comorbidities, and health care in advanced chronic obstructive pulmonary disease or chronic heart failure. J Palliat Med 2011;14(6):735–43.

25. Fitzsimons D, Mullan D, Wilson JS, et al. The challenge of patients' unmet palliative care needs in the final stages of chronic illness. Palliat Med 2007;21(4):313–22.

26. Incalzi RA, Corsonello A, Pedone C, et al. Construct validity of activities of daily living scale: a clue to distinguish the disabling effects of COPD and congestive heart failure. Chest 2005;127(3):830–8.

27. Janssen DJ, Franssen FM, Wouters EF, et al. Impaired health status and care dependency in patients with advanced COPD or chronic heart failure. Qual Life Res 2011;20(10):1679–88.

28. Janssen DJ, Wouters EF, Schols JM, et al. Care dependency independently predicts two-year survival in outpatients with advanced chronic organ failure. J Am Med Dir Assoc 2013;14(3):194–8.

29. Seamark DA, Blake SD, Seamark CJ, et al. Living with severe chronic obstructive pulmonary disease (COPD): perceptions of patients and their carers. An interpretative phenomenological analysis. Palliat Med 2004;18(7):619–25.

30. Pinnock H, Kendall M, Murray SA, et al. Living and dying with severe chronic obstructive pulmonary disease: multi-perspective longitudinal qualitative study. BMJ 2011;342:d142.

31. Habraken JM, Willems DL, de Kort SJ, et al. Health care needs in end-stage COPD: a structured literature review. Patient Educ Couns 2007;68(2):121–30.

32. Azad N, Molnar F, Byszewski A. Lessons learned from a multidisciplinary heart failure clinic for older women: a randomised controlled trial. Age Ageing 2008;37(3):282–7.

33. Nici L, Donner C, Wouters E, et al. American Thoracic Society/European Respiratory Society statement on pulmonary rehabilitation. Am J Respir Crit Care Med 2006;173(12):1390–413.

34. Vaes AW, Wouters EF, Franssen FM, et al. Task-related oxygen uptake during domestic activities of daily life in patients with COPD and healthy elderly subjects. Chest 2011;140(4):970–9.

35. Velloso M, Jardim JR. Study of energy expenditure during activities of daily living using and not using body position recommended by energy conservation techniques in patients with COPD. Chest 2006;130(1):126–32.

36. Janssen DJ, Spruit MA, Wouters EF, et al. Family caregiving in advanced chronic organ failure. J Am Med Dir Assoc 2012;15(4):447–56.

37. Hasson F, Spence A, Waldron M, et al. Experiences and needs of bereaved carers during palliative and end-of-life care for people with chronic obstructive pulmonary disease. J Palliat Care 2009;25(3):157–63.

38. Yamamoto-Mitani N, Ishigaki K, Kuniyoshi M, et al. Subjective quality of life and positive appraisal of care among Japanese family caregivers of older adults. Qual Life Res 2004;13(1):207–21.

39. Parker SM, Clayton JM, Hancock K, et al. A systematic review of prognostic/end-of-life communication with adults in the advanced stages of a life-limiting illness: patient/caregiver preferences for the content, style, and timing of information. J Pain Symptom Manage 2007;34(1):81–93.

40. Jones BW. Hospice disease types which indicate a greater need for bereavement counseling. Am J Hosp Palliat Care 2010;27(3):187–90.

41. Vanfleteren LE, Spruit MA, Groenen M, et al. Clusters of comorbidities based on validated objective measurements and systemic inflammation in patients with chronic obstructive pulmonary disease. Am J Respir Crit Care Med 2013;187(7):728–35.

42. Ferrer M, Alonso J, Morera J, et al. Chronic obstructive pulmonary disease stage and health-related quality of life. The Quality of Life of Chronic Obstructive Pulmonary Disease Study Group. Ann Intern Med 1997;127(12):1072–9.

43. Miravitlles M, Alvarez-Sala JL, Lamarca R, et al. Treatment and quality of life in patients with chronic obstructive pulmonary disease. Qual Life Res 2002;11(4):329–38.

44. Incalzi RA, Corsonello A, Pedone C, et al. Chronic renal failure: a neglected comorbidity of COPD. Chest 2010;137(4):831–7.

45. Nayak-Rao S. Achieving effective pain relief in patients with chronic kidney disease: a review of analgesics in renal failure. J Nephrol 2011;24(1):35–40.

46. Patel K, Janssen DJ, Curtis JR. Advance care planning in COPD. Respirology 2012;17(1):72–8.

47. Silveira MJ, Kim SY, Langa KM. Advance directives and outcomes of surrogate decision making before death. N Engl J Med 2010;362(13):1211–8.

48. Detering KM, Hancock AD, Reade MC, et al. The impact of advance care planning on end of life care in elderly patients: randomised controlled trial. BMJ 2010;340:c1345.

49. Janssen DJ, Engelberg RA, Wouters EF, et al. Advance care planning for patients with COPD: Past, present and future. Patient Educ Couns 2012;86(1):19–24.

50. Curtis JR, Wenrich MD, Carline JD, et al. Patients' perspectives on physician skill in end-of-life care: differences between patients with COPD, cancer, and AIDS. Chest 2002;122(1):356–62.

51. Janssen DJ, Spruit MA, Schols JM, et al. A call for high-quality advance care planning in outpatients with severe COPD or chronic heart failure. Chest 2011;139(5):1081–8.

52. Curtis JR, Engelberg RA, Nielsen EL, et al. Patient-physician communication about end-of-life care for patients with severe COPD. Eur Respir J 2004; 24(2):200–5.

53. Janssen DJ, Curtis JR, Au DH, et al. Patient-clinician communication about end-of-life care for Dutch and US patients with COPD. Eur Respir J 2011;38(2):268–76.

54. Grande GE, Farquhar MC, Barclay SI, et al. The influence of patient and carer age in access to palliative care services. Age Ageing 2006;35(3):267–73.

55. Habraken JM, Pols J, Bindels PJ, et al. The silence of patients with end-stage COPD: a qualitative study. Br J Gen Pract 2008;58(557):844–9.

56. Opasich C, Gualco A. The complex symptom burden of the aged heart failure population. Curr Opin Support Palliat Care 2007;1(4):255–9.

57. Bausewein C, Booth S, Gysels M, et al. Understanding breathlessness: cross-sectional comparison of symptom burden and palliative care needs in chronic obstructive pulmonary disease and cancer. J Palliat Med 2010;13(9):1109–18.

58. Bausewein C, Farquhar M, Booth S, et al. Measurement of breathlessness in advanced disease: a systematic review. Respir Med 2007;101(3):399–410.

59. Au DH, Udris EM, Fihn SD, et al. Differences in health care utilization at the end of life among patients with chronic obstructive pulmonary disease and patients with lung cancer. Arch Intern Med 2006;166(3):326–31.

60. Currow DC, McDonald C, Oaten S, et al. Once-daily opioids for chronic dyspnea: a dose increment and pharmacovigilance study. J Pain Symptom Manage 2011;42(3):388–99.

61. Jennings AL, Davies AN, Higgins JP, et al. A systematic review of the use of opioids in the management of dyspnoea. Thorax 2002;57(11):939–44.

62. Abernethy AP, Currow DC, Frith P, et al. Randomised, double blind, placebo controlled crossover trial of sustained release morphine for the management of refractory dyspnoea. BMJ 2003;327(7414):523–8.

63. Currow DC, Plummer J, Frith P, et al. Can we predict which patients with refractory dyspnea will respond to opioids? J Palliat Med 2007;10(5):1031–6.

64. Johnson MJ, Bland JM, Oxberry SG, et al. Opioids for chronic refractory breathlessness: patient predictors of beneficial response. Eur Respir J 2013;42(3):758–66.

65. Young J, Donahue M, Farquhar M, et al. Using opioids to treat dyspnea in advanced COPD: attitudes and experiences of family physicians and respiratory therapists. Can Fam Physician 2012;58(7):e401–7.

66. Rocker G, Horton R, Currow D, et al. Palliation of dyspnoea in advanced COPD: revisiting a role for opioids. Thorax 2009;64(10):910–5.

67. Eiser N, Denman WT, West C, et al. Oral diamorphine: lack of effect on dyspnoea and exercise tolerance in the "pink puffer" syndrome. Eur Respir J 1991;4(8):926–31.

68. Poole PJ, Veale AG, Black PN. The effect of sustained-release morphine on breathlessness and quality of life in severe chronic obstructive pulmonary disease. Am J Respir Crit Care Med 1998;157(6 Pt 1):1877–80.

69. Gott M, Gardiner C, Small N, et al. Barriers to advance care planning in chronic obstructive pulmonary disease. Palliat Med 2009;23(7):642–8.

70. Fried TR, Bradley EH, O'Leary J. Changes in prognostic awareness among seriously ill older persons and their caregivers. J Palliat Med 2006;9(1):61–9.

71. Knauft E, Nielsen EL, Engelberg RA, et al. Barriers and facilitators to end-of-life care communication for patients with COPD. Chest 2005;127(6):2188–96.

72. Heffner JE, Fahy B, Hilling L, et al. Attitudes regarding advance directives among patients in pulmonary rehabilitation. Am J Respir Crit Care Med 1996;154(6 Pt 1):1735–40.

73. Chittenden EH, Clark ST, Pantilat SZ. Discussing resuscitation preferences with patients: challenges and rewards. J Hosp Med 2006;1(4):231–40.

74. Reinke LF, Shannon SE, Engelberg RA, et al. Supporting hope and prognostic information: nurses' perspectives on their role when patients have life-limiting prognoses. J Pain Symptom Manage 2010;39(6):982–92.

75. Davison SN, Simpson C. Hope and advance care planning in patients with end stage renal

disease: qualitative interview study. BMJ 2006; 333(7574):886.

76. Curtis JR, Engelberg R, Young JP, et al. An approach to understanding the interaction of hope and desire for explicit prognostic information among individuals with severe chronic obstructive pulmonary disease or advanced cancer. J Palliat Med 2008;11(4):610–20.

77. Nava S, Santoro C, Grassi M, et al. The influence of the media on COPD patients' knowledge regarding cardiopulmonary resuscitation. Int J Chron Obstruct Pulmon Dis 2008;3(2):295–300.

78. Back AL, Young JP, McCown E, et al. Abandonment at the end of life from patient, caregiver, nurse, and physician perspectives: loss of continuity and lack of closure. Arch Intern Med 2009; 169(5):474–9.

79. Gerald LB, Sanderson B, Fish L, et al. Advance directives in cardiac and pulmonary rehabilitation patients. J Cardiopulm Rehabil 2000;20(6): 340–5.

80. Heffner JE, Fahy B, Barbieri C. Advance directive education during pulmonary rehabilitation. Chest 1996;109(2):373–9.

81. Heffner JE, Fahy B, Hilling L, et al. Outcomes of advance directive education of pulmonary rehabilitation patients. Am J Respir Crit Care Med 1997; 155(3):1055–9.

Program Organization in Pulmonary Rehabilitation

Chris Garvey, FNP, MSN, MPA[a],*, Brian Carlin, MD[b], Jonathan Raskin, MD[c]

KEYWORDS

- Pulmonary rehabilitation • Quality • Outcomes • Duration • Maintenance

KEY POINTS

- Longer pulmonary rehabilitation (PR) programs are associated with improved outcomes.
- PR is effective and safe when delivered in outpatient and inpatient settings and immediately following acute exacerbation of chronic obstructive pulmonary disease.
- Barriers to PR include clinician preferences and patient access. Technology may offer future options for those with access challenges.

INTRODUCTION

Pulmonary rehabilitation (PR) programs share essential features regardless of differences in available resources, staffing, program setting, structure, and duration. Although the optimal length of PR is unclear, longer programs generally translate into greater improvement and maintenance of benefits.[1,2] Contraindications to PR are few and include any condition that negatively impacts safe exercise or provision of PR. PR settings include inpatient and outpatient settings, with home exercise training as an option, based on adequate resources. PR translates into improved health care utilization, including when provided during or immediately following chronic obstructive pulmonary disease (COPD) exacerbations.[3] PR has historically been underutilized, and there are barriers to its enrollment and completion (**Box 1**). Those impacted by limited access (eg, patients who are homebound or living in rural or remote settings) may ultimately benefit from development of technological advances such as satellite PR and alternatives to PR.

PROGRAM DURATION

PR duration should be based on the individual's documented progress toward goals such as improved function, symptom control, and quality of life. However, this goal- and achievement-centered duration is not always feasible because of practical and financial considerations. Longer programs are generally associated with greater gains and maintenance of benefits, and a minimum of 8 weeks has been recommended to achieve benefit.[1,2,5] Importantly, improvements in daily physical activity levels may require a substantially longer program duration than improvements in exercise capacity, and may take 6 months or longer.[6,7] Outpatient PR programs are commonly provided 2 to 3 days a week, while inpatient programs usually occur 5 days a week. Each session length is generally 1 to 4 hours per day.[8–10]

REHABILITATION SETTING

PR is commonly provided in both outpatient and inpatient settings, with recent evidence suggesting effectiveness of exercise training in the home.[10–12] Factors influencing the choice of PR setting include disease severity and stability, the level of disability, comorbidities, transportation, program availability, and insurance or cost. Opportunities to potentially broaden the setting for PR include technology-assisted exercise training

a Cardiopulmonary Rehabilitation, Seton Medical Center, 1900 Sullivan Avenue, Daly City, CA 94015, USA;
b Drexel University School of Medicine, Lifeline Pulmonary Rehabilitation and Therapy, Pittsburgh, PA, USA;
c Pulmonary Rehabilitation, Beth Israel Medical Center, New York, NY, USA
* Corresponding author.
E-mail address: chrisgarvey@dochs.org

Clin Chest Med 35 (2014) 423–428
http://dx.doi.org/10.1016/j.ccm.2014.02.014
0272-5231/14/$ – see front matter © 2014 Elsevier Inc. All rights reserved.

Box 1
Potential barriers to enrollment and completion of PR

- Inconvenience for the patient
- Lack of perceived benefit
- Transportation/travel issues
- Parking issues
- Cost
- Inadequate insurance coverage
- Lack of support
- Illness severity
- Comorbidities
- Mood disorders
- Smoking
- Influence of the provider[4]

Box 2
Clinical staffing models for PR

- Coordinators
- Medical directors
- Respiratory therapists
- Nurses
- Exercise physiologists
- Physical therapists
- Occupational therapists
- Social workers
- Psychologists
- Dietitians

(including the use of home video games)[13–17] and strategies to augment physical activity such as feedback from pedometers[18,19] and other activity monitors.

STRUCTURE AND STAFFING

PR staffing models vary, with programs generally including a program coordinator and medical director. Other professional clinical staff may include respiratory therapists, nurses, exercise physiologists, physical therapists, occupational therapists, social workers, psychologists, and dietitians. The composition of this staff often depends on the resources of the facility. There is no clear-cut optimal staffing structure. However, staff-to-patient ratios must support efficacy and safety. PR staff members should have formal clinical education with certification in their specialty field, as well as experience and demonstrated competency in the care of persons with chronic lung disease in a rehabilitation setting. Evaluation of competency in skill performance such as formulating an exercise prescription in chronic lung disease and oxygen titration should regularly be evaluated. Additional skills include training in disease self management and symptom control (**Box 2**).

MEDICAL DIRECTOR

The medical director is the leader of the interdisciplinary rehabilitation team, providing a vital role in the development and management of the PR program. Minimum qualifications for the medical director in the United States are defined in current legislative and regulatory documents. The medical director must be a physician (MD or DO) who is licensed in the same state in which the PR services are performed and has expertise in respiratory physiology. He or she should be appropriately credentialed within the institution in which the rehabilitation program resides and should be contracted in a manner that allows appropriate time to devote to the responsibilities associated with direction of the program.

The medical director should have the skills to evaluate and manage patients with chronic lung disease as well as skills to direct data collection and analysis, outcome analysis, and quality improvement strategies. He or she needs to keep abreast of the research in the field of chronic lung disease and rehabilitation as well as the regulatory requirements and developments as applied to rehabilitative medicine.

The medical director must work with the team during the initial patient assessment process to help develop an individualized treatment plan. This plan should include the initial patient evaluation, including assessment of comorbid conditions, specific goals for improving self-management skills and exercise and activities of daily living performance, psychosocial and emotional support, and nutritional counseling. The medical director must oversee the patient's progress throughout the program at regular intervals and should adjust the rehabilitation plan as necessary. He or she should also oversee the communication between the rehabilitation staff and the patient's other health care providers.

The medical director should help the program staff develop protocols that facilitate individualized patient care. He or he should actively participate with the staff to develop the educational program and ensure that the program's policies and procedures are consistent with current guidelines and comply with regulatory and certification standards. One of the most important responsibilities of the medical director is awareness of reimbursement policies for the various third-party payers.

PROGRAM CERTIFICATION

In the United States, the American Association of Cardiovascular and Pulmonary Rehabilitation (AACVPR) PR program certification is the only peer review certification designed to review individual facilities for adherence to standards and guidelines developed and published by the AACVPR and other professional societies. Programs are required to demonstrate ongoing adherence to established measures of clinical performance, staffing, quality improvement, outcome measurement, and safety.

PROGRAM AUDIT AND QUALITY CONTROL

Program staff must ensure that high-quality care is being delivered for each patient in the rehabilitation program. Each program should use strict measurement of appropriate outcome measures, frequent auditing of the progress of the patients, and adherence to general safety standards. Various types of outcome measures that are program specific can be used in this assessment process, including program attendance, adherence to a home exercise program, patient satisfaction, health care resource utilization (eg, exacerbation rate and hospitalization rate), and translation of the program components into a self-management program, such as development of an action for the respiratory exacerbation. Throughout this assessment process, reorganization and modification of the program can then be successfully performed.

PATIENT SELECTION

PR is indicated for any individual with chronic respiratory disease who is receiving optimal medication management and who has persistent symptoms and/or functional status limitations.[20,21] It can be effective irrespective of age, disease severity, or disease stability.[22–24] Traditionally, PR has been reserved for stable patients with moderate-to-severe COPD. New data indicate its effectiveness in mild-to-moderate and very severe COPD and in the peri-exacerbation setting. Furthermore, recent evidence has demonstrated the effectiveness of PR for not only COPD, but also for other chronic respiratory diseases such as interstitial lung disease, pulmonary hypertension, and bronchiectasis. Contraindications to PR include any condition that precludes safe exercise training or would otherwise interfere with the rehabilitative process.

TECHNOLOGY-ASSISTED EXERCISE TRAINING

It is important for the patient to transfer those skills and adaptive behaviors learned during PR into his or her routine daily activities and maintain them on a long-term basis. Various types of technological advances, such as pedometers, videoconferencing, mobile phone, and Internet technology, have been evaluated over the last 2 decades to help facilitate the transfer of the exercise training benefits into the regular exercise and physical activity in the home environment.[13–19] A systematic review suggests that pedometer feedback employing a physical activity target (eg, 10,000 steps) is effective in promoting activity.[19] Further studies are needed to fully evaluate this approach in chronic respiratory disease.

The use of telemedicine for the management of patients with COPD has been demonstrated to improve health care-related outcomes in some studies,[13–19] although a recent study involving 256 patients showed no difference in health-related quality of life or COPD admissions.[25] Within the context of pulmonary rehabilitation, telehealth may assist in the maintenance of benefits and in translating adaptive behaviors into the home setting. Additionally, telehealth may eventually be useful in providing rehabilitation to those patients who might not otherwise be able to access a particular program due to travel or distance restrictions.

PROGRAM ENROLLMENT

Many patients who are offered PR will not enroll in the program for a variety of reasons, including a disruption to the patient's established daily routine, travel restrictions, lack of anticipated benefit, and inconvenient timing of the program. Those patients who are divorced, widowed, or living alone are also less likely to attend. The influence of the health care provider to an individual regarding the value of the rehabilitation program can help to play a role in greater enrollment. Further study into the barriers associated with enrollment in PR should be undertaken.

MAINTENANCE

Although most PR professionals believe that maintenance programs following the formal intervention provide benefit, there are few existing data to support this belief. Maintenance programs may be initiated at the rehabilitation center or at a local facility, which may be more convenient for the patient.

When a patient has completed formal PR, the medical director in coordination with the PR team should review the level of training the patient has achieved and write a discharge summary so that the receiving facility can resume exercise concordant with the patient's capacity. Description of appropriate oxygen usage as well as balance and orthopedic concerns should be clearly described in the discharge summary. Because the lifetime number of PR sessions is limited for Medicare patients in the United States, an early transition to maintenance when improvement has plateaued may save sessions and thereby allow for covered re-enrollment, when needed, at a later date.

Although there is no acknowledged formula for maintenance exercise sessions, it is customary to provide at least 2 to 3 sessions weekly to maintain benefits accrued during formal PR. Sessions should closely follow prior rehabilitation levels in intensity and duration to achieve and maintain as high a level of fitness as possible. Supervised versus unsupervised efforts appear to be less problematic when feedback strategies are implemented, ensuring enhanced compliance. One study[26] found that maintenance therapy (MT) was superior to usual care and determined that after 12 months those undergoing MT had a clinically and statistically significant improvement in 6-minute walk, all domains of the St. George Respiratory Questionnaire, as well as days spent in hospital. There was no difference in dyspnea scores and maximal work load between MT and usual care groups.

PROGRAM ADHERENCE

Program adherence is a significant issue in PR, as there is no clear framework for ensuring consistent attendance and subsequent adherence to exercise and behavioral modification.[6,27,28] Initially, the time commitment of the program should be made clear to patients so that they and their caregivers can consider schedule issues and can be sure they are able to make the appropriate commitment. When a time frame is agreed upon, the importance of attendance should be reinforced time and again, especially early on when patients are adapting to a change in their daily routines. The PR team should inquire about transportation issues, including relevant distance to the rehabilitation center and weight of the patient's portable oxygen equipment. These impediments should be addressed as best as possible, and the use of encouraging phone calls should be employed to demonstrate concern from the PR team as well as to facilitate attendance and adherence. If a patient has demonstrated poor efforts to commit to

the undertaking, he or she should be asked to reevaluate his or her motive and even encouraged to address participation at a later date.

HEALTH CARE UTILIZATION

PR in outpatients with COPD appears to reduce subsequent health care utilization.[29–31] More recently, PR provided in the peri-exacerbation period for hospitalized COPD patients, compared with usual care, has been associated with a reduction in subsequent hospital admissions as well as improved survival.[3] This finding suggests that PR can be added to a short list of interventions that improve survival in COPD, joining long-term supplemental oxygen use for hypoxemic patients, lung volume reduction surgery for patients with emphysema, and smoking cessation intervention.

PROGRAM COSTS AND REIMBURSEMENT ISSUES

As diminishing reimbursement has challenged the viability of PR programs, many centers no longer exist as freestanding entities. Rather, they have become incorporated into cost centers that include other programs such as cardiac rehabilitation. This allows an intelligent allocation of resources across various programmatic needs and creates needed financial synergies to allow PR programs to survive. It should be noted that despite such efforts PR programs continue to struggle. At the time of this writing, there is a substantial collaborative effort by pulmonary professional societies to remedy the inadequate reimbursements currently received. Reimbursement for PR varies across third-party payers. Those programs with a diverse payer mix potentially fare better financially than those completely dependent on Medicare reimbursement. Medicare provides PR for patients with moderate-to-very severe COPD (GOLD Stage 2–4, 2010 Global Initiative for Chronic Obstructive Lung Disease (GOLD) guidelines). There is 1 bundled fee or charge per session, which includes all services provided at the time of the session. It is mandatory that the session include exercise and that the rehabilitation session be least 31 minutes of rehabilitation to allow coverage for services. A second session may be provided and billed as long as the session includes exercise, and the total rehabilitation session (billed as 2 units) is at least 91 minutes in length. Under Medicare coverage rules, there is no component billing allowed.

Current Medicare billing for PR uses a limited number of 'G' payment codes. Billing restrictions include bundling all PR costs and services for

COPD under 1 code (G0424), with potential for coverage of other chronic lung diseases using codes GO237 through G0239. Restrictions for PR in COPD include prohibiting the use of physical therapy billing codes and bundling all costs of PR including medical director services and responsibilities into G0424 (currently reimbursed at approximately $39). Medicare coverage interpretation and payment of claims are provided by local Medicare administrative contractors (MAC) based on geographic regions. Many national associations are working to address PR reimbursement and coverage concerns. Information regarding Medicare coverage and MAC policy information is available at cms.gov and aacvpr.org.

SUMMARY

PR settings and delivery methods have the potential to be adapted to the needs of a diverse patient population. Indeed this adaptation must occur for the long-term success and viability of this intervention. This adaptation must include improving patient and clinician awareness of PR to enhance referrals, broadening the access to the intervention through exploring novel approaches such as telemedicine, eliminating barriers to enrollment, providing for the long-term maintenance of benefits, and addressing reimbursement limitations.

REFERENCES

1. Beauchamp MK, Janaudis-Ferreira T, Goldstein RS, et al. Optimal duration of pulmonary rehabilitation for individuals with chronic obstructive pulmonary disease—a systematic review. Chron Respir Dis 2011; 8:129–40.
2. Sewell L, Singh SJ, Williams JE, et al. How long should outpatient pulmonary rehabilitation be? A randomised controlled trial of 4 weeks versus 7 weeks. Thorax 2006;61:767–71.
3. Puhan MA, Gimeno-Santos E, Scharplatz M, et al. Pulmonary rehabilitation following exacerbations of chronic obstructive pulmonary disease. Cochrane Database Syst Rev 2011;(10):CD005305.
4. Keating A, Lee A, Holland AE. What prevents people with chronic obstructive pulmonary disease from attending pulmonary rehabilitation? A systematic review. Chron Respir Dis 2011;8:89–99.
5. Rossi G, Florini F, Romagnoli M, et al. Length and clinical effectiveness of pulmonary rehabilitation in outpatients with chronic airway obstruction. Chest 2005;127:105–9.
6. Ng LW, Mackney J, Jenkins S, et al. Does exercise training change physical activity in people with COPD? A systematic review and 34 meta-analyses. Chron Respir Dis 2012;1:17–26.
7. Pitta F, Troosters T, Probst VS, et al. Are patients with COPD more active after pulmonary rehabilitation? Chest 2008;134:273–80.
8. Brooks D, Sottana R, Bell B, et al. Characterization of pulmonary rehabilitation programs in Canada in 2005. Can Respir J 2007;14:87–92.
9. Yohannes AM, Connolly MJ. Pulmonary rehabilitation programmes in the UK: a national representative survey. Clin Rehabil 2004;18:444–9.
10. Maltais F, Bourbeau J, Shapiro S, et al. Effects of home-based pulmonary rehabilitation in patients with chronic obstructive pulmonary disease: a randomized trial. Ann Intern Med 2008;149: 869–78.
11. Güell MR, de Lucas P, Galdiz JB, et al. Home vs hospital-based pulmonary rehabilitation for patients with chronic obstructive pulmonary disease: a Spanish multicenter trial. Arch Bronconeumol 2008;44: 512–8.
12. Mendes de Oliveira JC, Studart Leitão Filho FS, Malosa Sampaio LM, et al. Outpatient vs. home-based pulmonary rehabilitation in COPD: a randomized controlled trial. Multidiscip Respir Med 2010;5:401–8.
13. Liu WT, Wang CH, Lin HC, et al. Efficacy of a cell phone-based exercise programme for COPD. Eur Respir J 2008;32:651–9.
14. Stickland M, Jourdain T, Wong EY, et al. Using telehealth technology to deliver pulmonary rehabilitation in chronic obstructive pulmonary disease patients. Can Respir J 2011;18:216–20.
15. Lewis KE, Annandale JA, Warm DL, et al. Does home telemonitoring after pulmonary rehabilitation reduce healthcare use in optimized COPD? A pilot randomized trial. COPD 2010;7:44–50.
16. Wewel AR, Gellermann I, Schwertfeger I, et al. Intervention by phone calls raises domiciliary activity and exercise capacity in patients with severe COPD. Respir Med 2008;102:20–6.
17. Hospes G, Bossenbroek L, Ten Hacken NH, et al. Enhancement of daily physical activity increases physical fitness of outclinic COPD patients: results of an exercise counseling program. Patient Educ Couns 2009;75:274–8.
18. Dallas MI, McCusker C, Haggerty MC, et al, Northeast Pulmonary Rehabilitation Consortium. Using pedometers to monitor walking activity in outcome assessment for pulmonary rehabilitation. Chron Respir Dis 2009;6:217–24.
19. Bravata DM, Smith-Spangler C, Sundaram V, et al. Using pedometers to increase physical activity and improve health: a systematic review. JAMA 2007; 298:2296–304.
20. Annegarn J, Meijer K, Passos VL, et al. Problematic activities of daily life are weakly associated with clinical characteristics in COPD. J Am Med Dir Assoc 2012;13:284–90.

21. Vogiatzis I, Terzis G, Stratakos G, et al. Effect of pulmonary rehabilitation on peripheral muscle fiber remodeling in patients with COPD in GOLD stages II to IV. Chest 2011;140:744–52.

22. Puhan MA, Spaar A, Frey M, et al. Early versus late pulmonary rehabilitation in chronic obstructive pulmonary disease patients with acute exacerbations: a randomized trial. Respiration 2012;83(6):499–506.

23. Ambrosino N, Venturelli E, Vagheggini G, et al. Rehabilitation, weaning and physical therapy strategies in the chronic critically ill patients. Eur Respir J 2012;39(2):487–92.

24. Rejbi IB, Trabelsi Y, Chouchene A, et al. Changes in six-minute walking distance during pulmonary rehabilitation in patients with COPD and in healthy subjects. Int J Chron Obstruct Pulmon Dis 2010;5: 209–15.

25. Pinnock H, Hanley J, McCloughan L, et al. Effectiveness of telemonitoring integrated into existing clinical services on hospital admission for exacerbation of chronic obstructive pulmonary disease: researcher blind, multicentre, randomised controlled trial. BMJ 2013;347:f6070.

26. Moullec G, Ninot G, Varray A, et al. An innovative maintenance follow-up program after a first inpatient pulmonary rehabilitation. Respir Med 2008;102: 556–66.

27. Nici L. Adherence to a pulmonary rehabilitation program: start by understanding the patient. COPD 2012;9(5):445–6.

28. Butts J, Belfer M, Gebke K. Exercise for patients with COPD: an integral yet underutilized intervention. Phys Sportsmed 2013;41(1):49–57.

29. Raskin J, Spiegler P, McCusker C, et al. The effect of pulmonary rehabilitation on healthcare utilization in chronic obstructive pulmonary disease: the northeast pulmonary rehabilitation consortium. J Cardiopulm Rehabil 2006;26:231–6.

30. California Pulmonary Rehabilitation Collaborative Group. Effects of pulmonary rehabilitation on dyspnea, quality of life, and healthcare costs in California. J Cardiopulm Rehabil 2004;24:52–62.

31. Rasekaba TM, Williams E, Hsu-Hage B. Can a chronic disease management pulmonary rehabilitation program for COPD reduce acute rural hospital utilization? Chron Respir Dis 2009;6:157–63.

Promoting Long-Term Benefits of Pulmonary Rehabilitation
The Role of Reducing the Impact of Respiratory Exacerbations

Bonnie F. Fahy, RN, MN, CNS

KEYWORDS

- Pulmonary rehabilitation • Chronic obstructive pulmonary disease • Maintenance program
- Exacerbation • Self-management • Hospital readmission

KEY POINTS

- Pulmonary rehabilitation generally provides substantial benefits in exercise capacity, dyspnea, and quality of life, but these positive outcomes tend to diminish gradually over time.
- Although a key focus of pulmonary rehabilitation is to provide strategies to maintain long-term benefits from the intervention, the most effective approaches to achieve this goal are not currently known.
- Extending the duration of pulmonary rehabilitation seems to prolong its benefits, but this may not be feasible in all areas.
- Exacerbations of COPD are associated not only with substantial deteriorations in symptoms, functional status, and health status, they also negatively impact long-term adherence with the adaptive behaviors achieved in pulmonary rehabilitation.
- Targeting the exacerbation through nonpharmacologic interventions, such as pulmonary rehabilitation or its components, should prolong the long-term benefits from pulmonary rehabilitation.

INTRODUCTION

Pulmonary rehabilitation arguably provides the most beneficial effects of any treatment in the outcome areas of dyspnea, exercise performance, functional status, health status, and health care use. Despite this impressive track record, there is often a gradual decline in benefit over time after the formal pulmonary rehabilitation intervention.[1] An example of this is given in **Fig. 1**.

There are multiple reasons for this drop-off in outcomes months after the formal pulmonary rehabilitation program has ended. These include the progressive nature of the underlying respiratory disease, the development of comorbidity, exacerbations of the respiratory disease, and suboptimal adherence to the long-term exercise prescription. Perhaps it is too much to administer what is often a short-duration, acute care intervention and expect it to achieve long-term benefits in a disease that can span several decades. Instead, pulmonary rehabilitation must be fitted into a chronic care model of disease management. Thus, this intervention must promote self-efficacy in its patients, with the adoption of healthy behaviors, such as regular exercise in the home or

Funding Sources: None.
Conflict of Interest: None.
Care Management, Mayo Clinic Hospital, 5777 East Mayo Boulevard, Phoenix, AZ 85054, USA
E-mail address: Fahy.bonnie@mayo.edu

chestmed.theclinics.com

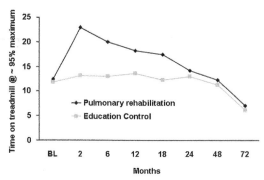

Fig. 1. Long-term effects of comprehensive pulmonary rehabilitation (x-axis) on submaximal exercise capacity (y-axis) in patients with COPD. Compared with a control group that was given didactic education, the pulmonary rehabilitation group had a significant increase in exercise capacity out to about 18 months. Thereafter, exercise capacity in both groups was similar and seemed to diminish gradually in time, possibly reflecting the progression of the disease. (*Data from* Ries AL, Kaplan RM, Limberg TM, et al. Effects of pulmonary rehabilitation on physiologic and psychosocial outcomes in patients with chronic obstructive pulmonary disease. Ann Intern Med 1995;122(11):823–32.)

Box 1
Initiatives aimed at prolonging the benefits of pulmonary rehabilitation

1. Extending pulmonary rehabilitation out for longer duration (lifetime would be best)[2]
2. Arranging for monthly patient visits to the rehabilitation center, supplemented by telephone calls in the interim[3]
3. Providing weekly telephone contacts and monthly supervised reinforcement sessions[4]
4. Giving repeated pulmonary rehabilitation at intervals (booster shots; these could be given in the periexacerbation period, which often leads to prolonged physical activity)[5]
5. Providing user-friendly pulmonary rehabilitation in the home setting, supplemented by visits to professionals in the center[6]
6. Offering structured daily self-monitored postrehabilitation walking exercise training at home, possibly incorporating feedback to the rehabilitation team[7]
7. Providing weekly supervised hospital-based exercise sessions[8]
8. Actively determining barriers to maintaining exercise by interview during formal rehabilitation, then working to reduce their impact[9]
9. Incorporating a home plan of exercise training early on in the formal rehabilitation program that fits the needs of the specific patient

community setting, and the use of collaborative self-management strategies at the time of the respiratory exacerbation.

There have been several systematic efforts to prolong the beneficial effects of pulmonary rehabilitation. These are listed in **Box 1**. Some of the approaches are clearly not practical or financially feasible, and none has unequivocally been shown to work. However, they provide current thinking on how the problem of drop off in outcomes might be approached.

These approaches either have had some success in maintaining the benefits or conceptually should do so. The remainder of this article discusses three additional approaches to prolong the beneficial effects of pulmonary rehabilitation. The first approach is to get patients to begin pulmonary rehabilitation in the first place. It should be obvious that prolongation of beneficial outcomes can be maintained only if the patient participates in pulmonary rehabilitation to achieve these initial positive outcomes. The second approach is to offer long-term postrehabilitation maintenance programs. To promote long-term gains, many pulmonary rehabilitation programs have set up maintenance programs. However, the benefits of participation in on-going, postrehabilitation exercise maintenance programs are not as widely researched, and consequently there is less awareness of this option among health care providers, hospitals, third-party payers, and most importantly

patients. The third approach is to prevent exacerbations of chronic obstructive pulmonary disease (COPD). It is known that respiratory exacerbations result in increased symptoms, decreased functional status, increased health care use, and increased mortality risk. Additionally, exacerbations play a prominent role in reducing long-term adherence to the adaptive behaviors (eg, regular exercise training) that had resulted from pulmonary rehabilitation. Thus, respiratory exacerbations should be discussed when dealing with long-term maintenance of benefits following pulmonary rehabilitation.

GETTING PATIENTS TO PARTICIPATE IN PULMONARY REHABILITATION

Initial patient enrollment into a pulmonary rehabilitation program can be challenging for several reasons. First, health care providers may not be aware of the effectiveness or availability of hospital-based, inpatient, community-based, or home-based pulmonary rehabilitation in their geographic area. Second, patients are often reluctant to begin the process, thinking "how can I possibly exercise if I cannot walk across the room?" This early inertia is a significant problem. Spouses or caregivers frequently share the same opinion, thereby offering little if any support. Third, logistic problems, such as missed work or transportation issues, may be substantial. Finally, insufficient third-party payment may make this therapeutic option too expensive for some patients. Once patients begin the process and begin receiving the individualized care characteristic of pulmonary rehabilitation they usually become motivated to continue. However, some of the previously mentioned issues reappear or the patient's medical condition changes, making continuation in the process problematic.

The beneficial effects of pulmonary rehabilitation have been demonstrated across all venues of delivery. However, the out-patient, hospital-based setting is most common in the United States. Canada has been the leader in assessing the effectiveness of home-based pulmonary rehabilitation. A recent study from that country demonstrated that 8 weeks of home-based exercise training following center-based education was not inferior to outpatient center-based pulmonary rehabilitation in improving dyspnea, exercise tolerance, and health status.[10] Additionally, rehabilitation given in both venues was safe. Additionally, a 12-week home-based program using computer-based exercise for patients with COPD was found to be an effective alternative to traditional pulmonary rehabilitation.[11] Giving pulmonary rehabilitation in the home setting might be expected to promote long-term adherence to positive health care behaviors, such as regular exercise training. However, there is little to suggest this in the literature.[10,12] What is not known is if the patients are choosing not to continue participating in maintenance programs, hospital-based or other, or if studies evaluating the effects of maintenance pulmonary rehabilitation are not being undertaken.

MAINTENANCE PROGRAMS FOLLOWING PULMONARY REHABILITATION

Pulmonary rehabilitation staff frequently tells their patients that the healthy behaviors learned and realized in the program must be continued indefinitely to ensure long-term benefits. However, in many health care systems only a limited number of pulmonary rehabilitation sessions are allowed, and adherence often falls off after the formal process has ended. A low-cost, ongoing exercise maintenance program should prove beneficial in this regard. Not only would patients exercise

regularly, but they would also have an ongoing interaction with the staff.

A recent study evaluated the feasibility and outcomes of a community-based, twice-weekly maintenance exercise program that followed a traditional hospital-based pulmonary rehabilitation program.[13] Transition to the community was facilitated by a case manager, and exercise was supervised by fitness consultants at a local community center. Although this was a single-arm study without a control group, the data suggested that for patients with moderate to severe COPD this type of case manager–facilitated maintenance exercise program in the community was feasible (70% adherence) and could maintain exercise capacity and health-related quality of life compared with baseline out to at least 1 year. Controlled trials using this approach are warranted.

Somewhat less encouraging long-term results came from a controlled trial evaluating community-based pulmonary rehabilitation study of patients with less severe COPD.[14] Patients in the intervention arm initially participated in 4 months of multidisciplinary pulmonary rehabilitation, exercising twice a week and receiving individualized education. This was followed by 20 months of exercise at home. This was supplemented by monthly home visits by a physical therapist that monitored exercise capacity and adherence to training and provided encouragement to continue exercising. Those patients having an exacerbation were allowed to have six additional training sessions with a physical therapist over 6 weeks. Compared with a usual care control group, the intervention group had significant improvements in quality of life, dyspnea, and exercise performance at 4 months. However, at the 2-year testing these favorable differences, although still significantly improved compared with usual care, had diminished in magnitude. Additionally, the intervention group did not have a decrease in exacerbation frequency compared with control subjects. Impressive was the finding that only 9% of the home exercise intervention group dropped out because of unwillingness to participate.

PROLONGING THE BENEFICIAL EFFECTS OF PULMONARY REHABILITATION INDIRECTLY THROUGH REDUCING THE FREQUENCY OF EXACERBATIONS
Reduced Hospital Admissions Rather than Reduced Number of Exacerbations as an Outcome in Pulmonary Rehabilitation

The long-term maintenance of functional outcomes after pulmonary rehabilitation is negatively affected by respiratory exacerbations.[3] Thereby, reducing the frequency of exacerbations may indirectly prolong the beneficial effects of pulmonary rehabilitation. The frequency of exacerbations in COPD can be reduced by pharmacologic and non-pharmacologic means. Reducing the total number exacerbations may not be an attainable outcome in pulmonary rehabilitation because of its emphasis on exacerbation identification in the self-management education. This type of education may actually increase the number of reported exacerbations, many of which may have gone unnoticed by the patient. However, a reduction in severe exacerbations, resulting in hospital admissions or readmission, through their early recognition and treatment is perfectly feasible from this intervention. Indeed, this may be considered a desirable goal of pulmonary rehabilitation.

In the United States in 2006, hospitalizations represented 52% to 70% of direct per patient costs to care for COPD, with exacerbations being the major contributor of 50% to 75% of the total disease costs.[15] The current estimated cost of care for the COPD exacerbation is $15 to $17 billion a year in the United States.[16] These costs, combined with the statistic that COPD contributes 22.6% of all Medicare readmissions, led to the estimate that $12 billion dollars a year is spent on potentially preventable hospitalizations for this disease.[17] As a consequence, the Centers for Medicare and Medicaid have added COPD to the list of diagnoses that are penalized if Medicare readmission rates within 30 days of discharge exceed a predetermined threshold. This monetary penalty to hospitals, contained in H.R. 3590: the Patient Protections and Affordable Care Act (Public Law 111-148, Section 3025), takes effect on October 1, 2014.

In addition to the financial burden of the hospitalization for COPD exacerbation, decreased functional status, impaired health-related quality of life, and increased mortality risk are prominent.[18] In the United Kingdom, 15% of patients admitted with exacerbations die within 90 days of admission,[19] and in France mortality over the 4 years following hospital admission was 45%.[20] Of note, nearly half of all emergency department visits by patients with COPD result in admission to the hospital.[21] Repeated hospitalizations for COPD exacerbations result in a rapid health decline and high mortality in the weeks after the events.[22]

Pulmonary Rehabilitation and COPD Exacerbations

Pulmonary rehabilitation has the potential to reduce severe exacerbations in COPD, and thereby reduce health care use for patients.

Potential components of the pulmonary rehabilitation intervention that may reduce severe exacerbations in COPD include (1) its promotion of physical activity; (2) its education program that stresses self-efficacy, including better adherence to instructions on adaptive behaviors and collaborative self-management in the periexacerbation period; and (3) its promotion of integrated care of the patient with chronic respiratory disease.

Promotion of Physical Activity During Pulmonary Rehabilitation

Patients with COPD are physically inactive compared with age-matched healthy control subjects,[23] and this inactivity seems to be an independent risk factor for hospitalizations[24] and mortality.[25] For example, patients sent home after a hospitalization for an exacerbation who report less than 20 minutes a day of moderate physical activity are at greater risk of readmission and mortality than those with higher self-reported activity. Additionally, those patients who walk 60 minutes or more a day reportedly have a reduction in the risk of readmission by almost 50%.[26] Finally, directly measured physical activity from an activity monitor has been demonstrated to be the strongest predictor of 4-year mortality in COPD, surpassing lung function, functional exercise capacity, and cardiovascular variables in this regard.[27]

Although a causal link between physical inactivity and health care use and mortality is not absolutely proved, the existing data are strongly suggestive of causality. Based on the strong association, higher levels of physical activity are now strongly promoted for patients with COPD, as it is indeed promoted for all individuals. Pulmonary rehabilitation, with its patient-centered approach, educational approach, and strong emphasis on self-efficacy promotion, provides a good platform to address this important issue. For example, in a Spanish study, only 25% of the patients with COPD followed recommendations to perform 30 or more consecutive minutes of moderate physical activity, 5 or more days a week.[28] Yet, almost 60% fulfilled the recommended duration of exercise when their exercise was accumulated by sessions of 10 or more minutes of exercise throughout the day, as is often the format of pulmonary rehabilitation. Furthermore, postrehabilitation exercise maintenance programs provide a venue to encourage exercise training and physical activity.

Because a lower level of physical activity is an important predictor of hospitalization, one of the goals of pulmonary rehabilitation has been to increase performance in this area. The concept is that increases in exercise capacity realized from pulmonary rehabilitation would eventually be translated into increased physical activity in the home or community settings. To date, nine controlled trials evaluating the effect of pulmonary rehabilitation or exercise training on activity have been published.[29,30] The results have been less than spectacular, with only a few demonstrating a positive effect on this outcome. Increasing the effectiveness of pulmonary rehabilitation on physical activity remains an important research area.

Promoting Self-Efficacy and Collaborative Self-Management in the Respiratory Patient

A core component of pulmonary rehabilitation, recognized in the newest American Thoracic Society/European Respiratory Society statement on pulmonary rehabilitation,[31] is behavioral change and collaborative self-management. With respect to reducing exacerbations and health care use in COPD, pulmonary rehabilitation could work favorably through improving adherence with pharmacologic and nonpharmacologic therapy and through promoting the use of collaborative self-management at the time of the exacerbation. Promoting adherence with the regular use of medications that have been demonstrated to reduce the exacerbation should, of course, prove beneficial. Additionally, the early recognition and prompt treatment of the exacerbation should reduce its impact.[32,33] Educating the patient to recognize the exacerbation earlier, begin treatment with an action plan (usually starting oral steroids and antibiotics via a preset plan), and contact the health care provider are part of this collaborative self-management strategy.[34]

For those hospitalized with an exacerbation, education about pulmonary rehabilitation could be provided and the patient could be referred to a program. Too often, priorities are placed on acute care, often overshadowing the importance of the management of chronic conditions. A recent study hypothesized that during a hospitalization for a respiratory exacerbation there are substantial missed opportunities for enhancing adherence to current guidelines and recommendations.[35] Their hypothesis was supported in that smoking cessation counseling was offered to only 48% of current smokers.

Pulmonary Rehabilitation and the Integration of Care of the Respiratory Patient at the Time of the Respiratory Exacerbation

Coordination of services is especially important at the time of the hospitalization for the COPD exacerbation, which is associated with substantial health care use, increased risk for readmission, and increased risk for mortality. The posthospital period is a time of generalized risk of physiologic impairment and deconditioning that diminishes a patient's ability to resume activities of daily living.[36] After hospital discharge, care is often fragmented among health professionals. Improving the integration of care in this setting may provide benefit through enhancing lines of communication and coordination among health care providers and patients. Integration in this setting includes proper assessment at the time of discharge, case management with discharge planning that provides the appropriate discharge services, a self-management plan for subsequent exacerbations, making sure this plan is available to all health care providers, and the use of modern information technology to facilitate transmission of this information.

The integration of care for the patient with COPD has been successful in some studies. In Quebec, comprehensive self-management instruction in the home after an exacerbation, with 2 months of weekly in-home visits, followed by monthly telephone follow-up for an additional 10 months, reduced hospitalizations by 39.8% over control subjects.[37] Additionally, visits to the emergency department were reduced by 41% and unscheduled visits to physicians were reduced by 58.9%. Without the inclusion of structured exercise in this program, it can only be hypothesized that the reduction in health care use might be even greater if exercise were a component of this home program.

A program consisting of a comprehensive evaluation of the patient at discharge, self-management education, development of an individually tailored plan, and accessibility of the specialized nurse to patients and primary care providers, facilitated through a World Wide Web–based process, led to a 50% reduction in subsequent hospital readmissions. This successful reduction in health care use was associated with better performance in self-management, including COPD knowledge, exacerbation identification, exacerbation early treatment, inhaler adherence, and correctness of inhaler technique.[38]

USING PULMONARY REHABILITATION OR ITS COMPONENTS TO OPTIMIZE CARE FOLLOWING HOSPITAL DISCHARGE

Optimizing health care use at the time of the hospital discharge for a respiratory exacerbation includes a scheduled follow-up visit with the primary care physician or pulmonologist; these can be facilitated by a pulmonary rehabilitation specialist. A follow-up visit within 30 days of discharge has been associated with 14% fewer emergency department visits and 9% fewer readmissions after discharge.[39] Possibly these numbers can be further reduced with on-going participation in rehabilitation in conjunction with timely patient-physician interaction.

The transition of care as a patient moves among providers and treatment settings as their medical condition and health care needs evolve can be facilitated by pulmonary rehabilitation professionals. This integration of care can be facilitated though formal or maintenance pulmonary rehabilitation, in which long-term, trusting relationships have been established between the patient and the rehabilitation staff.

The implementation of a COPD-specific discharge bundle has been shown to be successful in recent controlled trials. In the United Kingdom the discharge bundle was followed by 10.8% hospital readmissions, compared with 16.4% readmissions in the control group.[40] The investigators identified six practices that should be delivered to patients with COPD before hospital discharge: (1) notifying the respiratory clinical specialist of all admissions; (2) offering smoking cessation counseling if the patient is a smoker; (3) providing COPD-specific information, including a self-management booklet; (4) providing information, when needed, on supplemental oxygen, patient support groups, and the proper use of inhalers; (5) scheduling a follow-up appointment with a pulmonologist before discharge; and (6) referring to pulmonary rehabilitation. Additionally, at 48 to 72 hours after discharge, the clinical specialist made a brief, scripted telephone call to the patient to assess improvement or decline.

A second study[41] conducted in a general medical population in Boston and using a nurse discharge advocate resulted in a 30% lower rate of hospital use (readmissions and emergency department visits), improved self-perceived preparation for discharge, and increased physician follow-up after discharge in the treatment group. In the treatment group, a nurse advocate arranged follow-up visits, coordinated medication reconciliation, and prepared an after-hospital care plan. The care plan included medical provider contact information, dates for appointments and tests, medication schedule, list of tests with pending results, an illustrated explanation of the discharge diagnosis, and information on what to do if a problem arises (action plan). A pharmacist contacted the patient 2 to 4 days postdischarge to reinforce the discharge plan and review medications.

As a prominent component of integrated care, pulmonary rehabilitation provides or coordinates many of the previously mentioned services.[42] Pulmonary rehabilitation professionals can provide a transitional figure to review and update the patient's action plan to assist in identifying worsening symptoms[43] and support the patient in rebuilding strength and endurance, improving health-related quality of life, and optimizing health care use.[44] Virtually all the discharge services listed previously could have been coordinated by a pulmonary rehabilitation professional; indeed, a structured program might provide an ideal way to provide these services. Additionally, through organizing or providing these services, recruitment and retention of pulmonary rehabilitation candidates would be enhanced.

A systematic review of pulmonary rehabilitation started in the periexacerbation period reviewed nine randomized trials of 432 patients with COPD.[45] Pulmonary rehabilitation not only improved functional and exercise outcomes, but also reduced subsequent hospitalizations and mortality. It is not clear which component or components of pulmonary rehabilitation led to these positive results, because increased exercise capacity, increased physical activity, and improved self-management skills may have been responsible. Whatever the mechanism of action, based on this systematic review, the initiation of pulmonary rehabilitation (or return to a maintenance program) in the posthospitalization period seems appropriate.

Professional intervention in the home setting has also met with some success. A respiratory therapist initiated in-home COPD management of oxygen-dependent patients with COPD has been shown to improve proper medication use, increase daily exercise (even though no formal exercise instruction was given), and decrease hospitalizations.[46] For this program, at least three home visits were made, with the first occurring within 3 days of enrollment. The initial session assessed physical status, understanding of disease process, medication use, dietary habits, participation in daily exercise, support group attendance, and smoking history. Self-management instruction was provided at the first follow-up session, with participation in pulmonary rehabilitation encouraged.

An example of a program with more frequent patient contact comes from a disease management study of chronically critically ill patients.[47] An advanced practice nurse met with the 231 study participants before hospital discharge to develop a plan of care, met again within 48 hours of discharge, and had a third visit within the first week. Visits occurred weekly for the next 3 weeks, then every other week for the last 4 weeks, for a total of eight visits. Visits were also made any time there was a transition to another location of care, again illustrating the importance of a transition facilitator. When compared with control subjects, there was no difference in risk of readmission but the 93 subjects that were readmitted had fewer mean days of hospitalization (11.4 vs 16.7) for a cost savings of $481,811. Exercise was not specifically addressed in this study and patients with a pulmonary diagnosis comprised only 22.1% of the experimental group.

Many pulmonary rehabilitation professionals believe that their current patient care, especially when caring for long-term patients in maintenance programs, has characteristics of the case management model; a long-term, integrated approach of proactive and planned care. Two recent systematic reviews from the Netherlands[48,49] support the need to refocus pulmonary rehabilitation to be longer term, similar to the disease management model. This is based on findings that disease management, up to 24 months in duration, in primary, secondary, and tertiary care resulted in improved disease-specific quality of life, increased exercise tolerance, reduced hospital admissions, and reduced hospital days per person.

RECOMMENDATIONS

Lessons should be heeded from pulmonary rehabilitation in alternative venues (home), from alternative approaches to exercise (computer systems), and from our colleagues in disease management. Before advice is needed, patient enrollment must be optimized. Health care providers must be aware of the positive outcomes from pulmonary rehabilitation that assist in their care of the patient, including patients' improved ability to recognize an exacerbation and improved physical conditioning that can reduce hospitalizations and length of stay. Reduction in COPD readmissions should interest hospitals to fund maintenance rehabilitation. Third-party payers also benefit from reduced admissions but most of all, the patient benefits. Patients must be educated that pulmonary rehabilitation and maintenance programs increase exercise capacity and exacerbation awareness, both leading to a reduction in hospitalizations.

REFERENCES

1. Ries AL, Kaplan RM, Limberg TM, et al. Effects of pulmonary rehabilitation on physiologic and psychosocial outcomes in patients with chronic obstructive pulmonary disease. Ann Intern Med 1995;122(11):823–32.

2. Troosters T, Gosselink R, Decramer M. Short- and long-term effects of outpatient rehabilitation in patients with chronic obstructive pulmonary disease: a randomized trial. Am J Med 2000;109(3):207–12.

3. Brooks D, Krip B, Mangovski-Alzamora S, et al. The effect of postrehabilitation programmes among individuals with chronic obstructive pulmonary disease. Eur Respir J 2002;20(1):20–9.

4. Ries AL, Kaplan RM, Myers R, et al. Maintenance after pulmonary rehabilitation in chronic lung disease: a randomized trial. Am J Respir Crit Care Med 2003;167(6):880–8.

5. Foglio K, Bianchi L, Ambrosino N. Is it really useful to repeat outpatient pulmonary rehabilitation programs in patients with chronic airway obstruction? A 2-year controlled study. Chest 2001;119(6):1696–704.

6. Maltais F, Bourbeau J, Shapiro S, et al. Effects of home-based pulmonary rehabilitation in patients with chronic obstructive pulmonary disease: a randomized trial. Ann Intern Med 2008;149(12):869–78.

7. Ringbaek T, Brondum E, Martinez G, et al. Rehabilitation in COPD: the long-term effect of a supervised 7-week program succeeded by a self-monitored walking program. Chron Respir Dis 2008;5(2):75–80.

8. Spencer LM, Alison JA, McKeough ZJ. Do supervised weekly exercise programs maintain functional exercise capacity and quality of life, twelve months after pulmonary rehabilitation in COPD? BMC Pulm Med 2007;7:7, 8.

9. Hayton C, Clark A, Olive S, et al. Barriers to pulmonary rehabilitation: characteristics that predict patient attendance and adherence. Respir Med 2013;107(3):401–7.

10. Maltais F, Bourbeau J, Shapiro S, et al. Effects of home-based rehabilitation in patients with chronic obstructive pulmonary disease. Ann Intern Med 2008;149:869–78.

11. Albores J, Marolda C, Haggerty M, et al. The use of a home exercise program based on a computer system in patients with chronic obstructive pulmonary disease. J Cardiopulm Rehabil 2013;33:47–52.

12. Vieira D, Maltais F, Bourbeau J. Home-based pulmonary rehabilitation in chronic obstructive pulmonary disease patients. Curr Opin Pulm Med 2010;16:134–43.

13. Beauchamp M, Francella S, Romano J, et al. A novel approach to long-term respiratory care: results of a community-based post-rehabilitation maintenance program in COPD. Respir Med 2013;8:1210–6.

14. van Wetering C, Hoogendoorn M, Mol S, et al. Short- and long-term efficacy of a community-based COPD management programme in less advanced COPD: a randomized trial. Thorax 2010;65:7–13.

15. Perera P, Armstrong E, Sherrill D, et al. Acute exacerbations of COPD in the United States: inpatient burden and predictors of costs and mortality. COPD 2012;9:131–41.

16. Kallstrom T. COPD hospital readmissions: what challenges are on the horizon? AARC Times 2013.

17. Jencks S, Williams M, Coleman E. Rehospitalization among patients in the Medicare fee-for-service program. N Engl J Med 2009;360:1418–28.

18. Kon S, Canavan J, Man W. Pulmonary rehabilitation and acute exacerbations of COPD. Expert Rev Respir Med 2012;6:523–31.

19. Price L, Lowe D, Hosker H, et al. UK national COPD audit 2003: impact of hospital resources and organization of care on patient outcome following admission for acute COPD exacerbation. Thorax 2006; 61:837–42.

20. Piquet J, Chavaillon J, David P, et al. High-risk patients following hospitalization for an acute exacerbation of COPD. Eur Respir J 2013;42:946–55.

21. Lippmann S, Yeatts K, Waller A, et al. Hospitalizations and return visits after chronic obstructive pulmonary disease ED visits. Am J Emerg Med 2013; 31:1393–6.

22. Suissa S, Dell'Aniello S, Ernst P. Long-term natural history of chronic obstructive pulmonary disease severe exacerbations and mortality. Thorax 2012;67: 957–63.

23. Pitta F, Troosters T, Spruit MA, et al. Characteristics of physical activities in daily life in chronic obstructive pulmonary disease. Am J Respir Crit Care Med 2005;171:972–7.

24. Garcia-Aymerich J, Farrero E, Felez M, et al. Risk factors of readmission to hospital for a COPD exacerbation: a prospective study. Thorax 2003;58:100–5.

25. Garcia-Aymerich J, Lange P, Benet M, et al. Regular physical activity reduces hospital admission and mortality in chronic obstructive pulmonary disease: a population based cohort study. Thorax 2006;61: 772–8.

26. Revitt O, Sewell L, Morgan M, et al. A short outpatient pulmonary rehabilitation programme reduces readmission following a hospitalization for an exacerbation of COPD. Respirology 2013;18: 1063–8. http://dx.doi.org/10.1111/resp.12141.

27. Waschki B, Kirsten A, Holz O, et al. Physical activity is the strongest predictor of all-cause mortality in patients with COPD: a prospective cohort study. Chest 2011;140:331–42.

28. Donaire-Gonzalez D, Gimeno-Santos E, Balcells E, et al. Physical activity in COPD patients: patterns and bouts. Eur Respir J 2013;42:993–1002.

29. Casaburi R. Activity promotion: a paradigm shift for chronic obstructive pulmonary disease therapeutics. Proc Am Thorac Soc 2011;8:334–7.

30. Ng LW, Mackney J, Jenkins S, et al. Does exercise training change physical activity in people with COPD? A systematic review and meta-analysis. Chron Respir Dis 2012;9:17–26.

31. Spruit MA, Singh SJ, Garvey C, et al. Key concepts and advances in pulmonary rehabilitation based on

32. Seemungal TA, Donaldson GC, Bhowmik A, et al. Time course and recovery of exacerbations in patients with chronic obstructive pulmonary disease. Am J Respir Crit Care Med 2000;161:1608–13.

33. Seemungal TA, Wedzicha JA. Acute exacerbations of COPD: the challenge is early treatment. COPD 2009;6:79–81.

34. Morgan MD. Action plans for COPD self-management. Integrated care is more than the sum of its parts. Thorax 2011;66:935–6.

35. Yip N, Yuen G, Lazar E, et al. Analysis of hospitalizations for COPD exacerbation: opportunities for improving care. COPD 2010;7:85–92.

36. Krumholz H. Post-hospital syndrome: an acquired, transient condition of generalized risk. N Engl J Med 2013;368:100–2.

37. Bourbeau J, Julien M, Maltais F, et al. Reduction of hospital utilization in patients with chronic obstructive pulmonary disease. Arch Intern Med 2003;163: 585–91.

38. Garcia-Aymerich J, Hernandez C, Alonso A, et al. Effects of an integrated care intervention on risk factors of COPD readmission. Respir Med 2007;101: 1462–9.

39. Sharma G, Kuo Y, Freeman J, et al. Outpatient follow-up visit and 30-day emergency department visit and readmission in patients hospitalized for chronic obstructive pulmonary disease. Arch Intern Med 2010;17:1664–70.

40. Hopkinson N, Englebretsen C, Cooley N, et al. Designing and implementing a COPD discharge care bundle. Thorax 2012;67:90–2.

41. Jack B, Chetty V, Anthony D, et al. A reengineered hospital discharge program to decrease rehospitalization. Ann Intern Med 2009;150:178–87.

42. Nici L, ZuWallack R. An official American Thoracic Society workshop report: the integrated care of the COPD patient. Proc Am Thorac Soc 2012;9:9–18.

43. Currie G, Miller D. Action plans for patients with chronic obstructive pulmonary disease. BMJ 2012; 344:e1164. http://dx.doi.org/10.1136/bmj.e1164.

44. Wang Q, Bourbeau J. Outcomes and health-related quality of life following hospitalization for an acute exacerbation of COPD. Respirology 2005;10:334–40.

45. Puhan MA, Gimeno-Santos E, Scharplatz M, et al. Pulmonary rehabilitation following exacerbations of chronic obstructive pulmonary disease. Cochrane Database Syst Rev 2011;(10):CD005305.

46. Ramani A, Pickston A, Clark J, et al. Role of the management pathway in the care of advanced COPD patients in their own homes. Care Manag J 2010; 11:249–53.

the official 2013 American Thoracic Society/European Respiratory Society statement on pulmonary rehabilitation. Am J Respir Crit Care Med 2013; 188:e13–64.

47. Daly B, Douglas S, Kelley C, et al. Trial of disease management program to reduce hospital readmissions of the chronically critically ill. Chest 2005; 128:507–17.

48. Boland M, Tsiachristas A, Kruis A, et al. The health economic impact of disease management programs for COPD: a systematic literature review and meta-analysis. BMC Pulm Med 2013;13:40.

49. Kruis A, Smidt N, Assendelft W, et al. Integrated disease management for patients with chronic obstructive pulmonary disease. Cochrane Database Syst Rev 2013;(10):CD009437.

Pulmonary Rehabilitation
Future Directions

Linda Nici, MD[a],*, Richard L. ZuWallack, MD[b]

KEYWORDS

- Pulmonary rehabilitation • Chronic obstructive pulmonary disease • Self-management
- Physical activity

KEY POINTS

- Pulmonary rehabilitation appears to be effective in earlier stages of COPD severity and in chronic respiratory diseases other than COPD.
- Pulmonary rehabilitation appears to significantly reduce subsequent health care utilization in patients with an exacerbation of COPD; this has important implications to current health care systems.
- Pulmonary rehabilitation may be effective in the home and community settings, where telehealth may be a uniquely valuable adjunct.

PULMONARY REHABILITATION: STATE OF THE SCIENCE

As outlined in the preceding articles of this issue, pulmonary rehabilitation has certainly come of age! This interdisciplinary and patient-centered intervention, which includes structured exercise training and behavioral interventions aimed at promoting collaborative self-management, is now an established standard of care for patients with chronic obstructive pulmonary disease (COPD). Furthermore, an increasing body of evidence now indicates that it is also effective in other chronic respiratory diseases, probably because their disablement processes share common features addressed by pulmonary rehabilitation.

Pulmonary rehabilitation addresses the systemic effects of chronic respiratory disease, including peripheral muscle wasting and dysfunction, physical deconditioning, symptoms of anxiety and depression, and maladaptive behaviors such as a sedentary lifestyle and poor adherence to prescribed therapies. Often these systemic effects are complex and intertwined. As an example, the exercise training component of pulmonary rehabilitation in the COPD patient results in an increase in oxidative enzymes in ambulatory muscles, leading to less lactate production and consequently less ventilatory requirement at a given workload. In turn, this allows for a slower respiratory rate at that particular workload. The resultant longer expiratory time permits greater emptying of the lung at each exhalation, thereby reducing dynamic hyperinflation. The adaptive muscle changes and reduction in dynamic hyperinflation result in less exertional dyspnea. This decreased symptom burden, coupled with greater self-efficacy and less anxiety associated with dyspnea-producing activity, results in improved health-related quality of life.

The ascendancy of pulmonary rehabilitation for COPD to its current inclusion in major guidelines for this disease[1] reflects the fact that it works, and generally works very well. Although pulmonary rehabilitation has no appreciable direct effect on static measurements of lung function, it arguably provides the greatest benefit of any available therapy (including pharmacotherapy) across multiple outcome areas important to the patient with respiratory disease, including dyspnea, exercise

[a] Pulmonary Medicine/Critical Care Section, Providence VA Medical Center, 830 Chalkstone Avenue, Providence, RI 02908, USA; [b] Pulmonary Medicine, Critical Care-Medical, Department of Pulmonary Medicine, Saint Francis Medical Group, Inc, 114 Woodland Street, Hartford, CT 06105, USA
* Corresponding author.
E-mail address: linda_nici@brown.edu

Clin Chest Med 35 (2014) 439–444
http://dx.doi.org/10.1016/j.ccm.2014.02.015
0272-5231/14/$ – see front matter © 2014 Elsevier Inc. All rights reserved.

performance, and health-related quality of life. It also appears to be a potent intervention that reduces COPD hospitalizations, especially when given in the periexacerbation period. These beneficial effects have been summarized earlier in this issue (**Box 1**).

EXPANDING THE APPLICABILITY OF PULMONARY REHABILITATION
Pulmonary Rehabilitation for the Non-COPD Respiratory Patient

Traditionally, most patients beginning outpatient pulmonary rehabilitation have had COPD as a primary diagnosis. However, as outlined in detail in a previous article in this issue by Rochester and colleagues, a considerable body of evidence has accumulated showing that pulmonary rehabilitation, always modified to meet the needs of the individual patient, has benefits in respiratory diseases other than COPD. To date, the evidence supporting pulmonary rehabilitation for the non-COPD respiratory patient is similar to that for COPD in the early 1990s. Undoubtedly, this body of evidence will continue to grow. Research in this area will include building on the body of evidence demonstrating its effectiveness in various respiratory diseases, determining the specific mechanisms underlying this effectiveness, and then determining the best ways to adapt the pulmonary rehabilitation intervention to maximize benefits.

Pulmonary Rehabilitation in Earlier Stages of COPD

Most studies evaluating the effectiveness of pulmonary rehabilitation in COPD have enrolled patient groups with a mean forced expiratory volume in 1 second (FEV_1) less than 50% of predicted.[2] Although reasoning from this observation may lead to the conclusion that it is not effective in milder disease, this thinking represents a fallacy in informal logic (argumentum ad ignorantiam). In fact, a recent study demonstrated that community-based pulmonary rehabilitation is effective in COPD patients with mild and moderate spirometric severity and concurrent impaired exercise performance.[3] This finding brings to the forefront a concept that the pulmonary rehabilitation professional community has always held: that symptoms and functional status limitation, not FEV_1 thresholds, are the relevant inclusion criteria. It is anticipated that this principle will lead to a shift in referral patterns, with patients with less severe disease (and a greater potential for disease-modifying therapies to work) referred for pulmonary rehabilitation. For this to occur, clinicians and third-party payers must realize this widened applicability, which to date has not yet occurred.

Pulmonary Rehabilitation in the Periexacerbation Period

Providing pulmonary rehabilitation during or shortly after a serious exacerbation of COPD, often at the time of hospitalization, is an exciting new application of this comprehensive intervention. Interest in this application is heightened by the knowledge that exacerbations are very costly in terms of morbidity, mortality, and dollars, and that pulmonary rehabilitation has a demonstrable benefit in this clinical situation. Pulmonary rehabilitation can be beneficial when provided before, during, and immediately after the exacerbation. These benefits, which have been documented in a

---

Box 1
Pulmonary rehabilitation in 2014

- Pulmonary rehabilitation is defined as "a comprehensive intervention based on a thorough patient assessment followed by patient-tailored therapies, which include, but are not limited to, exercise training, education and behavior change, designed to improve the physical and emotional condition of people with chronic respiratory disease and to promote the long-term adherence of health-enhancing behaviors"[1]

- It has become standard care and is now incorporated into major COPD guidelines

- Its effectiveness depends on its ability to reduce the systemic consequences of chronic respiratory disease and its ability to promote adaptive behavior change through promoting self-efficacy

- It is typically provided in a hospital-based, outpatient setting, but can be effectively provided in inpatient, home, and community settings

- Its effectiveness has been demonstrated across multiple patient-centered outcome areas in COPD, including dyspnea, exercise performance, and health-related quality of life; it arguably provides the greatest benefits in these areas in comparison with any other therapy

- It appears to significantly reduce subsequent health care utilization in patients discharged following an exacerbation of COPD; this obviously has important implications to current health care systems

- Evidence suggests it is effective in earlier stages of COPD severity and in chronic respiratory diseases other than COPD

systematic review,[4] include better adherence to prescribed therapies, improved collaborative self-management skills (especially centered on an exacerbation action plan), and higher levels of exercise capacity and (potentially) physical activity. Exactly which of these factors are responsible for subsequently lower health care utilization are not known. In addition, pulmonary rehabilitation in the post-hospitalization period can help coordinate the health care of the often complex, multimorbid patient, thereby fostering integration of care for these individuals. Future research in this general area will take 2 paths: (1) increasing the scientific knowledge base, including that of the optimal timing and the best ways to provide the intervention; and (2) increasing knowledge among clinicians and hospitals of benefits of pulmonary rehabilitation in the periexacerbation period, notably its potential to reduce subsequent hospitalizations.

Pulmonary Rehabilitation During Critical Illness

The application of pulmonary rehabilitation early in the course of a critical illness is promising[5] and has some support from guidelines,[6] although relatively little research on outcomes and feasibility is available in this area. Exercise training can begin with range of motion and limited mobility exercises, progressing in intensity, duration, and generalization as the patient's condition permits. Neuromuscular electrical stimulation of the ambulatory muscles may also serve as a useful adjunct to improve muscle function in severely disabled critically ill patients.[7]

Pulmonary Rehabilitation in the Home and Community Settings

Pulmonary rehabilitation is typically provided either in hospital-based, outpatient settings or in inpatient settings, reflecting the availability of trained personnel and space in these locations. Despite this practical reality, these venues limit the availability of pulmonary rehabilitation and can be costly. Because of these considerations, clinicians and investigators have evaluated pulmonary rehabilitation provided in the home or in the community. Home-based and community-based pulmonary rehabilitation offer the advantages of greater convenience and accessibility and, if provided under minimal supervision, lower cost. The drawback is that the interdisciplinary support needed for the typically complex, multimorbid respiratory patient is not readily available in these settings. Therefore, in most cases they can be considered training interventions rather than comprehensive pulmonary rehabilitation programs. Another potential disadvantage of the home or community setting is that direct supervision of exercise typically is not present, so there is a potential for safety issues in these unsupervised settings. However, a systematic review of home-based rehabilitation[8] and one large randomized trial[9] demonstrated that, with respect to improvements in exercise capacity and changes in health status, the home-based setting was not much different from the traditional setting. Similarly, pulmonary rehabilitation provided in a community-based setting has also been proved to be effective when compared with usual care.[3] Further research is needed in determining which patients would be best suited for rehabilitation provided in these nontraditional venues, whether they provide real cost savings, and whether they can reduce subsequent health care utilization.

Technology-Assisted Pulmonary Rehabilitation

Telemonitoring has already been implemented in COPD as an adjunctive method to help patients self-manage their disease in collaboration with health care providers. This approach often involves having patients report symptoms or physiologic measurements electronically to a health care team on a regular basis, with the idea that this might promote the early recognition of exacerbations and subsequent early initiation of appropriate therapy. Although this approach has yet to be unequivocally proved to be successful in reducing health care utilization,[10] the potential use of telemonitoring as an adjunct to pulmonary rehabilitation would seem to have benefit in several areas. For example: (1) telemonitoring could provide useful feedback to the patient and rehabilitation staff on adherence to daily exercise and physical activity in the home, potentially augmenting or sustaining long-term benefits; (2) computer-based education workbook modules can provide feedback and practice time for patients to successfully self-manage; and (3) in rural communities or when transportation is an obstacle, pulmonary rehabilitation education may be delivered through Internet-based programs.

FURTHER DEFINING THE EFFECTIVENESS OF PULMONARY REHABILITATION
Self-Management Education

The educational component of pulmonary rehabilitation has evolved from a didactic approach to collaborative self-management to elicit positive and sustained behavior change.[11] This new emphasis includes, among other properties, the promotion of healthy behaviors and lifestyle changes including smoking cessation, fostering adherence to recommended pharmacologic and nonpharmacologic therapies, and striving to have the patient incorporate increased exercise and physical activity into the home and community settings. In addition, collaborative self-management focuses on the development of an action plan aimed at the early recognition and appropriate treatment of the exacerbation.

At first thought, collaborative self-management in COPD, with resultant better communication and close collaboration between the patient and health care provider, would seem to be a straight-forward concept. Unfortunately, the results from the clinical trials thus far have not been convincing. For instance, 2 large, multicenter Veterans Administration research studies run independently (and nearly simultaneously) to compare rational, collaborative self-management strategies (called disease management) with usual care in COPD patients at risk for exacerbations and increased health care utilization had polar opposite results. One study showed a substantial reduction in its combined end point of hospitalization and emergency department visits for COPD exacerbations in the treatment group, whereas the other had to be terminated by its Data Safety Board because of an increased mortality signal and no health care benefit in its treatment group![12,13]

The reason or reasons behind the discordant results regarding self-management in the COPD patients described are not known, but it is reasonable to assume that for self-management to work in the respiratory patient, more information is needed with regard to selecting the appropriate patient (ie, the one who would be helped, not harmed), the optimal setting, and the best techniques for the intervention. Pulmonary rehabilitation, with its emphasis on collaborative self-management, its interdisciplinary staffing, its success across multiple patient-centered outcome areas, and its relatively long duration (several weeks), would seem to be ideal for implementing and testing collaborative self-management strategies. Unfortunately, because pulmonary rehabilitation has multiple components, it is likely to be difficult or impossible to separate out the effects of exercise training, psychosocial support, and other interventions from those effects resulting from its self-management component. Nonetheless, this promises to be a fertile area for research.

Maintaining the Benefits of Pulmonary Rehabilitation

Although pulmonary rehabilitation arguably provides substantial beneficial effects in dyspnea, exercise performance, and health-related quality of life for COPD, these gains tend to diminish in the months to years following the formal intervention.[14] These declines probably stem in large part from progression of the respiratory disease and its comorbidities and intervening exacerbations, and the fact that clinicians are delivering an acute intervention (ie, pulmonary rehabilitation provided over several weeks) for a chronic disease.[15] With respect to the latter, more research is needed to determine which modifications to the pulmonary rehabilitation approach would lead to longer-term benefits. Prolonging the pulmonary rehabilitation intervention would help in this regard and has some supporting data,[16] but is not feasible in the current health care climate. In all likelihood, a successful approach would center on behavior change through promoting self-efficacy for exercise and physical activity. This area is also fertile ground for research and development.

Translating Gains in Exercise Capacity into Meaningful Physical Activity

Lower levels of exercise performance and reduced daily physical activity both predict poor outcome in patients with COPD, independent of other measures of disease severity.[17–19] While higher levels of exercise capacity are permissive of increased physical activity in the home and community settings, other factors such as motivation, self-efficacy for walking, and cultural issues undoubtedly play a role in modulating baseline physical activity. Illustrating this point, gains in exercise capacity realized in the pulmonary rehabilitation setting do not necessarily translate into increased physical activity.[20,21] Acknowledging this discord in outcomes and emphasizing the prominent behavioral component of physical activity, one editorial glibly stated that "one needs 3 months to train the muscle, but 6 months to train the brain."[22] Pulmonary rehabilitation must look beyond simply providing exercise training for the muscles, and develop better ways to train the brain. Clinicians must focus on physical activity as an important outcome in pulmonary rehabilitation, and find better ways to increase it.

PROMOTING ACCESSIBILITY TO PULMONARY REHABILITATION
Increasing the Awareness of Pulmonary Rehabilitation

A significant barrier to the effective use of pulmonary rehabilitation in the community is a lack of awareness among many health care providers of the nature and benefits of this intervention.[23] This information gap is probably slowly decreasing, perhaps through the incorporation of pulmonary rehabilitation into major guidelines for respiratory diseases such as COPD. However, more could be done to enhance its awareness. Although education on pulmonary rehabilitation is required in pulmonary fellowship training in the United States, based on the Accreditation Council for Graduate Medical Education requirements, this education varies widely among training programs and remains open to enhancement and standardization. The same holds for the education of other health professionals, including nurses, nurse practitioners, physical therapists, occupational therapists, and respiratory therapists. In addition, newer data demonstrating the effectiveness of pulmonary rehabilitation in reducing health care utilization,[4] and the gradual incorporation of pulmonary rehabilitation (or its components) into the integrated care for COPD,[23,24] should enhance its awareness.

Fair Reimbursement for Pulmonary Rehabilitation

Payment for pulmonary rehabilitation varies widely among health care systems worldwide. In the United States, reimbursement depends on third-party payer coverage of the individual patient. In 2010, for patients covered under Medicare (generally individuals ≥65 years), the Centers for Medicare and Medicaid Services (CMS) began directly reimbursing for pulmonary rehabilitation for COPD patients who had moderate to very severe disease. Because no baseline data were initially available, reimbursement had to be based on assumptions from proxy information. However, beginning in 2012, reimbursement was reduced based on new claims data and cost-to-charge ratios. This new reimbursement, which represents a gross underpayment, undoubtedly reflects initial underreporting by hospitals of charges that were then used as a basis for CMS reimbursement. The eventual establishment of fair reimbursement for pulmonary rehabilitation services will require education of hospital administrators and pulmonary rehabilitation staff to thoroughly report all services, supplies, and equipment necessary for this intervention.

PULMONARY REHABILITATION AND INTEGRATED CARE OF THE RESPIRATORY PATIENT

The acute care model, with its major goal of curing an acute disease with an intervention of short duration, does not fit into the management strategy of patients with chronic respiratory diseases such as COPD.[24] Rather, a chronic disease management model is necessary, which would integrate the multiple dimensions of care needed for optimal and sustained benefits for patients with chronic illness and complex comorbidities. The World Health Organization has defined integrated care as "a concept bringing together inputs, delivery, management and organization of services related to diagnosis, treatment, care, rehabilitation and health promotion."[25] Integration of care has the potential to enhance access, quality, efficiency, and satisfaction.

Pulmonary rehabilitation, with its interdisciplinary, patient-centered approach and its emphasis on partnering, communication, and coordination among health care professionals, is an excellent platform for the implementation of integrated care. This integration becomes even more imperative at the time of the respiratory exacerbation. Pulmonary rehabilitation in this setting can facilitate communication among health care providers, foster timely and regular follow-up, and provide a means for a more seamless transition into the community.[24] Integrated care at the time of discharge for a COPD exacerbation generally includes: (1) a comprehensive assessment; (2) an self-management plan to deal with new exacerbations; (3) sharing this individually tailored plan with health care providers across the system; and (4) accessibility to a specialized case manager, perhaps facilitated by information technology.[26] The role of pulmonary rehabilitation within the larger schema of integrated care certainly represents a fruitful area for further research and development.

REFERENCES

1. Spruit MA, Singh SJ, Garvey C, et al. An official American Thoracic Society/European Respiratory Society statement: key concepts and advances in pulmonary rehabilitation. Am J Respir Crit Care Med 2013;188(8):e13–64.
2. Qaseem A, Wilt TJ, Weinberger SE, et al. Diagnosis and management of stable chronic obstructive pulmonary disease: a clinical practice guideline update from the American College of Physicians, American College of Chest Physicians, American Thoracic Society, and European Respiratory Society. Ann Intern Med 2011;155(3):179–91.
3. van Wetering CR, Hoogendoorn M, Mol SJ, et al. Short- and long-term efficacy of a community-based COPD management programme in less advanced COPD: a randomised controlled trial. Thorax 2010;65(1):7–13.
4. Puhan MA, Gimeno-Santos E, Scharplatz M, et al. Pulmonary rehabilitation following exacerbations of

chronic obstructive pulmonary disease. Cochrane Database Syst Rev 2011;(10):CD005305.

5. Rochester CL. Rehabilitation in the intensive care unit. Semin Respir Crit Care Med 2009;30(6):656–69.

6. Tan T, Brett SJ, Stokes T, Guideline Development Group. Rehabilitation after critical illness: summary of NICE guidance. BMJ 2009;338:b822.

7. Sillen MJ, Franssen FM, Gosker HR, et al. Metabolic and structural changes in lower-limb skeletal muscle following neuromuscular electrical stimulation: a systematic review. PLoS One 2013;8(9):e69391.

8. Vieira DS, Maltais F, Bourbeau J. Home-based pulmonary rehabilitation in chronic obstructive pulmonary disease patients. Curr Opin Pulm Med 2010; 16(2):134–43.

9. Maltais F, Bourbeau J, Shapiro S, et al. Effects of home-based pulmonary rehabilitation in patients with chronic obstructive pulmonary disease: a randomized trial. Ann Intern Med 2008;149(12):869–78.

10. Pinnock H, Hanley J, McCloughan L, et al. Effectiveness of telemonitoring integrated into existing clinical services on hospital admission for exacerbation of chronic obstructive pulmonary disease: researcher blind, multicentre, randomised controlled trial. BMJ 2013;347:f6070.

11. Bourbeau J. The role of collaborative self-management in pulmonary rehabilitation. Semin Respir Crit Care Med 2009;30(6):700–7.

12. Rice KL, Dewan N, Bloomfield HE, et al. Disease management program for chronic obstructive pulmonary disease: a randomized controlled trial. Am J Respir Crit Care Med 2010;182(7):890–6.

13. Fan VS, Niewoehner DE, Lew R. A comprehensive care management program to prevent chronic obstructive pulmonary disease hospitalizations. Ann Intern Med 2012;157(7):530–1.

14. Ries AL, Kaplan RM, Limberg TM, et al. Effects of pulmonary rehabilitation on physiologic and psychosocial outcomes in patients with chronic obstructive pulmonary disease. Ann Intern Med 1995;122(11): 823–32.

15. Nici L. Can we make it last? Maintaining benefits achieved with pulmonary rehabilitation. Lung 2007; 185(5):241–2.

16. Troosters T, Gosselink R, Decramer M. Short- and long-term effects of outpatient rehabilitation in patients with chronic obstructive pulmonary disease: a randomized trial. Am J Med 2000;109(3):207–12.

17. Garcia-Aymerich J, Lange P, Benet M, et al. Regular physical activity reduces hospital admission and mortality in chronic obstructive pulmonary disease: a population based cohort study. Thorax 2006; 61(9):772–8.

18. Garcia-Rio F, Rojo B, Casitas R, et al. Prognostic value of the objective measurement of daily physical activity in COPD patients. Chest 2012;142(2): 338–46.

19. Zanoria SJ, ZuWallack R. Directly measured physical activity as a predictor of hospitalizations in patients with chronic obstructive pulmonary disease. Chron Respir Dis 2013;10(4):207–13.

20. Ng LW, Mackney J, Jenkins S, et al. Does exercise training change physical activity in people with COPD? A systematic review and meta-analysis. Chron Respir Dis 2012;9(1):17–26.

21. Casaburi R. Activity promotion: a paradigm shift for chronic obstructive pulmonary disease therapeutics. Proc Am Thorac Soc 2011;8(4):334–7.

22. Polkey MI, Rabe KF. Chicken or egg: physical activity in COPD revisited. Eur Respir J 2009;33(2): 227–9.

23. Nici L, Raskin J, Rochester CL, et al. Pulmonary rehabilitation: what we know and what we need to know. J Cardiopulm Rehabil Prev 2009;29(3): 141–51.

24. Nici L, ZuWallack R, American Thoracic Society Subcommittee on Integrated Care of the COPD Patient. An official American Thoracic Society workshop report: the integrated care of the COPD patient. Proc Am Thorac Soc 2012;9(1):9–18.

25. Grone O, Garcia-Barbero M. Integrated care: a position paper of the WHO European Office for Integrated Health Care Services. Int J Integr Care 2001;1:e21.

26. Casas A, Troosters T, Garcia-Aymerich J, et al. Integrated care prevents hospitalisations for exacerbations in COPD patients. Eur Respir J 2006;28(1): 123–30.

Index

Note: Page numbers of article titles are in **boldface** type.

Clin Chest Med 35 (2014) 445–449
http://dx.doi.org/10.1016/S0272-5231(14)00033-1
0272-5231/14/$ – see front matter © 2014 Elsevier Inc. All rights reserved.

chestmed.theclinics.com

Moving?

Make sure your subscription moves with you!

To notify us of your new address, find your **Clinics Account Number** (located on your mailing label above your name), and contact customer service at:

Email: journalscustomerservice-usa@elsevier.com

800-654-2452 (subscribers in the U.S. & Canada)
314-447-8871 (subscribers outside of the U.S. & Canada)

Fax number: 314-447-8029

Elsevier Health Sciences Division
Subscription Customer Service
3251 Riverport Lane
Maryland Heights, MO 63043

*To ensure uninterrupted delivery of your subscription, please notify us at least 4 weeks in advance of move.

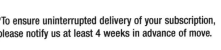
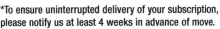

Printed and bound by CPI Group (UK) Ltd, Croydon, CR0 4YY

03/10/2024

01040366-0007